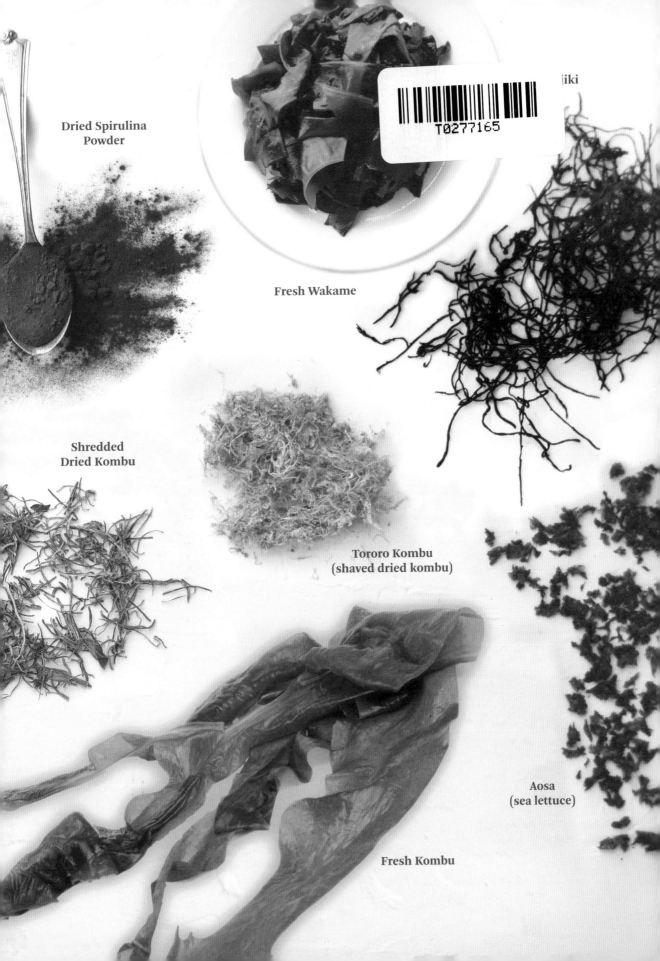

Dried Spirulina
Powder

iki

Fresh Wakame

Shredded
Dried Kombu

Tororo Kombu
(shaved dried kombu)

Aosa
(sea lettuce)

Fresh Kombu

T0277165

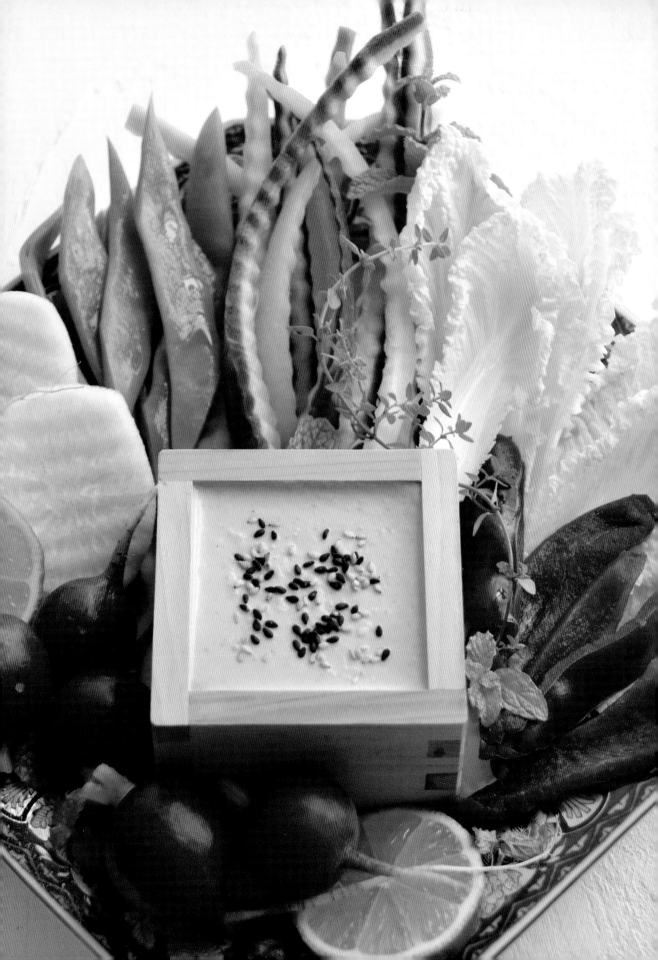

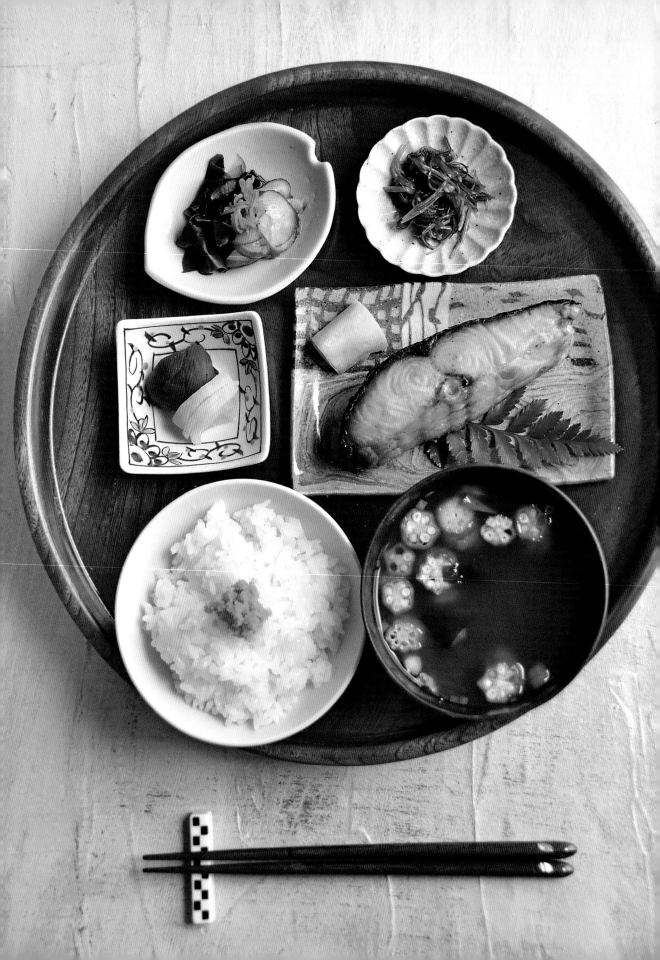

Japanese
SUPERFOODS

Learn the Secrets of Healthy Eating
and Longevity—the Japanese Way!

YUMI KOMATSUDAIRA

TUTTLE Publishing

Tokyo | Rutland, Vermont | Singapore

Contents

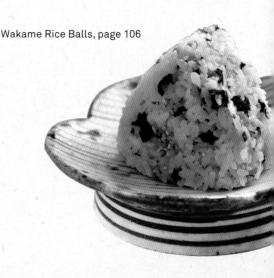

Wakame Rice Balls, page 106

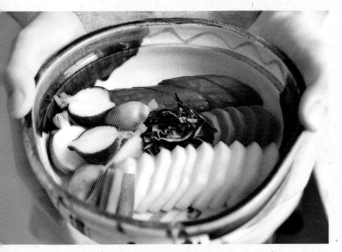

Quick Miso Yogurt Pickles, page 43

My Go-to Superfood Seaweed Recipes

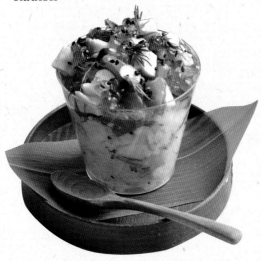

Cup Sushi, page 92

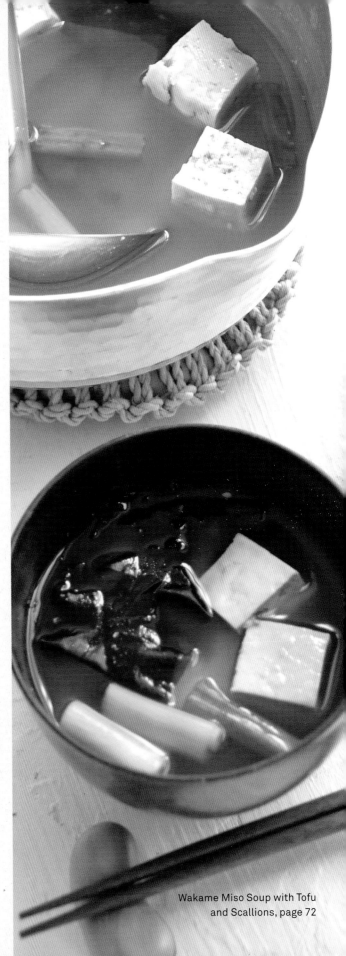

Wakame Miso Soup with Tofu and Scallions, page 72

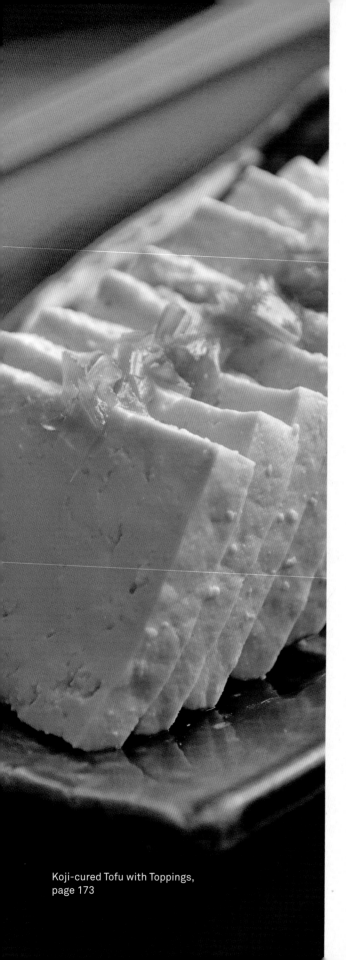

Koji-cured Tofu with Toppings,
page 173

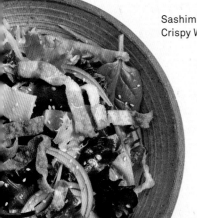

Sashimi and Wakame Salad with Crispy Wonton Chips, page 128

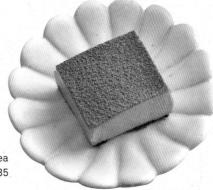

Matcha Green Tea Cheesecake, page 235

Welcome to the World of Japanese Superfoods

The earth's best foods are now increasingly available to all of us. The news isn't news any more: plant-based, nutrient-dense whole foods energize, nourish and, most importantly, they're easily transformed into a range of delicious dishes. Superfood-based recipes combine natural ingredients that deliver powerful amounts of antioxidants, omega-3 fatty acids, vitamins and minerals. They'll make you feel as good as they taste!

Nature's Most Powerful Foods

It's no wonder more and more people are turning to the Japanese diet as a model for maintaining health and sustaining well-being. Life expectancy in Japan is consistently at the top of the charts. Low levels of obesity and cardiovascular disease add to the attractions and benefits of the Japanese superfoods that lie at the heart of the nation's cuisine. Nutrient-rich, low-calorie superfoods boast a long list of benefits: extending life, boosting immunity, reducing inflammation and helping restore and maintain gut health. The cumulative benefits of healthful superfood-centered eating are irrefutable.

What Are Japanese Superfoods?

Many are foods you're already familiar with and have been integrating into your diet for years. The benefits of probiotic "ferments" are an increasing reason Japanese superfoods play more and more of a starring role on contemporary tables. Tofu is not only low in fat and calories, it contains all the essential amino acids that help our bodies to function properly, as well as iron, calcium and other vitamins and minerals.

Miso is another ingredient enjoying wider exposure. A fermented paste, it's a great source of probiotics and high in bone-building minerals like calcium. The bright green hues of matcha green tea powder have surfaced beyond teatime. Adding its distinctive flavor to a range of desserts, drinks and dishes, matcha contains antioxidants, specifically L-theanine, an amino acid that helps you to stay alert.

Natto may be the new kid on the block for many. With its pungent smell, sticky texture and musty taste, it's often described as an acquired taste, despite its ardent proponents. Made from whole soybeans that have been soaked then boiled or steamed, and then fermented, it's low-carb, high-protein, high-fiber and packed with a range of nutrients, including extremely high levels of vitamin K2, which plays an important role in bone mineralization, cancer prevention and cardiovascular health. Natto also contains an enzyme that helps break down proteins involved in blood clotting to reduce the risk of heart attacks and stroke.

The Power of Sea Greens

But if I had to choose one true star of Japanese superfoods, it would have to be seaweed (also called sea greens or sea vegetables.) They come in a variety of guises. Wakame is nutrient-dense, low in fat as well as an amazing source of omega-3s, which lower the risk of heart disease, depression and arthritis. Seaweed is rich in minerals and iodine, supports thyroid hormones and improves skin health.

I spent my youth playing and working in my family's seaweed factory, so I've long known the benefits of a superfood diet. And in this book, I present my affordable, accessible and reinvented versions of family favorites and classic comfort dishes. You'll look at Japanese food in new ways after reading this book, and but best of all, you'll learn to unlock the power of Japanese superfoods.

Clockwise from top: An array of superfood goodness, including a selection of pickled vegetables; matcha powder; miso and soybeans; enoki mushrooms; and two forms of wakame. The superfood superstar, seaweed, does double duty not only as a nutritious powerhouse, but also removes large amounts of carbon dioxide from the atmosphere.

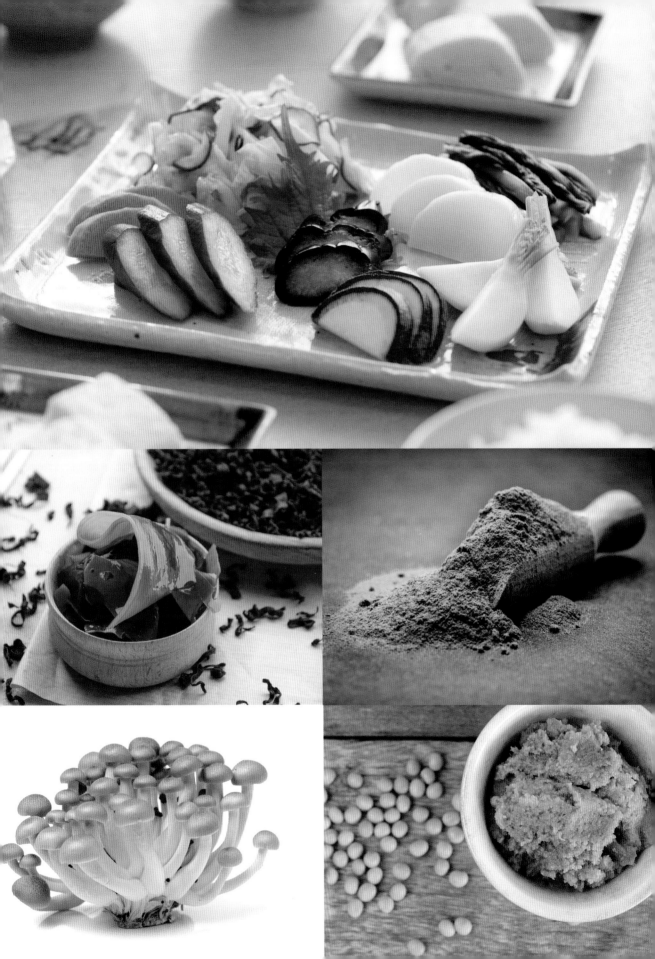

The Power of Sea Vegetables: Japan's Most Super Ingredient

Like terrestrial plants, seaweed performs photosynthesis and grows by absorbing water and nutrients. Seaweed mostly thrives in rocky areas with a strong current, and breeding is carried out by spores transmitted through the water. Seaweed is divided into three categories based on leaf color: green algae (chlorella and spirulina), brown algae (wakame, kombu and hijiki) and red algae (nori and dulse). The difference in color is a result of the depth of the waters in which the seaweed grows. The color ranges from green in shallow waters (where more sunlight reaches), to brown and red in deeper, darker waters. There are approximately 20,000 kinds of seaweed in the world, of which 50 are regularly eaten today—most notably brown algae such as wakame, kombu and hijiki in Japan. Let's learn more about these.

Kombu

The word "kombu" is similar to the Japanese word for joy (*yoro kobu*), contributing to the idea that consuming kombu brings joy. Kombu contains a great deal of iodine and amino acids, both of which support healthy thyroid function. The body tends to be acidic as a result of the processed foods in today's diet. In order to maintain a healthy body, we need to maintain an alkaline state, keeping the body close to its natural pH level. Eating alkaline foods such as kombu, helps to achieve that. When boiled, kombu acquires a slippery texture indicative of its water-soluble dietary fibers such as alginate and fucoidan. These suppress the absorption of carbohydrates and lipids and help reduce blood-cholesterol levels. The mineral content of kombu is highly digestible and is easily absorbed into the body, with about an 80% absorption rate. The main source of umami found in kombu dashi is glutamate, a type of amino acid. When there is umami, it's possible to reduce the amount of salt in a dish. In addition, glutamate acts on sensors in the stomach to improve the function of the gastrointestinal tract and prevent overeating. Fiber and natural sugars found in kombu support healthy bacteria, which helps to improve your gut health.

How to prepare dried kombu

1. Wipe the kombu with a dry paper towel, but don't remove the white powder that's on the surface. This is called mannitol, which is sweet and adds to the flavor.
2. Soak the kombu in room-temperature water for 30 minutes or according to the package directions.
3. Squeeze out the excess water. The kombu pieces are now ready to be sliced and added to your recipes.

How to store dried kombu

In an airtight container, store it in a cool, dry place. Hidaka-kombu (named for the part of Hokkaido where it's harvested) should be trimmed into rectangles from 3 to 5 inches (about 8–13 cm) on each side. The shelf life of dried kombu is approximately one year.

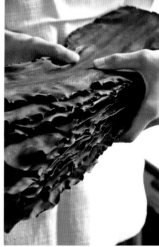

Right and below: A ripple effect: kombu in its natural state (full leaves after drying) and after being cut into pieces.

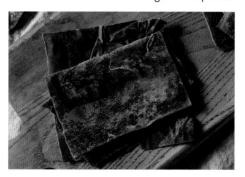

Wakame

The Japanese word "wakai" means young, and in the old days wakame was prized for its powers of rejuvenation. In the Nara period (C.E. 710–784), harvesting seaweed such as wakame required a Shinto ritual. Wakame has the medicinal effect of preventing aging and its slimy components cleanse the blood and promote good circulation. It is rich in water-soluble dietary fiber, so foods eaten with it are absorbed more slowly. Because blood glucose levels increase more slowly as a result, wakame is beneficial for diabetes prevention. In addition, it helps lower blood pressure. At the same time, because it helps to reduce the absorption of cholesterol, it also prevents arteriosclerosis.

Wakame contains a wide range of vitamins, minerals, iron and calcium including vitamin B12. It is a great source of plant-based omega-3 fats which regulate healthy cell function as well as helping to prevent strokes and heart disease. Wakame promotes urination, while the slime components promote healthy bowel movements. Finally, wakame is rich in fucoxanthin, which reduces fat by heating adipose tissue, thus promoting weight loss. In addition, fucoxanthin is an antioxidant with properties that contribute to beautiful skin and hair.

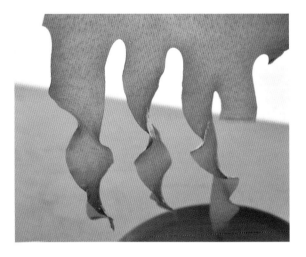

How to prepare dried wakame

1. Place the dried wakame in a small bowl and fill it with plenty of water.
2. Let the wakame rehydrate for 5 minutes, or until it softens.
3. Drain and quickly rinse under water in a colander, then squeeze out the excess water.
4. Wakame will expand as much as eight to ten times in volume after being soaked. Most dried wakame is precut into bite-sized pieces, so follow the instructions on the package.

How to store dried wakame

Store in an airtight container or a resealable plastic bag in a cool, dry place away from heat and moisture. The shelf life for dried seaweed is one year.

Top: A sheet of wakame
Left: Fresh wakame
Bottom: Dried precut (left) and after rehydration (right)

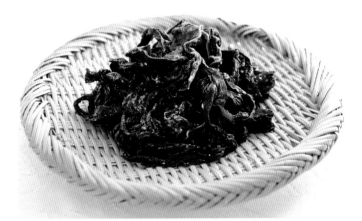

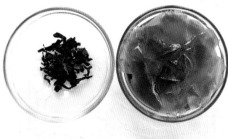

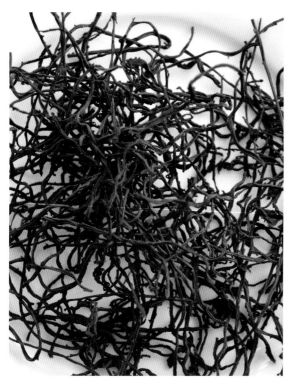

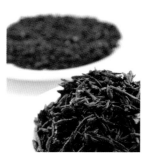

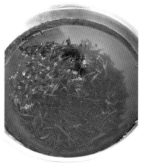

Dried (back), fresh (front)

A thorough soaking

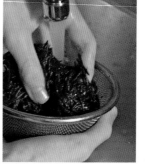

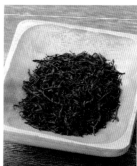

Thin strands of dried hijiki

Rinse several times

The end results

Hijiki

Dried hijiki is known for its high nutritional value—with about 12 times more calcium than milk, seven times more dietary fiber than burdock root and twice as much magnesium as almonds. There are two different types of hijiki: me hijiki (sprouts), which looks like black tea and has a tender texture, and naga hijiki (long), which is the stem part of the plant and has a crispy texture. Hijiki contains high amounts of folic acid, an important nutrient before and during pregnancy that helps prevent major birth defects. It contains more folic acid than spinach and beef liver. Calcium promotes the formation of strong bones and teeth, and dietary fiber helps to shape the intestinal environment. In addition, magnesium helps maintain good blood circulation, while a rich iron supply serves to carry oxygen to cells as a component of hemoglobin in red blood cells. Hijiki is also rich in vitamins for healthy skin and hair. It is also rich in water-soluble plant fibers that lower blood cholesterol levels and slow the absorption of sugars. Overall, hijiki is one of the best ways of adding iron, minerals and calcium to our daily diets—elements that are often under-represented.

How to prepare dried hijiki

1. Place dried hijiki strands in a bowl and fill with plenty of water. Let sit until softened, about 15 to 20 minutes at room temperature, or in hot water (about 190°F/80°C) for 4 to 5 minutes, or follow the manufacturer's instructions on the package. The water will initially turn brown.
2. Drain the water in a colander. Repeat this process five or six times, rinsing each time with fresh water, until the water runs clear.
3. Squeeze out the excess water. The hijiki is now ready to add to your recipe. Hijiki will expand as much as five to eight times in volume after being soaked.

How to store dried hijiki

Store in an airtight container or resealable plastic bag in a cool, dry place away from heat and moisture. The shelf life for hijiki is one year.

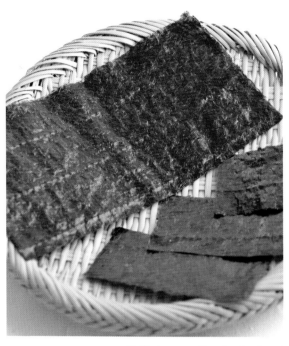
Delicate paperlike sheets of nori

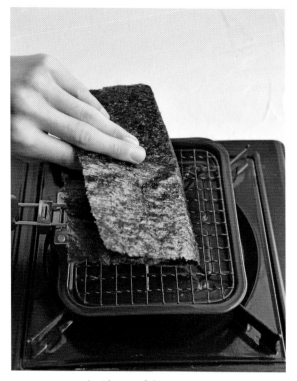
Just be careful not to overtoast the sheets

Nori

Nori has approximately 40% protein by weight, which is why it is called "ocean soybeans" in Japan. It not only contains more protein than soybeans, but also all the essential amino acids needed to support a healthy body. It is rich in vitamin C, containing 210 mg per 100g (vs. 100 mg in lemons).

Nori is sensitive to moisture. You need to re–fresh it by toasting it before serving, which gives it a crispy texture and a great smoky aroma. Depending on the type of dishes you are serving, different kinds of nori are available, ranging from powdered nori (such as aonori flakes), to shredded nori (kizami nori). The most common type, however, are the sheets used for making sushi.

How to toast nori

1. Heat a wire toasting pan, griddle or grill pan over medium heat.
2. Fold a piece of nori in half with the glossy surface on the inside.
3. Toast the rough outer side of the nori for about 5 to 7 seconds on each side.
4. Toast until the nori becomes crispy and the color turns slightly greenish.

How to store dried nori

Keep it in an airtight container or double reseal-able plastic bags and store in the refrigerator or freezer. You can also store in a cool, dry place away from heat and moisture. Unopened, the shelf life is about six months to a year; after opening, about one to two months. Nori has a glossy, smooth side and a rough side. The glossy side is the front.

Vegetable-based rolls wrapped in dried nori

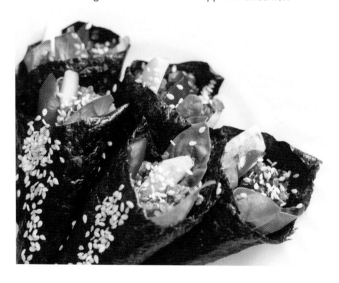

The Magical Soybean

Beans and soy products are key ingredients in the Japanese diet. They are rich in nutrients essential for maintaining our health, such as polyunsaturated fat and vitamins, and they can also help reduce cholesterol, improve immunity and prevent lifestyle-related diseases. Beans contain high amounts of dietary fiber, which promotes the growth of beneficial gut bacteria. Buddhist monks follow a strict vegan diet, receiving essential amino acids and high quality plant proteins mainly from soybeans and soy products. The Japanese have long recognized the benefits of processing soybeans through fermentation and other techniques, transforming them into tofu, miso, soy sauce and many other delicious ingredients. The Japanese were already eating processed and fermented soybean products such as miso and natto by the Nara period (C.E. 710–784), a healthful tradition that continues to this day.

Soybeans have been one of the most important crops grown in Japan since the Jyomon era (300 B.C.E.). There are different kinds of soybeans, including yellow, blue and black. Soy is one of the most common crops to be genetically modified, so I make sure that the beans used are organic and/or non-GMO when I purchase soy products such as tofu and natto.

Edamame are green when immature and in the pod (these are steamed and served with a sprinkling of sea salt as a popular snack in Japan). Once the edamame are fully matured, hardened and dried, they turn yellow.

Yellow soybeans are grown throughout the country and are used to make a variety of soybean products such as tofu, natto, soy sauce and miso paste. Yellow soybeans are simply matured edamame.

Blue soybeans, which are actually green in color, are a rare variety also called "emerald soybeans." Because they're difficult to grow, the production volume is small. While most soybeans turn yellow or black when ripe, these remain green when ripe. Blue soybeans have less fat than yellow or green soybeans, but contain high amounts of natural sugar. A popular dish in the northern Tohoku region is *hitashi-mame*, in which boiled blue soybeans are marinated in dashi soy sauce.

Black soybeans are the biggest, sweetest and firmest of all soybeans. They're widely eaten at special celebration meals, such as the New Year's Day dish *kuro mame*, in which the beans are simmered in sugar. The color black has long been regarded as providing protection against evil spirits in Japanese culture. In addition, the word *mame* means beans as well as high energy with good health and strength, which represents good luck.

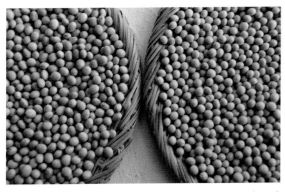

Blue soybeans (left) and yellow soybeans (right)

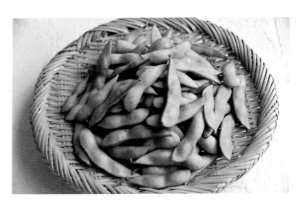

Edamame

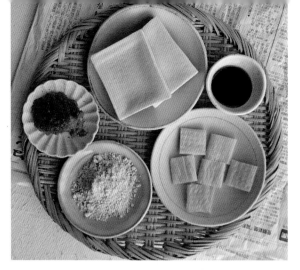

Clockwise from top: koyadofu (freeze-dried tofu), soy sauce, dried yuba, kinako (roasted soybean powder), miso

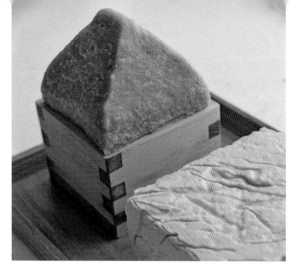

Miso and tofu, two key Japanese ingredients

Processed foods made with soybeans

In recent years, Japan has become the country with the greatest longevity in the world, according to the World Health Organization. One of the reasons for this is that the Japanese diet has a good nutritional balance and we have successfully incorporated a wide variety of soy products into our daily diet. Here are some of the popular soybean products that we enjoy on a daily basis.

Aburaage (thin sheets of tofu) and **atsuage** (thick slices of tofu) are both deep-fried until golden brown and crispy on the outside. Aburaage forms a pouch when the top is sliced off. Seasoned sushi rice mixed with vegetables is stuffed into the pouch to make the well-loved Inarizushi. Both types of fried tofu are either sliced or shredded to add to soups, stews, salads and stir-fries with other ingredients.

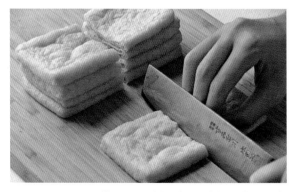

Aburaage: thin slices of deep-fried tofu

Kinako roasted soybean powder is widely used as a healthy alternative to sugar to sweeten Japanese desserts. It contains vitamins, dietary fiber and a high amount of isoflavones which lowers cholesterol levels. Kinako is also added to beverages as a plant-based protein powder. It is often served swith mochi rice cakes as a powdered topping.

Koyadofu or freeze-dried tofu is a traditional preserved food in Japan that originated in a small mountaintop Buddhist community south of Kyoto. Koyadofu is easier to digest than plain tofu and is an excellent source of protein, iron and calcium. It is a versatile pantry staple found in almost every Japanese household.

Miso fermented soybean paste is made with salt and koji (a mold called Aspergillus oryzae.) It is used to make soups, dressings and sauces, and as a seasoning to add umami flavor to meat or fish. Miso is classified by its three main types of ingredient combinations: rice miso, barley miso and bean miso. Miso varies in color from white (shiro), the mildest, to red (aka), the strongest and a combination of red and white (awase miso). They can be used interchangeably in most recipes.

Moyashi sprouted soybeans, one of the most popular Asian vegetables, are grown in a dark place until the roots are long. Despite being low in fat and calorie-free, they are a rich source of protein. This is a great ingredient to add to stir fries, salads and as a topping for noodles.

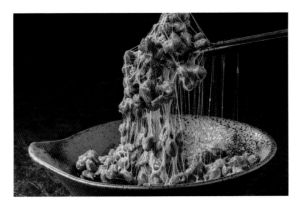

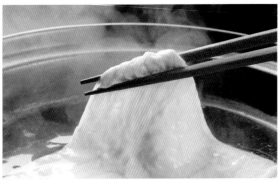

Top: natto; **bottom**: yuba

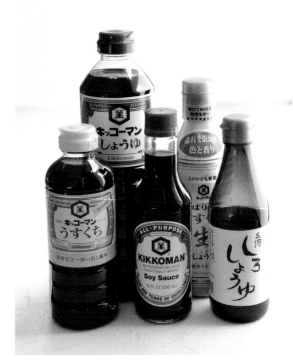

Try different soy sauces and note the subtle differences.

Sprouted soybeans have a crunchy texture and a mild soybean flavor that goes well with any dish.

Natto is made with soybeans that have been fermented with Bacillus subtilis. It has a sticky texture with a strong fermented aroma and is a highly nutritious probiotic food that's uniquely delicious (although it's an acquired taste for many, and even some Japanese do not like it.) Natto is served as part of a traditional Japanese breakfast.

Okara is the leftover soy pulp from making tofu. It is used in a popular sidedish called unohana, which is made with soy sauce, mirin and vegetables. It is hard to find at general supermarkets, even in Japan today, but if you find a specialty tofu shop, they normally carry it. Okara contains both soluble and nonsoluble fiber, which is more nutritious than most soybean products.

Soy sauce is a familiar fermented seasoning liquid made from soybeans, wheat, salt and koji (a fungus called Aspergillus oryzae). It's the most popular condiment in Japanese cuisine and is categorized into five different types based on the percentage of ingredients and the length of the fermentation process used. These are dark and light, tamari (gluten-free), twice-brewed and white.

Tofu is made from soy milk that is coagulated and pressed into solid white blocks by using the coagulant nigari, a bitter-tasting sea salt. Tofu is one of the most popular and versatile soybean products and is eaten in a variety of dishes with many different flavors and cooking methods. It has a variety of textures ranging from soft to firm.

Tonyu is soy milk produced by soaking and grinding soybeans. Used for sweet desserts as well as a soup base for healthy hot pots, it's a great alternative to cow's milk. Freshly made tonyu is great for making homemade tofu, which has a naturally sweet flavor and extra creamy texture.

Yuba is a film created on the surface of soy milk when it is heated. It can be consumed either fresh or dried. Fresh yuba has a smooth, silky consistency. When dried, yuba takes on a chewy texture. Yuba has a unique nutty, sweet flavor that goes well with salads, simmered vegetables, soups and hot pots.

Five Healthful Japanese Vegetables

The Japanese have long known that fresh seasonal ingredients are a source of necessary nutrients. For example, watermelon eaten in the summer hydrates and cools the body due to its high water content. Since Japan has such diverse topography, a wide variety of vegetables are grown to suit the regional climate and terrain.

Spring Vegetables
Spring vegetables, which grow slowly in the soil over the winter, are characterized by a slight bitterness. Common vegetables are bamboo shoots (takenoko), wild herbs such as butterbur (fuki), slightly bitter rapeseed plant (nanohana), soft and tender spring cabbage and sweet onions.

Summer Vegetables
Vegetables with a high moisture content cool the body during summer heat. Some examples are cucumbers (kyuri), tomatoes, eggplants (nasu), corns, edamame, Japanese ginger (myoga), shiso (a basil-like herb) and bitter melon (goya).

Fall Vegetables
Fall vegetables contain protein and starch to provide energy. Examples include potato varieties such as taro yams (satoimo), sweet potatoes (satsumaimo) and mountain yams (nagaimo), pumpkins (kabocha) and mushrooms such as matsutake.

Winter Vegetables
Winter root vegetables are sweet because they store sugar as protection from the cold. Leafy vegetables such as Japanese mustard spinach (komatsuna) and green onions (negi) are also popular in winter miso soup and hot pots. Root vegetables such as daikon, burdock (gobo) and lotus roots (renkon) are widely available. Yuzu citrus abounds. Winter vegetables are also popular for pickling.

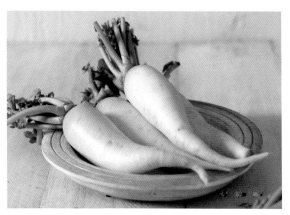

Daikon

Daikon
This versatile radish pops up in a range of main and sidedishes and is great cooked or raw.

Preparation
Grated daikon is a popular condiment served with grilled fish, tamagoyaki egg omelette, tempura, soba noodles, hot pots and sauces to enhance the flavor of the dish. It's slightly spicy 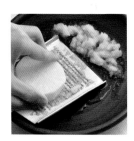 with a refreshing aftertaste. Raw daikon contains natural digestive enzymes so that eating it with oily food helps promote digestion and better gut heath. For mild to sweet grated daikon, use the top portion closer to the leaves rather than the bottom as that tends to be spicier and harder in texture. Cut off the amount you want to use, then peel it and shred it using the fine holes on a grater.

How to store daikon:
Wrap daikon in newspaper and keep it in the refrigerator for up to 2 weeks.

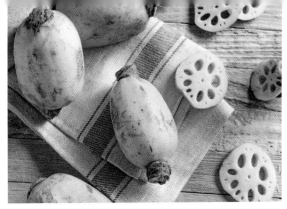
Whole and sliced lotus root

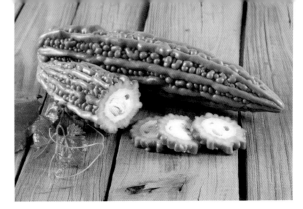
Bitter melon, or goya

Lotus Root (Renkon)

Lotus root, a popular vegetable throughout Asia, is full of fiber, vitamins and minerals. It's available fresh, uncooked, whole, vacuum packed in slices, or whole in water at any Asian market. I prefer to use uncooked lotus root because it's fresher and has a crunchier texture.

Preparation:

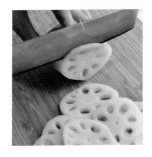

1. Look for lotus root that is heavy and firm without any bruising or soft spots. When it's fresh, the color is whitish-light brown. When it matures, the color tends to change to darker brown, so look for a lighter flesh color. Do not eat raw lotus root as it has an unpleasant tannic quality.
2. To prepare the lotus root: peel it, slice it, soak for 10 minutes in water, then rinse under cold water. Fresh lotus root will start to darken immediately so it needs to be kept in cold water before cooking.
3. For pickling or salads: boil for a couple of minutes in vinegar and water. Then add it to your pickling brine or salad. Use an aluminum or stainless-steel pot to retain the root's light color.
4. For stir-frying or soups, pair it with meat, seaweed or vegetables for a crunchy yet tender texture. You don't need to boil it first. Simply add raw lotus root to the dish you're cooking after soaking it in a vinegar solution for 15 minutes.

How to store it:
Wrap lotus root in newspaper and keep it in the refrigerator for up to 1 weeks.

Bitter Melon (Goya)

As the name suggests, this is a bitter-tasting vegetable, though one with a delicious and somewhat addictive flavor. It's a source of powerful antioxidants that boosts our immune system and reduces blood sugar levels. The skin of bitter melons is uneven and rough. Once largely produced in the Okinawa and Kyushu regions of southern Japan, today it's grown all over the country. My family in the Honshu region grows bitter melon in our garden which we enjoy during the summer. A famous Okinawan dish is *goya-chanpuru*, which combines tofu, pork, eggs and bitter melon in a stir fry.

Preparation:

1. Cut it in half lengthwise and remove the seeds with a spoon.
2. Cut it into thick slices for a stir fry or into thin slices for a salad. You can eat it raw or cooked. If it's too bitter in flavor, sprinkle it with some salt and let it sit for a couple of minutes. Rinse with water and drain. Now it's ready to be added to a salad or simply eaten with katsuobushi bonito flakes and soy sauce on top.

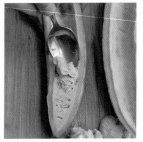

How to store it:
You can store it in a plastic bag in the refrigerator for 2 to 3 days. If you don't use it right away, seeded and cut pieces will keep well-wrapped in the freezer for up to 1 month.

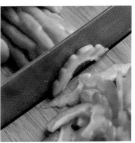

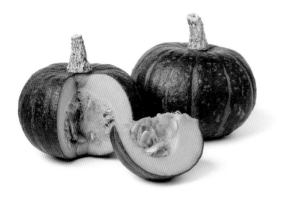

Kabocha is an increasingly common sight on Western tables

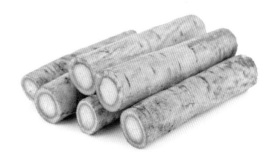

Burdock root or gobo

Japanese Pumpkin (Kabocha)

Kabocha, a type of squash, is a staple vegetable during the fall and winter seasons in Japan. It's increasingly popular and available in the United States and Europe. It tastes similar to sweet potato or chestnut and has a silky texture when cooked. The skin is edible. Due to its versatility, it's used in soups, simmered dishes, tempura and desserts. As an added benefit, it's loaded with beta-carotene, which transforms into vitamin A, a powerful antioxidant that boosts immunity.

Preparation:
1. Cut it in quarters and scoop out the seeds.
2. Cut it into 2-in (5-cm) chunks. You can peel the skin or keep it on, depending on the dish you're making.

How to store it:
Wrap it whole in newspaper and keep it in a cool, dry place for up to 1 month. Once cut, store it in the refrigerate and use it within 5 days.

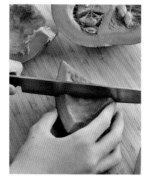

Burdock Root (Gobo)

Burdock root, a long thin root vegetable about 3 feet (1 m) long and 1 inch (2.5 cm) in diameter, is very common in Japan. Available at any Asian market or health food store, it's also increasingly appearing at many well-stocked American supermarkets. Burdock root is used in kinpira gobo, a very popular Japanese sidedish. Burdock root contains powerful health benefits—it helps to detox the liver, balances and maintains stable hormones and improves the blood circulation throughout the body.

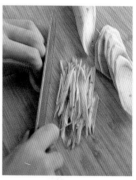

Preparation:
1. Peel it then thinly slice it on the diagonal. Then cut it into thin strips about 2 inches (5 cm) in length.
2. Soak in water for 10 minutes, changing the water a couple of times to get rid of the bitterness. Drain well.

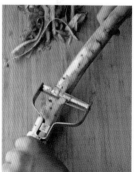

How to store it:
Wrap whole roots in newspaper and keep in the refrigerator for up to 2 months.

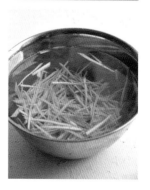

Fresh and Dried Mushrooms

Mushrooms are a popular ingredient in Japanese cuisine. Many different varieties of mushrooms are sold throughout Japan, both at supermarkets as well as at local vegetable stands (often located near rural train stations). Whenever I travel back to Japan, it is a treat to cook aromatic dishes using fresh local mushrooms. Mushrooms contain large amounts of vitamin B, fiber and protein—which support a strong immune system—and an abundance of antioxidants. Studies show that foods with high antioxidant content help lower blood pressure and reduce cholesterol, which helps fight cancer and prevent diabetes. Mushrooms also support a healthy digestive system. Due to a toxin found in most mushrooms, it is unsafe to eat them raw (with the exception of white mushrooms) and most mushrooms should be cooked before serving. Some of the most popular Japanese mushrooms are profiled here. Try them all!

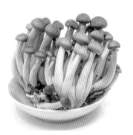
Buna shimeji

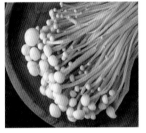
Enoki

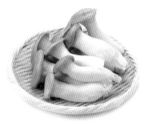
Eringi

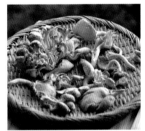
Hiratake

Buna shimeji has a great aroma and is packed with umami flavor. This spindly specimen is often cooked with steamed rice or found accompanying dashi-infused dishes. Buna shimeji is considered an all-purpose mushroom in Japanese cuisine, one that is versatile with a rich, nutty flavor, beautiful shape and a firm cap.

Enoki is the second most popular type of mushroom in Japan (after shiitake). It has been cultivated since 1928 and is now the most widely-grown mushroom. It is either white or brown, has a mild flavor and slippery noodle-like texture that is unique.

Eringi is originally from the Mediterranean and was introduced to Japan in 1993. The thick stem has a meaty texture that is often referred to as "abalone of mushrooms" because of its chewy, tender texture. Its mild flavor makes it adaptable to many types of dishes, both Japanese and western. You can slice the stem into thin or thick slices depending on the dish you are making.

Hiratake or oyster mushrooms have a high moisture content, making them suitable for stock-based dishes, such as soups and hot pots. They have a mild flavor and delicate, leafy caps and are great to serve in kombu-based soups.

Maitake is a recent addition to the scene, known for its distinctive shape. It's a large bulky mushroom (known in other countries as "Hen of the Woods") that is cut into smaller pieces for the convenience of home cooks. There is interesting folklore behind the name "Maitake." Because it was historically extremely rare, it was called the "phantom mushroom." Thus, when people found it in the woods, they would jump up and down with joy, a movement that resembles floating or dancing, and the word *mai* means to dance or move in Japanese.

Matsutake is the king of all mushrooms in Japan. You can find them at high-end department stores where they are sold as a gift item that comes with a high price tag. I often think

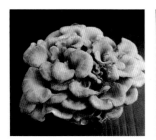
Maitake

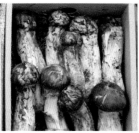
Matsutake

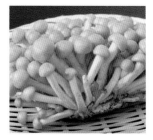
Nameko

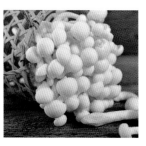
Shiro shimeji

matsutake are similar to truffles because of their distinctive aroma and unique pine-like, nutty flavor. My uncle, who lived in Iwate prefecture in northeastern Japan, often picked them in his own backyard in the mountains and sent some to us in the fall. They were a treat that we enjoyed eating with steamed rice and a simple soup to truly enjoy the beautiful fall flavor.

Nameko is well known for its earthy, silky and natural gelatin-like, slippery texture. It's commonly served with tofu in red miso soup as a breakfast staple. It has a brownish-orange color and is commonly sold in convenient pre-cut pieces packed in a small plastic bag. Nameko easily oxidizes, resulting in a sour taste, so I recommend buying it with the stems attached so it will have a longer shelf life.

Shiitake (fresh) is the most widely sold and consumed mushroom in Japan. It's available in a variety of sizes and thicknesses and is popular in hot pots or as tempura or grilled and simmered and in stir fries. Popular since the Edo period, its main characteristics are its thickness and meaty texture.

Shiitake (dried) There are 2 types of dried shiitake mushrooms available for cooking.

Donko has a thick and meaty texture with a stronger mushroom flavor and makes a darker brown dashi stock than koushin. The unique cracked pattern on the caps are a result of being air-dried in a cold climate during the winter months, which creates the most delicious and high-priced mushrooms in the market today.

Koushin are grown between spring and fall during the short humid summer months. They have much thinner caps and a smooth texture that makes a light brown dashi stock, with a more delicate flavor. It works well in any type of dish.

Shiro shimeji or white beech mushrooms have a soft and tender texture. They're popular among non-mushroom lovers because they have a very mild flavor. It's common to boil them and add them to salads and simple marinade dishes and it lend an elegant shape to any meal.

White mushrooms were introduced to Japan in 1922, popular due to their versatility in both Western and Japanese cooking. This is the only type of mushroom that can be eaten raw, so it has become a popular ingredient in salads. It often comes with dirt clinging to it, so make sure to wipe it with a dry towel. You can wash it, but some of the rich flavor will then be lost.

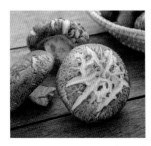
Shiitake (fresh)

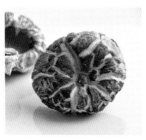
Shiitake (dried), donko,

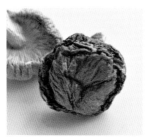
Shiitake (dried), kouchin

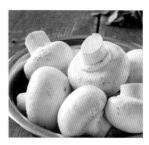
White mushrooms

The Superpowers of Green Tea

Japanese tea has become one of the most popular drinks in the world. Japanese Buddhist monks first brought green tea back from China to Japan in the early 9th century, C.E. In the 12th century a Buddhist monk named Eisai founded Japan's first Zen temple and introduced green tea as a medicinal beverage with health benefits, which was the beginning of a popular green tea culture that has since spread throughout Japan. Today, people around the world cannot get enough green tea, especially matcha—from hip neighborhood coffee shops serving matcha lattes to local grocery stores selling matcha-flavored snacks. Why has green tea become so popular in recent years? One major reason is its wide range of health benefits. Green tea, known to be one of the healthiest beverages in the world, is loaded with powerful catechin, natural antioxidants that help protect against cancer, lower the risk of heart disease and support healthy brain function.

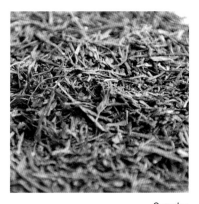
Sencha

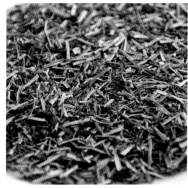
Gyokuro

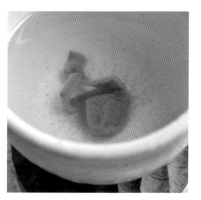
Daifukucha or Oubukucha

Sencha When Japanese people talk about green tea they generally mean sencha, which is widely consumed and dominates the green tea market in Japan. In the 18th century, distinctive new styles of sencha green tea were developed in Japan. Sencha is made from tea plants grown under strong sunlight, which results in a darker color and a stronger, more savory flavor. The process of making sencha includes steaming (to prevent the tea from oxidizing), then rolling, drying and sorting the leaves according to their sizes and shapes. I drink sencha every morning, either before or after my breakfast so that I feel energized and ready to start my day. Sencha provides caffeine, but one-third less than coffee, making it a great alternative for anyone wanting an energy boost from a less-caffeinated beverage.

Gyokuro This type of green tea, the first in the market, is grown in the shade in the spring-time when the young leaves are developing, resulting in larger amounts of chlorophyll being produced to compensate for the lower amount of sunlight available. This results in a brighter green color and a higher level of amino acids known as L-theanine, which gives gyokuro a well-balanced, sweet flavor and an elegant aroma. At New Year, an important holiday in Japan, a special green tea drink called *daifukucha* (or *oubukucha*) is served representing good luck and good health for the upcoming year. Oubukucha is made with green tea and kombu kelp with umeboshi pickled plums added. It originated in Kyoto over 1,000 years ago. The first crop of tea, called *shincha*, is only available between mid-April to mid-May, when the young tea leaves have less astringency, a sweeter taste and a bright green color, giving the tea greater flavor and nutrition.

Matcha green tea powder is made from tencha, a shade-grown tea with increased chlorophyll due to

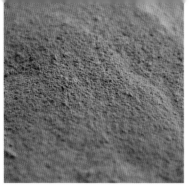

Matcha

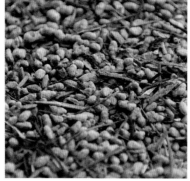

Genmaicha

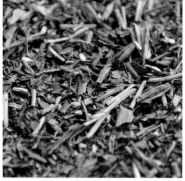

Hojicha

the lack of sunlight. This results in an intensified sweet flavor and a vivid green color. This is a result of increased L-theanine, an amino acid with a range of health benefits including a boost to the immune system and stress relief. Matcha also has a rich umami flavor due to the glutamate in the young green tea leaves. Matcha was developed in the 16th century among tea growers in Uji, near Kyoto, and has made high-quality green tea more widely available. Both matcha and gyokuro contain the same level of caffeine as coffee, making them the most caffeinated of all green teas. This is because the young tea leaves used to produce matcha and gyokuro contain more caffeine than the stems and mature leaves used to make other teas. They also help deliver longer-lasting effects of the caffeine—the L-theanine amino acid, which slow the release of caffeine in your body, providing a calming effect. Matcha is made by removing the stems and veins from the green tea and then stone grinding the leaves into a fine green powder. Because matcha is green tea consumed in a more conventional form, it provides maximum health benefits. The method of preparing and drinking matcha is completely different from other types of green tea. A special

bamboo whisk is used to mix the matcha powder with hot water in a special tea bowl until it becomes foamy. The Japanese tea ceremony has become a cultural activity revolving around the ceremonial preparation of matcha green tea.

Genmaicha is made by blending green tea with roasted brown rice in approximately a 50:50 ratio. This makes genmaicha relatively inexpensive compared to other Japanese teas. It has a smaller amount of caffeine, making it suitable for children and pregnant women. Genmaicha can also be blended with matcha or gyokuro, resulting in a more expensive type of tea with slightly different tastes and aromas. The brown rice imparts a nutty aftertaste, making it a popular tea to drink after meals. The best way to bring out the aroma and flavor is to brew it using very hot water—hotter than making sencha. High-quality tea can also be brewed slowly with cold water as cold brew, but in the case of genmaicha, hot water is recommended (about 200°F/95°C, or slightly higher), so the tea gives off its unique savory flavor and aroma after steeping for 1 to 2 minutes in a teapot.

Hojicha is a type of caffeine-free roasted green tea that originated in Kyoto in 1920. The tea leaves, stems and twigs are all steamed, then roasted in a special pan over high heat until the tea turns a reddish-brown color. This process removes the caffeine and gives hojicha an earthy and smoky-sweet flavor, making it the most popular caffeine-free tea. Although the color of hojicha is quite dark compared to other types of green tea, it's not bitter and is the perfect beverage to drink before going to bed or for relaxation. For hojicha, hot water is highly recommended, about 200°F (95°C) or slightly higher, so the tea gives off its sweet and smoky flavor after steeping for 1 to 2 minutes, similar to genmaicha.

Matcha is prepared using special implements in Japan and forms the basis for the Japanese tea ceremony.

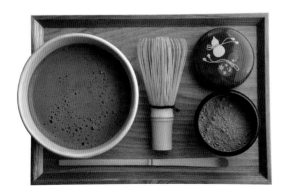

Green tea storage tips

The main cause for the deterioration of the quality of green tea, including the aroma, is oxidation. Other factors that can cause oxidation are light, oxygen, moisture and temperature. So the best way to store these teas is to keep them away from heat or moisture in a dark, cool area in an air-tight container. The shelf life of green tea varies depending on the type and manufacturer. In the case of sencha, for example, it is often labeled as six months to one year. However, since the deterioration begins as soon as the package is opened, it's recommended to use the tea within 2 to 3 weeks of opening in order to enjoy the full taste and aroma.

Preparation tips for sencha

Sencha may become bitter or lose its flavor if you are not careful with the temperature of the hot water. Warming up the teacups as well as cooling the hot water down are important steps in brewing aromatic and delicious sencha tea. Here is the step-by-step process for making sencha at home, Japanese style.

1. Bring the water to a boil and cook for 5 minutes without a lid (this helps remove any chlorine odors). Remove from the heat and allow to cool down to about 155°F (70°C), the perfect temperature for sencha. Pour the hot water into the teacups to keep them warm and to cool the water.

2. Add the tea leaves to the teapot. For 4 people, you will need about 1½ tablespoons of sencha, or follow the guidelines on the packet. When the water is at the correct temperature (you should be able to hold

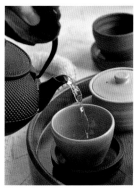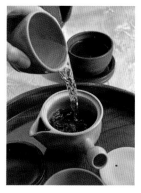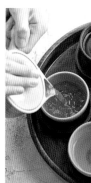

Homemade Hojicha Roasted Tea

When I have leftover sencha that has expired, I often make my own hojicha by roasting the old tea leaves in a pan at home. It's very easy to make. Here is how to make my hojicha.

COOKING TIME: 10 minutes

4 oz (100 g) leftover sencha green tea that has expired

1. Heat a small-sized heavy saucepan or Dutch oven over medium heat. Spread the tea leaves evenly in the pot, cover and cook for 2 minutes. Shake the pan frequently to prevent burning.
2. Remove the lid and raise the heat to medium-high. Using a wooden spoon, constantly stir the tea leaves to prevent burning for about 2 to 3 more minutes.
3. When smoke starts to rise from the tea leaves, turn the heat to low and continue roasting for another 3 to 5 minutes. When the tea leaves have turned from green to brown, turn off the heat.

4. Remove the tea from the pan and quickly spread it on a tray. Let it stand for about 10 minutes, until the leaves are completely cooled. Store in a tightly sealed glass jar or other type of airtight container and keep it in a cool, dark place away from moisture. The shelf life is 30 days.
5. To brew the hojicha (4 servings): combine 2 to 3 tablespoons of tea leaves with 4 cups of boiling water, (200°F/95°C), steep in a teapot for 1 to 2 minutes and serve.

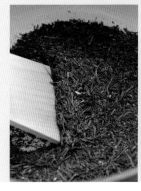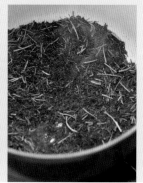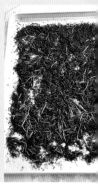

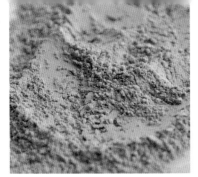
Kobucha

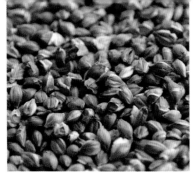
Mugicha

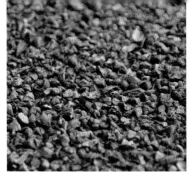
Kuromamecha

the cups), transfer it from the teacups to the teapot, then cover and let the tea steep for 2 minutes. Be mindful of the timing—if you steep too long, the tea will get bitter, and if you steep too little, the flavor will not develop.

3. If there are multiple cups, pour it little by little in several round to fill each cup. After pouring one round, pour the tea in the reverse order the next time so that the flavor of tea distributes evenly. Only fill the teacups about 70 to 80 percent full.

Other healthy "teas"

Japanese people are obsessed with healthy teas that have strong medicinal properties. Here are other kinds of popular healthy beverages that are treated as "tea," even though they do not contain any tea leaves. The Japanese word for tea is *cha*, and although these teas do not use traditional tea leaves, they have become important parts of the Japanese diet and are treated as teas. So I want to introduce them to you. The best way to store these teas is to keep them away from heat or moisture, and keep them in a dark, cool area in an air-tight container. The shelf life of these teas is from 6 months to one year. As always, check the label on the package for more information.

Kobucha literally means "kombu kelp tea," not to be confused with kombucha, the fermented black tea known in the West (called "mushroom tea" in Japan). Kobucha is made from kombu kelp powder, sometimes with green tea powder or umeboshi plum powder added, along with some seasoning salts that give it a savory, salty flavor. Because kobucha comes in a fine powder, it dissolves quickly in water. It's packed with minerals, vitamins and fiber, and the glutamic acid found in kombu gives a natural umami flavor to the tea. In addition to drinking kobucha as tea, it can also be used in food preparations,

like soups and quick pickles, as a source of extra umami flavor.

Mugicha is a common summertime drink in Japan, a roasted barley tea that is caffeine-free and therefore a popular choice for children and pregnant women. It reduces constipation and stomach pain and promotes sound sleep. Mugicha is widely available in convenient tea bags, but the traditional method of making it is to boil and steep the grains in a big teapot, resulting in an amazing roasted nutty aroma. I love the smell of roasted barley in my kitchen—so much so that I still make my mugicha in this traditional way. I strain it and store it in a pitcher in the refrigerator to drink cold as iced tea year-round.

Dokudamicha is a caffeine-free tea made from the leaves of the dokumai plant (this name means "poison blocker.") It is known to have medicinal properties that support the immune system, as well as containing the powerful antioxidant polyphenol and acts as a detoxifier too. Native to Asia, dokudami grows in dark, moist areas. While it has a strong, unpleasant odor, I've come to appreciate it as an adult both for its health benefits and its nutty flavor. The plant, which has heart-shaped leaves and pretty little white flowers, grew in the backyard of my childhood home.

Kuromamecha This is a tea made from black beans that originated in Hokkaido. It is available as whole black beans or ground powder form and is caffeine-free. If you're brewing whole black beans, you can use the leftover softened beans for cooking. Kuromamecha has a naturally sweet and slightly nutty flavor that children like. It's packed with fiber, high in vitamins that reduce blood pressure, has anti-aging properties that foster healthy skin and nails and also improves metabolism.

Japanese Rice

Perfectly-cooked rice is the foundation of the Japanese diet. Brown rice, *genmai*, is considered special due to its health benefits as a non-processed food. When we talk about rice within Japanese cuisine, however, we are referring to machine-polished white rice, *uruchimai*. *Uruchimai* when cooked is called *gohan* in Japanese. It is a Japanese short-grain variety, known as japonica, which becomes sticky when cooked. Sushi Rice is also made with *uruchimai*. The two most popular brands are Koshihikari and Sasanishiki, preferred by most Japanese, myself included, for their high-quality flavor and texture. They are the perfect rice for a bento box, as the rice remains moist and chewy for a long time at room temperature.

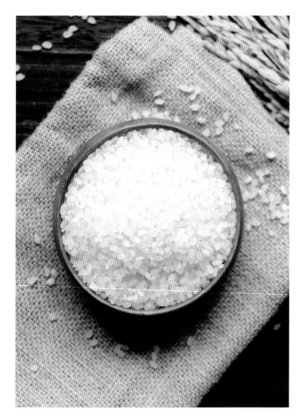

Another popular Japanese rice is *mochigome* or glutinous rice. *Mochigome* is best known for its very sticky texture and is eaten as a staple in many Asian countries. Compared to *uruchimai*, it is whiter in color and rounder in shape. The best known traditional mochigome dish is *sekihan*, red bean rice, which is steamed together with red adzuki beans. Because the dish is dyed red (which is a symbol of celebration) by the adzuki beans, it is served on special occasions such as weddings, holidays and birthdays.

Another popular ingredient is mochi rice cakes (see photo on page 29), which have a chewy sticky texture and a naturally sweet flavor. Glutinous rice is often referred to as "sweet rice"

Left: Rice is much more than a simple staple. Try adding different Japanese rice varieties to your pantry. You'll soon discover that there are subtle differences!

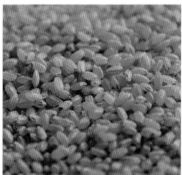

Genmai (brown rice)

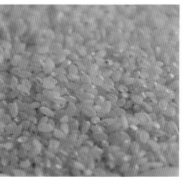

Uruchimai (polished white rice)

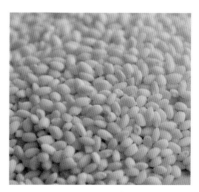

Mochigome (glutinous rice)

because it is so often used in desserts and sweet snacks. Traditionally, mochi is made by steaming mochigome and pounding it with a mallet in a wooden barrel until it becomes a sticky, elastic dough with a soft, smooth consistency.

The difference between the two types of rice is the type of starches they contain. Uruchimai contains 80% amylopectin, which is the starch that makes rice sticky, and 20% amylose, which makes rice harder. On the other hand, mochigome contains 100% amylopectin, so it is very sticky and moist after being cooked. In addition, uruchimai and mochigome look different.

Uruchimai is semi-translucent, while mochigome is milky-white and opaque. Both types of rice absorb water while being stored. Since the quality of rice deteriorates quicker after it is polished, it is important to check the date on the bag indicating when the rice was milled, and buy only small amounts. In Japan, the "best before" date (expiration date) is about one to two months in the winter, one month in the spring and two weeks in the summer, depending on the year of milling. Keep uncooked rice in a cool, dark place or in the vegetable compartment of the refrigerator in an airtight container or resealable plastic bag.

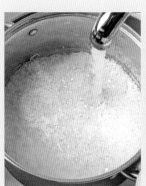 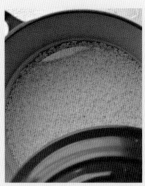 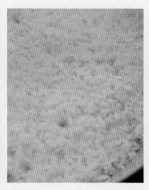 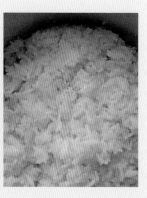

How to Cook Japanese Rice in a Pot

PREPARATION TIME: 10 minutes
SOAKING TIME: 30 minutes
COOKING TIME: 50 minutes
SERVES 4

1½ cups (330 g) uncooked Japanese
  short-grain white rice
1½ cups (375 ml) water

1. Place the rice in a large bowl or pot and cover with water. Lightly stir the rice with your hand five to six times, then drain the cloudy water immediately. Do not leave the rice in the cloudy water after the first wash as it will absorb the bran, resulting in an undesirable taste.
2. Cover the rice with water again. Use the palms of your hands to gently press the rice about 10 times, then drain the cloudy water. Repeat this process three to four times, until the water runs clear. Then, refill the bowl with the washed rice and 1½ cups water and soak for 30 minutes.
3. Drain the rice completely in a colander.
4. Combine 1½ cups water and the rice in a small (2.5 quarts/2.4 liters) heavy pot or Dutch oven (or in a rice cooker, if using.)
5. Cook, covered, over medium-high heat for 8 to 10 minutes, until the water comes to a boil. (If you are not sure if the water is boiling, you can quickly open the lid at this point to check.) If there is still water inside, close the lid and continue cooking for a few more minutes.
6. Turn the heat to low and continue cooking, covered, for 13 to 15 minutes. (From this point onward, do not open the lid until the rice is fully cooked.)
7. Turn off the heat and let the rice steam in the covered pot for another 15 minutes. Do not remove the lid. If using a rice cooker, follow the instructions.
8. When the rice is done cooking, fluff the rice quickly by using a wet rice paddle and serve in individual bowls.

Other rice products

Sake is made from a mixture of steamed rice, rice malt and water that goes through a fermentation process, producing alcohol. "Alcoholic fermentation" refers to the conversion of sugar into alcohol, but the rice used to make sake contains no sugar; therefore, it cannot be fermented. To solve this problem, koji (cooked rice that has been inoculated with a mold called Aspergillus oryzae) is used to convert rice starch into sugar (glucose) using koji enzymes (saccharification), and alcoholic fermentation is carried out by yeast. The technique of performing saccharification and alcoholic fermentation, two chemical reactions that occur simultaneously in the same tank, is called parallel double fermentation. It's a unique Japanese brewing method that produces a high-alcohol-content beverage. Under Japanese liquor laws, sake is labeled with the word *seishu*, meaning clear liquor. Sake has been made for over 1,000 years ago, and there are over 10,000 types—with slight differences in the brewing methods. For example, sake brewed with locally-grown rice and water is called jizake. The alcohol content in sake is, at most, about 20 percent. As sake lovers know, it can be enjoyed both hot and chilled and sake has a wider range of drinking temperature compared to other alcoholic beverages, from 41ºF (5ºC) to 131ºF (55ºC). Depending on the temperature, the aroma and flavor of sake changes.

Rice vinegar refers to a liquid seasoning made by fermenting rice to create alcohol and then to acetic acid. The flavor of rice vinegar is mellow, sweet and less acidic than distilled white or malt vinegars. Rice vinegar is the best choice of when making sushi rice due to its sweetness and umami flavor. When white rice is fermented and processed into vinegar, 15 kinds of amino acids and more than 70 kinds of organic acids are produced. In particular, rice vinegar contains a lot of citric acid, which helps to burn off amino acid fats, which is beneficial in weight loss. Since the aroma disappears when it's heated, rice vinegar is better suited for marinades and dressings that are used without heating them to high temperatures.

Rice crackers (senbei) are made by steaming and crushing leftover cooked rice, then forming it into rounds and drying it. The crispy texture and the natural sweet flavor of rice is often seasoned with umami-packed soy sauce, salt, sugar or other flavorings such as curry or wasabi. The flavors become more intense when baked. While senbei are typically baked, in recent years, they are also fried, resulting in a thin, flat shape and a moderately hard and crispy texture.

Rice flours, which are gluten-free, are a great alternative to wheat flours. There are three major types of rice flour made from Japanese short grain rice that are popular for making savory and sweet dishes.

Shiratamako is made from *mochigome* glutinous rice. The coarse granules lend a chewiness and elastic texture to many traditional desserts called

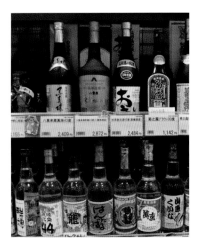

Sake comes in hundreds of varieties

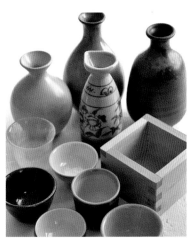

Traditional sake flasks and cups

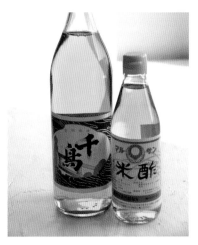

Rice vinegars

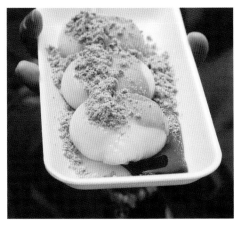
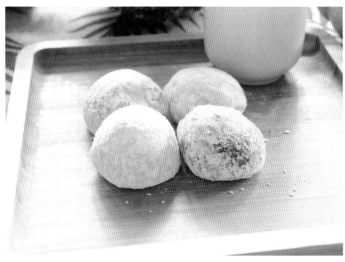

Above and right: Two mochi favorites are *shiratama dango* and adzuki-stuffed *daifuku*.

wagashi. The best known, *shiratama dango* (mochi dumplings), are made from *shiratamako* dough that is boiled for a few minutes in water until tender. Shiratamako has a satisfying bouncy texture and is the most popular type of rice flour used for Japanese home cooking. It maintains its softness the next day better than mochi made with other rice flours, which get hard if not eaten right away. *Shiratamako* is also used to make a popular dessert called *daifuku mochi* which has a smooth and soft texture and is filled with sweet adzuki red bean paste.

Mochiko is a finely milled flour that is also made from *mochigome* glutinous rice, but is used differently in cooking. It is more suitable for baking due to being softer and more pliable than *shiratamako*, which lends a satisfying chewiness to baked dishes. It is widely used as an alternative to wheat flour since the texture is perfect for making cakes and cupcakes.

Joshinko is rice flour made from common *suruchimai* white rice. It is white in color and has a powdery texture like all finely milled flours, making it perfect for gluten-free breads and creamy white sauces. Since *joshinko* is made from *uruchimai*, it has less elasticity and chewiness than glutinous rice flour. A popular dessert made with *joshinko* is *yomogi mochi* with adzuki beans. Since *joshinko* can be slightly tough due to its less elastic nature, it is commonly mixed with *shiratamako* to make it chewier and softer. It's used to make bite-sized mochi rice balls, the traditional molded and steamed treat called uiro and the oak-leaf-wrapped confection, kashiwa mochi.

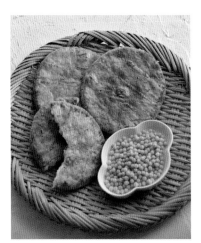

Rice crackers

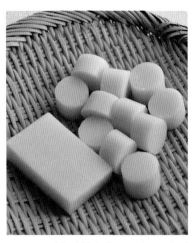

Mochi (glutinous rice cakes)

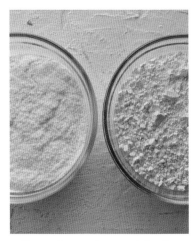

Fine and coarsely ground rice flours

Japanese Noodles
Healthy Comfort in a Bowl

Wheat began to be cultivated in western Asia around 7000 B.C.E. It then migrated via the Silk Road to China, where the original noodles were born. It is said that the history of Japanese noodles began in the Nara period (C.E. 710–794), when a type of somen noodle, called *muginawa*, was made by combining salt water with wheat and rice flour, mixing it into a dough, stretching it into a rope and baking it into a confection. During that time, noodles were only eaten by wealthy aristocrats. Today, noodles such as soba, udon and ramen have become staples of Japanese cuisine. They are made from a variety of ingredients including wheat, buckwheat, konjac yam and seaweed, and are packed with vitamins, minerals and dietary fiber that support the healthy Japanese diet. Since Japanese noodles are made with salt, unlike Italian pasta, it is not necessary to add salt to the water when you boil them. The salt activates gluten in the wheat flour making the noodles chewy. Here is a survey of the most popular noodles you can find in Japanese cuisine.

Soba Buckwheat as a plant was introduced to Japan quite early, but only transformed into soba noodles from the late Muromachi period onward. It was initially eaten in special places, such as tea rooms, and then later spread more widely in the 17th century. The highest quality soba, both fresh and dried, is made only with buckwheat flour and water, which is what I love about soba because of its distinctive nutty buckwheat aroma and flavor. It is considered good manners in Japan to enjoy soba served in soup, either hot or cold, by noisily slurping the entire noodles up in a continuous motion without biting them. This custom is not considered polite outside of Japan, however. The importance of slurping the noodles is that it allows the aroma of the buckwheat to waft up into one's nose, enhancing the flavor. However, because buckwheat flour is fragile, soba are often made with wheat flour added to help bind the dough, with the added gluten resulting in a more durable noodle. If you are looking for gluten-free soba be sure to check the package ingredients for buckwheat only, and note that it is more expensive. Beside wheat flour, you might find soba with mountain yam, seaweed or egg added as binders. Common labels for soba with wheat flour added might say, *Hachi-wari soba*, which means buckwheat flour is used in an 8:2 proportion with wheat flour. Various types of flavored soba are also available, such as matcha soba—which has a green color and a slight green tea taste. Buckwheat contains powerful polyphenols called rutin that help reduce blood sugar levels, prevent blood clots and reduce heart disease. Rutin has powerful antioxidant properties that are more effective when taken with vitamin C. Thus soba in soup with grated daikon radish is a nutritious way to serve it. Rutin dissolves in water and so after eating the soba, *sobayu* (the leftover water in which the soba was boiled) is served in a tea pot so you can drink it together with the soy and ponzu dipping sauce to finish off your meal.

Different varieties of soba

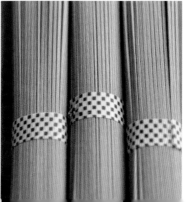
Matcha green tea soba

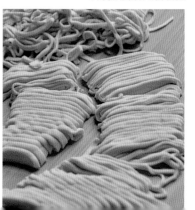
Fresh udon noodles

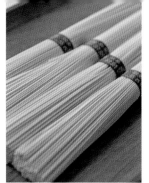
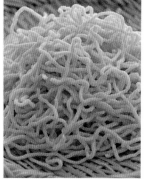
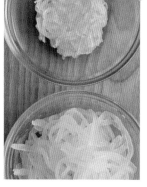
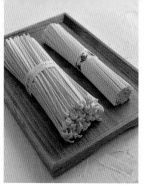

| Somen | Fresh ramen | Shirataki yam noodles | Dried udon |

Somen Smooth and refreshing, somen wheat noodles are a summertime tradition in Japan. They are dried noodles with a smooth and pleasant texture. After boiling, they are cooled under cold running water and flavored with a soy-based dipping sauce which provides a refreshing taste to the dish. Japan is a heavily forested mountainous country with many great sources of soft water which make delicious noodles. Somen are extremely thin wheat noodles that are kneaded and carefully stretched to about ¹⁄₁₆ in (1.5 mm) in diameter as dictated by a Japanese manufacturing standard. There are two methods of manufacturing somen noodles: *tenobe*, the traditional hand-stretching method or by machine. They look the same, but tenobe somen has a unique chewy texture that is considered to be the best quality. Since somen are very thin noodles, keep the cooking time short, about 2 to 3 minutes, and then immediately rinse the noodles under cold running water to retain their chewy texture.

Ramen have become popular all around the world today. They were introduced to Japan from China during the Meiji period in the late 19th century. Ramen are eaten both dried (often as the ubiquitous instant noodles) and fresh. They are made with wheat flour, salt water and kansui, which is an alkaline water similar to baking soda that helps the dough rise and gives it a chewy, firm texture. Ramen noodles have a wavy shape and a yellow color, though they are made without eggs—rather, it is the kansui that turns the noodles yellow naturally. Ramen are served with various kinds of soups such as soy sauce (shoyu), miso (fermented soybean paste), salt (shio) and pork bone stock(tonkotsu), to name a few popular choices; andtoppings, such as boiled eggs, sliced pork chashu, nori and wakame seaweed, bamboo

shoots and chopped green onions. Ramen is typically served with a delicious flavored stock that is unique to each ramen shop. Some shops only use bone broths, while others might add kombu or katsuobushi, creating a synergistic effect between the natural amino acids, such as glutamate and inosinate, and packing lots of umami flavor!

Shirataki (the name literally means "white waterfall.") are thin and translucent, jelly-like noodles. They are also called *konnyaku* noodles, because they're made from the *konjac* yam, and can be either white or dark brown in color. They are mainly composed of water (97%) and dietary fiber (3%) and are low in calories and carbohydrates, making them a healthy, low-carb form of pasta. They're sold as fresh noodles (soft, packed in water and kept in the refrigerated section), or as dried noodles. The noodles have no flavor on their own, so we season them with flavorful dressings or sauces and serve them with vegetables in light and refreshing salads. They are also added to popular hot pot dishes such as shabu shabu, sukiyaki and oden.

Udon are thick and chewy wheat noodles that have been eaten since the Muromachi period (1337–1573) as a substitute for rice, and were often served as a celebratory foods. They are made from a wheat flour and salt water dough which is kneaded and stretched out to about ¹⁄₁₀ in (2.5 mm) diameter. Udon is the basis for unique local dishes in every region of Japan, each using different production methods, shapes and sizes of noodles, as well as different preparation styles. It's at its most delicious when freshly cooked, either served cold with a dipping sauce or hot with a soy-sauce dashi broth made with kombu and katsuobushi.

Dashi and Umami
The "Secret Sauce" of Japanese Cooking

Dashi is perhaps the most important ingredient in Japanese cuisine. Packed with umami, it's a flavorful, traditional broth made of seaweed and dried and smoked tuna fish flakes. But beyond this classic form of dashi, there are other full-flavored versions made with kombu, shiitake mushrooms, noboshi (dried sardines) or awase miso. Dashi is the most important Japanese superfood hiding in plain sight—the most singular and definitive of all Japanese ingredients, and a ubiquitous presence in the Japanese diet. Miso, ramen, stews, omelettes—the list goes on and on. The key ingredients are normally kombu and katsuobushi—simmered, smoked, fermented and flaked skipjack tuna. Together they produce a strong and distinctive umami flavor. Katsuobushi contains inosinic acid and essential amino acids and is rich in minerals. High in protein, low in calories and fat—it strikes all the right superfood notes.

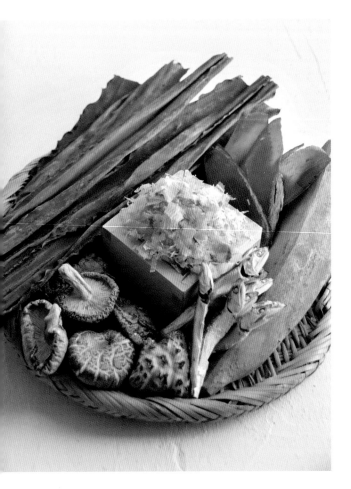

The raw ingredients for dashi (**clockwise from top**): kombu seaweed, thick katsuobushi slices, whole katsuobushi skipjack tuna, niboshi dried baby sardines, dried shiitake mushrooms and shaved katsuobushi flakes.

Kombu makes its own ultra-nutritive contributions, while shiitake mushrooms are another often overlooked superfood. The stems of shiitake mushrooms are a good source of beta-glucans, linked to lower blood cholesterol levels. Mushrooms, in general reduce the risk of cancer and type 2 diabetes and contribute to cardiovascular health. They contain protein, vitamins, minerals and antioxidants, which help eliminate free radicals from the body. Among the antioxidant agents in mushrooms is choline. It can help facilitate muscle movement, learning and memory, and assists in maintaining the structure of cellular membranes while playing a role in the transmission of nerve impulses.

Discovering dashi

Dashi is a clear broth which lies at the heart of Japanese cuisine as one of the most important ingredients in most recipes. Dashi differs from condiments that add flavor, such as soy sauce or miso. Instead, dashi helps bring out the flavors of the ingredients you are cooking with to their full potential. The source of umami in dashi stock most commonly comes from the following ingredients: kombu or kelp (glutamic acid), katsuobushi or dried bonito flakes (inosinic acid), niboshi or small dried sardines (inosinic acid), and dried shiitake mushroom (guanylic acid). The combination and heating of these ingredients results in the umami being intensified by as much as seven or eight times.

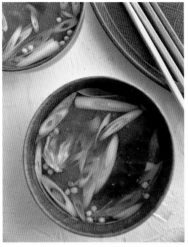
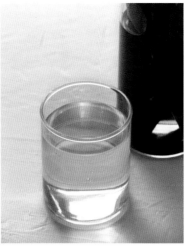
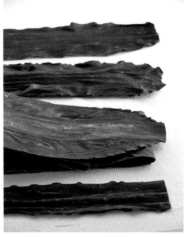

It all starts with dashi | Kombu cold brew | Strips of wavy-edged dried kombu

Today, commercial powdered dashi is available and popular for its convenience; however, it is not the same as handmade dashi since it's loaded with MSG, preservatives and other artificial flavors. Homemade dashi on the other hand is very easy to make once you know how. And it is much flavorful *and* more healthy.

More about umami

In 1908, Professor Kikunae Ikeda of Tokyo University discovered that the main source of the flavor in kombu is glutamic acid and amino acid. This compound makes any dish naturally more tasty. He decided that this unique taste ought to be called umami—which refers to any food with an inherent savoriness. Umami is said to be one of the five basic tastes—along with sweetness, saltiness, sourness and bitterness. It is the natural flavor of amino acid and proteins. You can find umami flavor in a variety of foods, such as parmesan cheese, meat, tomatoes, mushrooms and miso, which contains high levels of the amino acid glutamate. Newborn babies typically have their first taste of umami in breast milk, which also contains large amounts of glutamate. So, there is a sense of familiarity in all umami flavors, as it is among our earliest taste memories. Western and Chinese cooking normally use soup stocks made with fresh meat and vegetables. By comparison, Japanese dashi stock uses dry ingredients containing almost no fat however with not as much umami flavor. That is why dashi stock is characterized by a clean and light flavor. If you want to cook healthier food with reduced sodium, fat and sugar, these umami ingredients not only contribute a savory, delicious flavor, they also make your food light and satisfying. When you combine these umami components in a balanced way, the taste of the ingredients stands out with only a little extra seasoning to help them along. That is the secret of Japanese cuisine, which is known for it light and clean yet complex flavors.

The basics of dashi making

Two ingredients, then add water. Does it get any simpler than that? For some, making dashi is like brewing a delicate tea as opposed to other cuisines where you need to simmer a stock for many hours. Smoky and simple, it's a flexible concoction that serves as a building block for so much of Japanese cuisine.

There are two types of dashi: natural dashi, made with natural ingredients without any added flavorings; and processed dashi, made with food additives (synthetic preservatives, synthetic colors and antioxidants). This book focuses on dashi made from natural ingredients. All of the dashi ingredients are readily available at Asian grocery stores, health food stores and online. By learning the basic methods of making dashi, you can cook authentic Japanese food at home that is healthy and wholesome for you and your family. Now let's talk about the key ingredients.

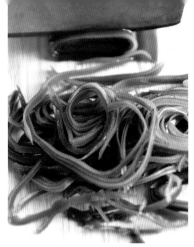
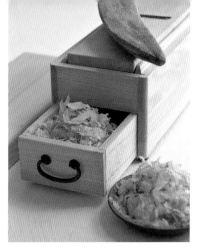
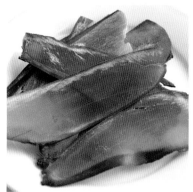

| Sliced kombu | A shaving box used to shave whole pieces of katsuobushi into flakes | Thicker slices of katsuobushi |

Kombu

Historically, Japanese soil was lacking in minerals and it was difficult to get much nourishment from eating vegetables. Therefore, the tradition of eating seaweeds such as kombu arose. Kombu is an ocean vegetable that grows by photosynthesis. It's one of the richest sources of minerals, vitamins, fiber and protein—vital nutrients that are indispensable in any diet. Kombu is also low in calories, rich in glutamic acid (one of the sources of umami) and contains lots of nutrients along with soluble plant fiber, fucoidan, alginate and iodine. The most popular, high-quality types of kombu get their prefixes from the areas in Hokkaido where they're harvested: Ma-kombu, Rishiri-kombu, Rausu-kombu and Hidaka-kombu.

Katsuobushi

Katsuobushi (dried skipjack tuna) is often classified as a fermented food; however, not all katsuobushi is fermented. It's broadly divided into two types: ara-bushi (not fermented) and honkare-bushi (fermented). Depending on the production process, skipjack tuna is filleted into pieces, boiled and then smoked to create ara-bushi, which is then shaved into flakes. Ara-bushi is not fermented as it does not undergo the molding process and is the most common type of katsuobushi (sold under the name of hana-katsuo.)

After the ara-bushi is made, the surface is scraped off with a grinder to remove the tar and it is then covered with a mold and dried in the sun to transform into honkare-bushi, a fermented form of katsuobushi that is more expensive than ara-bushi. Honkare-bushi is fermented with a healthful bacteria (Eurotium herbariorum),

adding to its nutritional benefits and flavor. The mold absorbs moisture from the tuna, so the water content drops to less than 15%. This hardens the katsuobushi and breaks down the fat content, which gives the dashi stock made with it a more elegant, refined flavor. This process also increases its shelf life and concentrates the umami flavor.

Most katsuobushi production is located in Kagoshima and Shizuoka prefectures. The main umami component of katsuobushi is inosinic acid, which is found in animal products such as meat and fish; but the amount of inosinic acid in katsuobushi is by far the highest of any foods (at over 600 mg per 100 grams). It takes up to six months for a single batch of katsuobushi to be made, as over ten manufacturing steps are required to create this unique product. Traditionally, every time katsuobushi is prepared, it must first be shaved into flakes using a wooden box with a sharp blade attached (like a mandolin), which is how I grew up eating it as a child.

Today, however, packaged katsuobushi flakes are widely available, with options that include thinly shaved (hana-katsuo), thicker shaved (atsukezuri) and powdered (kezuri-ko). The type to buy depends on the type of dish you are making. Katsuobushi is also used as a topping for cold and hot dishes and is delicious sprinkled on tofu and over okonomiyaki pancakes.

How to select and store katsuobushi

Choose a light pinkish color for thinly shaved katsuobushi flakes, or slightly shiny ones with a dark color for the thickly shaved slices. Freshly-shaved katsuobushi has much more aroma than

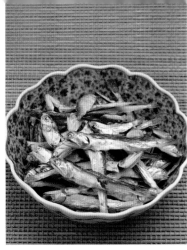
Niboshi

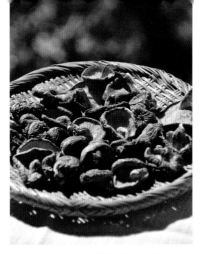
Shiitake mushrooms

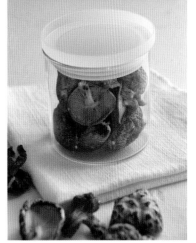
Store away from heat and moisture

preshaved, however if you want to try it, then you need to get a shaving box. Once the package has been opened, the flakes begin to oxidize and the color will start to dull. So store open flakes in the refrigerator or freezer in an airtight container or resealable bag and consume it within six months of opening the package.

Niboshi (small dried sardines)

Niboshi, also called iriko are boiled and dried baby sardines. They are mainly harvested in the coastal regions of Kyushu and Shikoku islands, where the Kuroshio current, known as the Black Stream, is filled with these tiny fish. Blue fish such as sardines are rich in unsaturated fats and contain high amounts of DHA (docosahexaenoic acid) and EPA (eicosapentaenoic acid), as well as calcium and vitamin D, which helps to maintain low blood pressure and good brain function. Dashi made from niboshi contains plenty of umami (from the inosinic acid). Niboshi dashi is often used for ramen and udon noodle broths, and is also used to enhance the flavor of miso soup.

Shiitake mushrooms

Historically, shiitakes were very expensive and used only by samurai and the wealthy. They also factor heavily in Shojin cuisine (plant-based Zen Buddhist cooking). Shiitake mushrooms cultivation began in the Edo period (1603–1868) and spread widely during the 1970s as a result of popular health fads. Dashi made from dried shiitake has an intense flavor and aroma and is highly nutritious. It is umami-rich as a result of containing guanidyl acid (guanylate), one of the three major umami ingredients in Japanese cuisine. It's also rich in eritadenine (an element that makes blood smooth) and lentinan, (which strengthens the immune system). When shitake mushrooms are sundried, the proteins are broken down into amino acids, which increase the umami to a level ten times greater than fresh shiitake mushrooms. Shiitake dashi is widely used to make simmered and rice-based dishes.

How to select and store shiitake mushrooms

Choose well-dried shiitake mushrooms that have beautiful, brown-colored caps with a slightly shiny surface. The underside of the caps should be light beige-yellow in color with short stems. Store them in an airtight container or resealable bag in a cool, dry place away from heat and moisture. You can also dry them by laying them flat on a tray and setting them in the sun for 2 to 3 hours before cooking, increasing the amount of vitamin D.

Soft vs. hard water?

Water, an important element of cooking, has characteristics—such as flavor and mineral content, or hardness—that varies greatly by location. Water in Japan is naturally soft, which helps in effectively extracting the umami components of glutamic acid and inosinic acid. High levels of minerals such as calcium and magnesium over 120 ppm (parts per million), result in hard water which causes the umami to be trapped inside the ingredients. My recommendation is to use soft water, if possible, for the best results when making dashi at home. Living in New York City, I use the tapwater (which is considered soft to moderately hard at 65 ppm), and I always let the water sit overnight to remove the chlorine odors, which evaporate.

Making Dashi Stock

Dashi stock is the foundation for most Japanese cooking—whether it's made with dried fish or with purely vegetarian ingredients like kombu or shiitake. Dashi is used not only in soups but in many other dishes as a seasoning. It will make any dish taste better once you know how to use it. Dashi plays a different role from other seasonings like salt, sugar, soy sauce and miso. It is an umami-rich liquid made from kombu and katsuobushi flakes. It gives a dish a deep, satisfying flavor and the umami effect reduces the amount of salt needed. In combination with other ingredients, dashi offers unlimited possibilities. Various dashi recipes are given here along with ways to use the dashi and to reuse the dashi ingredients.

Basic Dashi Stock (First-Brew Dashi)

This is the most popular type of dashi stock, made with a combination of kombu and katsuobushi. Basic Dashi Stock has an intense flavor and elegant aroma that goes well with clear soups, delicate dishes such as steamed egg custard (chawanmushi), and vinaigrette dressings (sunomono). It adds deep and savory umami flavors to any dish. The primary umami ingredients, glutamic acid from the kombu and inosinic acid from the katsuobushi, are combined here, making any dish naturally more delicious and satisfying simply by incorporating this stock.

YIELD: approx. 4 cups (1 liter)

Three 5-in (13-cm) squares of dried kombu (about ½ oz/15 g)

1¼ cups (15 g) katsuobushi flakes

4 cups (1 liter) water

1. Gently wipe the surface of the kombu with a dry paper towel. Do not remove or wash off the white powdery substance on the surface of the kombu, which is a source of umami flavor called mannitol.

2. Soak the kombu in the water in a saucepan for at least 15 minutes, or more, at room temperature.

3. Heat the kombu and soaking liquid in the same saucepan over medium-low heat just until you start to see small bubbles forming around the edges of the pot (150°F/65°C). Do not allow the water to boil.

4. Remove the kombu from the saucepan.

5. Add the katsuobushi flakes and turn off the heat. Let the katsuobushi sit for 2 to 3 minutes.

6. Line a colander or a strainer with a layer of paper towel and place it in a bowl. Strain the broth without squeezing the katsuobushi. Once it has cooled, store it in a resealable plastic bag in the refrigerator for up to 2 days or in the freezer for up to a month. You can reuse the kombu and katsuobushi by repeating the process one more time, adding more katsuobushi to the pan (see Second Brew Dashi Stock on the next page).

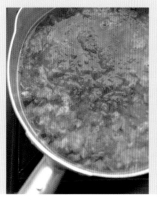 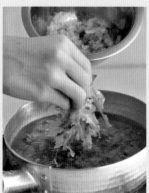 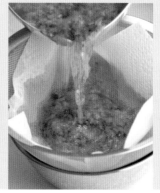 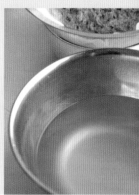

Second-Brew Dashi Stock

You can reuse the kombu and katsuobushi used to make First-Brew Dashi by repeating the same process one more time with this recipe by adding more katsuobushi flakes to the pot. Second Brew Dashi Stock has a less intense flavor, but is still a good soup base for noodles, simmered dishes and miso soups.

YIELD: approx. 4 cups (1 liter)
Leftover kombu and katsuobushi from First-Brew Dashi (previous page)
¾ to 1 cup (10 g) additional katsuobushi flakes
4 cups (1 liter) water

1. Combine the leftover kombu and katsuobushi with the water in a small saucepan. Turn the heat on until you just start to see small bubbles around the edge of the pan.

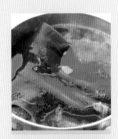

2. Add the new katsuobushi to the saucepan and turn off the heat.

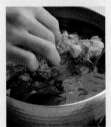

3. Let the mixture sit for 2 to 3 minutes.

4. Line a colander or a strainer with a paper towel and place in a bowl. Strain the broth without squeezing the katsuobushi. Store in a resealable plastic bag in the refrigerator for up to two days or in the freezer for up to a month.

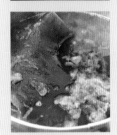

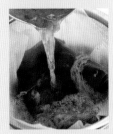

Quick Dashi Stock in a Teapot

This is my quick version of Basic Dashi Stock for times when I only need a small amount, just enough to make a bowl of soup or noodles or a few condiments. This is an easy way for you to incorporate dashi into your daily cooking. It only requires kombu, katsuobushi, a teapot and boiling water. It is the same as brewing a pot of tea—simply place all the ingredients into the teapot and steep them for 1 to 2 minutes. For a basic dashi stock, use both kombu and katsuobushi. For a plant-based version, use kombu and/or shiitake mushrooms only. This quick method is perfect to make miso soup in the morning for breakfast, a dish enjoyed by many Japanese. Simply add miso paste, diced tofu, wakame seaweed and/or chopped green onions to a cup/bowl of hot dashi stock from the teapot.

YIELD: approx. 2 cups (500 ml)
SHELF LIFE: Store in an airtight container in the refrigerator for up to 2 days, freezer for 1 month
RECIPE IDEAS: Soups, dressings, sauces and condiments

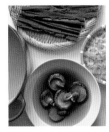

2 small squares (3 in/8 cm) dried kombu
½ cup (7 g) katsuobushi flakes
2 cups (500 ml) boiling water, about 175°F (80°C)

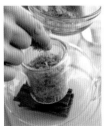

1. Combine the kombu and katsuobushi in a teapot.

2. Pour the boiling water into the teapot and steep, covered, for 1 to 2 minutes.

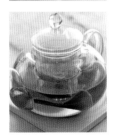

3. Pour the stock into a cup and use as needed, or strain through a colander or strainer into a bowl. Strain the broth without squeezing the katsuobushi.

4. Transfer any unused broth to a sterilized glass bottle or jar with a lid. Let it cool to room temperature before storing, tightly covered, in the refrigerator.

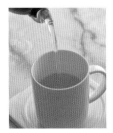

5. For ways to use the leftover kombu and katsuobushi, check out the other recipes and suggestions in this section.

Kombu Dashi Stock (Hot Brew)

Kombu dashi is a vegetarian stock made by soaking pieces of kombu in water then gently heating the liquid, but not to boiling (150°F/65°C), then removing it from the heat and allowing it to steep. This stock has a stronger umami flavor than Kombu Water (Cold Brew), the other recipe on this page, as the gentle heat helps release more flavor into the liquid. Use it for miso soups and noodle broths, as well as dressings, sauces, stir-fries and simmered dishes. Kombu Dashi Stock has a savory flavor with a hint of the ocean.

YIELD: approx. 4 cups (1 liter)
Three 4-in (10-cm) squares dried kombu
4 cups (1 liter) water

1. Gently clean the surface of the kombu with a dry paper towel. Do not remove or wash off the white powdery substance on the surface of the kombu, which is a source of umami flavor called mannitol.

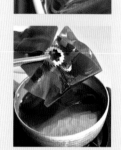

2. Soak the kombu in the water in a saucepan for 15 minutes or more, as long as overnight, at room temperature. If soaking overnight, keep the saucepan in the refrigerator.

3. Heat the kombu and the soaking liquid in the same saucepan over medium-low heat until you start to see tiny bubbles forming around the edges of the pot (150°F/65°C). Be sure not to boil the water. Remove from the heat.

4. Remove the kombu from the saucepan. Once it has cooled, store the dashi in a resealable plastic bag or a container with a lid in the refrigerator for up to 2 days, or in the freezer for up to a month. You can reuse the kombu by repeating the same process with 50% less water.

Kombu Water (Cold Brew)

Kombu Water is the cold-brew version of Kombu Dashi Stock—a simple method for extracting the natural umami flavor from kombu by soaking pieces of kombu in water overnight. You can drink Kombu Water as a beverage, or add it to smoothies, soups, dressings and sauces. Kombu Water has a clean and fresh oceanic flavor and is full of nutrients. It will keep for up to 3 days in the refrigerator.

YIELD: approx. 4 cups (1 liter)
Three 4-in (10-cm) squares dried kombu (¾ oz/20 g)
4 cups (1 liter) water

1. Gently clean the surface of the kombu with a dry towel. Do not remove or wash off the white powdery substance on the surface of kombu, which is a source of umami flavor called mannitol.

2. Place the kombu and the water in a container and let it steep in the refrigerator overnight.

3. Remove the kombu from the water the following day.

4. Store the liquid in a resealable plastic bag or a container with a lid in the refrigerator for up to 3 days, or in the freezer for up to a month. You can reuse the kombu pieces by repeating the process using half the amount of water.

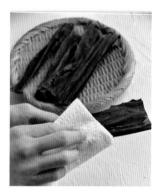
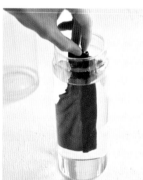
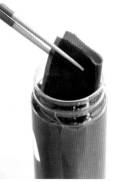
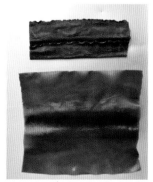

Shiitake Dashi Stock

This is a cold brew stock that is very simple to make; you just soak the dried mushrooms in water overnight. Or, if you are in a hurry, soak them in hot water for 20 minutes before removing the stems. After soaking them to obtain the liquid, you can cook and eat the caps and stems. Shiitake Dashi Stock is a key ingredient in Shojin-style Buddhist temple vegetarian cooking.

YIELD: approx. 2 cups (500 ml)
4 dried shiitake mushrooms, with stems attached
2 cups (500 ml) cold water

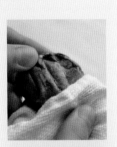

1. Gently wipe the surface of the shiitake mushrooms with a dry paper towel.

2. Place the shiitake and water in a small container or jar.

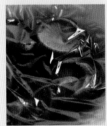

3. Cover the container and place it in the refrigerator to steep overnight. Remove the shiitake the next day and reserve the liquid.

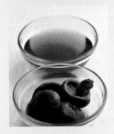

4. Store the liquid in a resealable plastic bag in the refrigerator for up to 3 days, or in the freezer for up to a month.

Niboshi Dashi Stock (Hot Brew)

This is the dashi stock that I grew up drinking in our daily miso soup. It's made by soaking dried baby sardines in water then simmering the liquid gently. It's a popular dashi to use for ramen, udon and soba noodle dishes. It has an immensely powerful and deep savory flavor, with a rich oceanic aroma.

YIELD: approx. 4 cups (1 liter)
8–10 pieces (½ cup/15 g) niboshi dried baby sardines (see page 35)
4 cups (1 liter) water

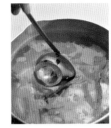

1. Remove the heads and innards, if necessary, of the niboshi then break them in half lengthwise.

2. Soak the niboshi in the water in a saucepan for at least 15 minutes, or more, at room temperature.

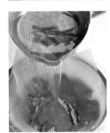

3. Heat the niboshi and the soaking liquid in the same saucepan over medium-high heat. When bubbles begin to appear (175°F/80°C), reduce the heat to low and cook for 3 to 4 more minutes. Skim the foam from the surface of the liquid using a ladle or sieve.

4. Turn off the heat. Line a colander or strainer with a paper towel and set it in a bowl. Strain the broth without squeezing the niboshi. Store the liquid in a resealable plastic bag in the refrigerator for up to two days, or in the freezer for up to a month.

Niboshi Dashi Stock (Cold Brew)

This is another version made using the cold-brew method, which is an easy way of extracting natural umami flavor from the niboshi. It simply requires soaking the niboshi in water overnight. You can use this stock to make miso soup and noodle soup broths. It will keep for up to 2 days in the refrigerator.

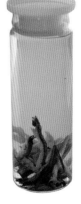

YIELD: approx. 4 cups (1 liter)
1½ cups (15 g) niboshi dried baby sardines (see page 35)
4 cups (1 liter) water

1. Remove the heads and innards from the niboshi, then break them in half lengthwise.

2. Place the niboshi and water in a container and let it steep in the refrigerator overnight.

3. Remove the niboshi from the water. Store the liquid in a resealable plastic bag in the refrigerator for up to two days, or in the freezer for up to a month.

Ponzu Sauce

Surprise! I'm using orange juice in this all-purpose sauce instead of Japanese yuzu citrus. If you prefer a tarter ponzu, use lemon or a combo of the two. You can buy bottled ponzu, but it is fun to make your own!

YIELD: approx. 1¼ cups (300 ml)
SHELF LIFE: Store in an airtight container in the refrigerator for up to one week.

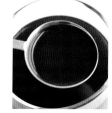

⅓ cup (80 ml) soy sauce
⅓ cup (80 ml) rice vinegar
⅓ cup (80 ml) Basic Dashi, Kombu or Shiitake Stock (pages 36, 38–9)
⅓ cup (80 ml) fresh-squeezed orange juice (see headnote)

Combine the soy sauce, rice vinegar, Dashi Stock and orange juice in a sterilized glass bottle or jar with a lid. Shake it well to combine all the ingredients and then store, tightly covered, in the refrigerator.

Goma Sesame Salad Dressing

Here I use Basic Dashi Stock, but if you want an extra-creamy plant-based dressing, you can replace the stock with soy milk for a satisfyingly rich texture.

YIELD: approx. 2 cups (500 ml)
SHELF LIFE: Store in an airtight container in the refrigerator for up to one week.

¼ cup (65 ml) soy sauce
¼ cup (65 ml) mirin sweet rice wine
1 cup (250 ml) Basic Dashi Stock (page 36)
¼ teaspoon grated garlic
2 tablespoons maple syrup or granulated sugar
¼ cup (65 ml) neri goma sesame paste or tahini
3 tablespoons toasted white sesame seeds

1. Add soy sauce, mirin, Basic Dashi Stock, garlic, and maple syrup to a small saucepan and bring to a boil over medium heat.

2. Reduce the heat to low and add the neri goma and sesame seeds to the pot and cook, while stirring with a spatula until the ingredients are well-combined and the sauce has a smooth consistency, 3 to 5 minutes.

3. Transfer to a sterilized glass bottle or jar with a lid. Let it cool to room temperature before storing, tightly covered, in the refrigerator.

Kaeshi Sauce

Kaeshi is a thick soy-based sauce that is one of the most popular condiments in Japanese cooking. Many people buy premade Kaeshi because of its convenience—you would be surprised how many different brands are on the shelves of Japanese supermarkets—but it is extremely easy to make, using a few basic ingredients that you may already have in your pantry. What is unique about this family recipe is that we add a piece of kombu to the jar once the sauce is made for an extra boost of rich umami flavor. Having ready-made Kaeshi in the refrigerator allows you to make so many different dishes by adding it to your dashi stocks, vinegar, oil, miso, spices or simply using it to season meats, fish, tofu and vegetables. Once you become familiar with how to make Kaeshi, you can control the sweetness to your liking by adjusting the amount of mirin sweet rice wine and granulated sugar.

YIELD: approx. 1½ cups (375 ml)
SHELF LIFE: Store in an airtight container in the refrigerator for up to one month.
RECIPE IDEAS: For fish, meat, vegetables

½ cup (125 ml) mirin sweet rice wine (or ½ cup [125 ml] sake or white wine mixed with 2 tablespooons sugar)
4 tablespoons granulated sugar
1 cup (250 ml) soy sauce
One 6-in (15-cm) square dried kombu

1. Add the mirin and sugar to a small saucepan and bring to a boil over medium-high heat.

2. Reduce the heat to medium-low and add the soy sauce to the pan. Cook for 2 to 3 minutes, or until the sugar is dissolved and you start seeing small bubbles around the edges of the pan.

3. Transfer to a sterilized bottle or glass jar with a lid and add the kombu. Let it cool to room temperature before storing, tightly covered, in the refrigerator.

4. To use the leftover kombu, cut into small pieces, to add to soups.

Simmered Kombu and Katsuobushi Tsukudani

Tsukudani is seafood, meat, seaweed or vegetables simmered in a sweet and soy-based sauce. A delicious appetizer or sidedish, it will keep in the refrigetator for up to 2 weeks.

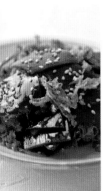

3 or 4 pieces rehydrated or leftover
   kombu (from making Basic Dashi Stock)
1 or 2 cups leftover katsuobushi
2 tablespoons Kaeshi Sauce (page 40)
1 teaspoon brown sugar
1 teaspoon rice vinegar
1 tablespoons sake
1 teaspoon toasted white sesame seeds
½ cup (125 ml) Second-Brew Dashi Stock
   (see page 37)

1. Cut the kombu into 1-in (2.5-cm) squares.

2. Combine the kombu, katsuobushi, Kaeshi Sauce, brown sugar, rice vinegar, sake, sesame seeds and dashi in a small saucepan, cover, and set over medium-low heat. Cook until the kombu is soft, about 20 minutes. If the liquid starts to evaporate during cooking, add some more dashi and cook until the water is almost gone, and the kombu has become soft and tender. Serve with steamed rice, noodles or in a bento box.

3. Store leftover Tsukudani in a container or a resealable plastic bag in the refrigerator for up to seven days, or in the freezer for up to a month.

Kombu Marinated in Ponzu

Citrus-based sauces and preparations are ideal for marinades, dipping and on salads. With its mildly tangy flavor, ponzu adds a flash of acid, pairing perfectly with marinated tomatoes. Here, strips of kombu come to life when bathed in citrusy ponzu.

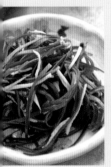

3 or 4 large pieces rehydrated or leftover kombu
½ cup (125 ml) Ponzu Sauce (page 40)
1-in (2.5-cm) piece fresh ginger, peeled and
   cut into thin strips

1. Slice the kombu into thin strips by first rolling the kombu up (see photo.)

2. Combine the kombu, ponzu and ginger in a bowl or container and mix well. Cover and marinate overnight, or up to seven days in the refrigerator. Serve as is, or added to salads, tofu, steamed rice or noodles.

Stirfried Kombu and Niboshi

Sweet, spicy and with umami undertones, this sidedish pulls in all the flavor notes, the perfect fusion of superfood goodness.

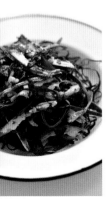

3 or 4 pieces leftover kombu from
   Basic Dashi Stock (pages 36–37)
1½ cups leftover niboshi from Niboshi
   Dashi Stock (page 39)
1 tablespoon sesame oil
1 tablespoon Kaeshi Sauce (page 40)
½ teaspoon fish sauce
½ teaspoon minced garlic
1 tablespoon maple syrup
¼ teaspoon red pepper (optional)

1. Cut the kombu into thin strips (see photo above.)

2. Heat a nonstick skillet over medium-high heat and add the kombu and niboshi. Stir them with a spatula continually for two to three minutes to revive them.

3. Add the sesame oil, Kaeshi Sauce, fish sauce and garlic to the skillet and contimue to cook over medium-high heat for 4 to 5 minutes. Add the maple syrup, stirring continually, and cook for an additional 2 to 3 minutes, or until the liquid has completely evaporated. Serve with steamed rice, bento box or appetizers and sprinkle with chili pepper, if you like.

4. Store in the refrigerator for up to 7 days, or the freezer for up to a month.

Super Japanese Pickles

In Japan there are many different kinds of umami-rich pickles that utilize fresh seasonal vegetables. There are many different pickling methods, including pickling with salt, with fermented rice koji, salted rice bran, sweetened sake, seasoned vinegar and miso. Since fermented pickles contain probiotics, beneficial to maintaining gut health, they have been an important part of the Japanese superfood diet over the centuries. Japanese pickles are always included in traditional ichijyu-sansai, set meals consisting of rice, soup and three main dishes. Here, I show you how to make various Japanese-style pickled vegetables (called *tsukemono* in Japanese), made with fermented ingredients such as miso and yogurt, and umami-rich ingredients such as kombu. There are also several quick and easy pickles that can be eaten immediately like a salad by simply cutting up vegetables and dressing them with a pickling liquid or sauce.

Umeboshi are pickled plums that are dried in the sun, then matured for three years in barrels. Traditionally they are pickled in 25-30% salt to give them a long shelf life, making them very salty. However, with the growing trend of eating less salt, the salt content has dropped to less than 20% During the pickling process, the mineral content (especially calcium and iron) increases. Umeboshi are popular in bento boxes as the citric acid prevents the growth of bacteria. Umeboshi are also an acidic food, keeping our bodies alkaline—and as the body becomes more alkaline, it is said that the immune system is strengthened. Other benefits include recovery from fatigue, improvement of bowel movements, prevention of blood clots, stimulation of sugar metabolism and strengthening of liver functions.

Nukazuke are seasonal vegetables pickled in rice bran, to which about 15 percent salt and the same amount of water are added. Other additions are red pepper for an antiseptic effect and kelp for umami flavor. Pickling has been used for 2,000 years as a way of not only keeping vegetables from spoiling, also adding great flavor and increased nutrition to foods. Raw vegetables provide the body with their full dose of vitamins, fiber and carotene without compromising their nutritional value. This, provides vitamin B for beautiful skin, lactic acid bacteria to relieve constipation, boosts immunity, improves sleep and helps to relieve fatigue.

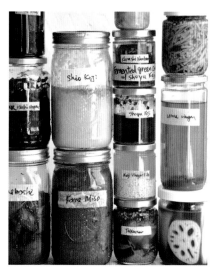
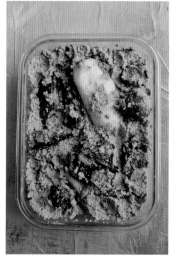

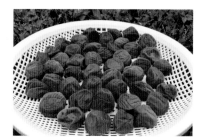

Far left: Assorted Homemade Japanese Pickles, Vinegars and Koji. **Left**: Nukazuke, vegetables fermenting in a bed of seasoned rice bran. **Below:** Umeboshi.

Quick Miso Yogurt Pickles

There is nothing better than freshly pickled seasonal vegetables with a bowl of steamed rice for a tasty Japanese-style breakfast! While the most popular Japanese pickles are made in the nukazuke style—by fermenting the vegetables in a bed of rice bran—this approach requires a lot of attention. The contents need to be stirred by hand once or twice a day to ensure proper pickling and to avoid mold. I wanted to create similar pickles without all the work. So I asked my mom. I was very surprised when she suggested mixing awase miso with yogurt. She thought it would create a flavor very similar to nukazuke with no effort required, and she was right. Mom knows best. Fermented foods such as miso and yogurt are a great source of probiotics because they contain live bacteria, which support your gut heath. If you're lactose intolerant, substitute a plant-based yogurt (such as coconut, cashew or soy milk) for the Greek yogurt. These pickles are ready to eat within a day, or less.

PREPARATION TIME: 10 minutes
PICKLING TIME: half day to one day
SERVES 4 servings

1 medium carrot, peeled
2 Japanese or baby cucumbers
4 small red radishes
1½ teaspoons sea salt
6 tablespoons miso paste
6 tablespoons whole milk Greek yogurt
1 piece of dried kombu, 2 x 6 in (5 cm x 15 cm)

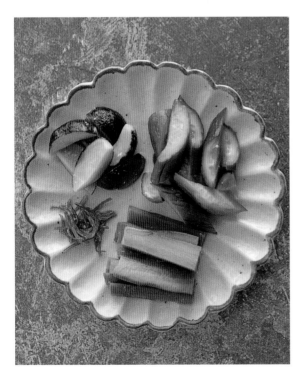

1. Cut the vegetables in half lengthwise. Sprinkle the salt on them and let them sit for 10 minutes at room temperature. The salt draws the water out and seasons the vegetables. Remove it by wiping and dabbing the vegetables with paper towels.

2. Place the miso, yogurt and kombu strips in a resealable bag or a glass container with a lid and mix well.

3. Add the vegetables to the miso mixture. Gently massage the vegetables through the bag for a couple of minutes, or if using a glass container, massage with your hands inside the container. Remove the air and close the bag tightly or put a lid on the glass container.

4. Let the vegetables pickle in the refrigerator overnight. They will be ready in anywhere from 12 hours to a day, depending on the vegetables and the type of miso you're using.

5. Remove the vegetables from the bag or glass container. If you like a strong umami flavor, leave the sauce on the vegetables. For a milder flavor, wipe the excess sauce off with a paper towel. To serve, cut the vegetables into bite-sized pieces and the kombu into thin strips. The kombu will rehydrate in the pickling liquid. You can store the pickles in the refrigerator for up to 7 days.

Koji Pickled Vegetables

I often watched my mom make the pickling for fermented rice pickles by combining 3 parts salt, 5 parts rice koji and 8 parts steamed rice. It took her ten days! And as much as I love pickles, I wanted to be able to make something similar that was fast and easy. So I developed this recipe, which uses amazake and sea salt to create a similar pickling base, but in much less time. Amazake, which means "sweet sake," is a naturally sweet rice drink with a thick and creamy texture made from fermented rice koji. It contains a high amount of amino acids, vitamins and probiotics, and is known to improve digestion. For this recipe, you will need amazake made from rice koji (or brown rice or oat koji). The vegetables are ready to be eaten after 8 hours to a day of pickling. Don't remove or rinse off the sauce, as it's packed with malty, savory umami flavor!

PREPARATION TIME: 15 minutes
PICKLING TIME: half day to one day
SERVES 4

½ carrot, peeled
1 Japanese or baby cucumber
1 large bok choy stem
1 piece, 1 x 2 in (2.5 x 5 cm) peeled
  daikon
1 cup (250 ml) amazake sweet sake
1½ tablespoons sea salt, divided

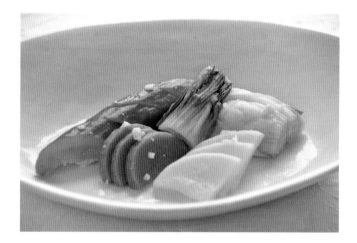

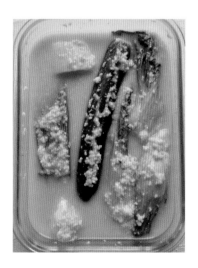

1. Cut the vegetables in half lengthwise and place on a plate. Sprinkle ½ tablespoon of the salt on the vegetables and let them sit for 10 minutes at room temperature, allowing the salt to draw out the water from the vegetables. Remove the salt by wiping the vegetables with a paper towel.

2. Place the amazake and the remaining 1 tablespoon of salt into an airtight glass container with a lid or a resealable plastic bag, and mix well.

3. Add the vegetables to the amazake mixture. Gently massage the vegetables with your hands in the container, or through the bag for a couple of minutes. Put the lid on the glass container or remove the air and seal the bag tightly.

4. Let the vegetables pickle in the refrigerator overnight. They will be ready in anywhere from 8 hours to 1 day, depending on the vegetables you're using.

5. Remove the vegetables from the glass container or the bag. Leave the sauce on the vegetables. To serve, slice the vegetables into bite-sized pieces and serve with steamed rice and miso soup as a complete meal, or serve as an appetizer paired with tea or alcoholic beverages.

Quick Mixed Vegetable Pickles

These pickles are made using a homemade pickling salt recipe that has been passed down in my family for generations: sea salt, kombu, dried shiitake mushroom and dried red chili pepper. This recipe is truly simple and quick—the pickles are ready to eat in only 15 minutes! By sprinkling some salt on the vegetables, the water is drawn out while preserving and concentrating their flavors. In Japan we generally use a pickling container with a press for this dish, but here we use a resealable plastic bag with a weight of some kind. The weight helps squeeze out excess water and heightens the natural flavors of the vegetables. A mix of green and white napa cabbage leaves, along with colorful carrots and cucumbers, will give you a beautiful presentation. The result is a great crunch and clean taste without too many pungent, overpowering flavors.

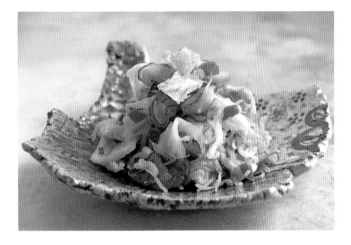

PREPARATION TIME: 15 minutes
PICKLING TIME: 15 minutes to two days
SERVES 4

¼ head napa cabbage, cut lengthwise
1 Japanese cucumber or baby cucumber
½ carrot
1 piece of dried kombu, 2-in (5-cm)
  square
1 small dried shiitake mushroom
1½ tablespoons sea salt
1 small red chili pepper, seeds removed
Peel of ¼ yuzu or lemon

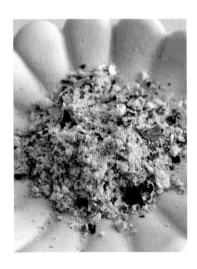

1. Remove the core of the cabbage and cut the leaves into bite-sized pieces, about 2 inches (5 cm). Thinly slice the cucumber. Peel and julienne the carrot.

2. Using scissors, cut the kombu and shiitake into a couple of smaller pieces. Put the kombu, shiitake, salt and chili pepper in a blender or food processor and coarsely chopped by pulsing for 10 to 12 seconds. Do not overblend into a powder. You want to see small bits and pieces of kombu, shiitake and chili pepper in the salt.

3. Put all the vegetables and the pickling salt mixture into a resealable plastic bag and massage the bag with your hands until the vegetables begin to soften and are well-coated, about 1 minute. Remove the air from the bag and seal it tightly. Put the bag on a plate and place another heavy plate or pot on top of it to weigh it down. Place it in the refrigerator and leave it to pickle for at least 15 minutes. The salt will draw the liquid out of the vegetables and turn it into a brine. You can let the vegetables pickle for up to two days in the refrigerator.

4. Squeeze the liquid from the vegetables with your hand. Or lightly rinse them in cool water to remove the salt, if needed. Garnish with the grated yuzu peel on top.

Tangy Pickled Daikon and Carrot with Yuzu

This sweet and tangy pickled daikon called *namasu* is a traditional New Year's dish. Raw vegetables are thinly sliced and marinated in sweet vinegar. We always make these cool and crunchy pickles in big batches at home and mix in some fresh crabmeat or ikura salmon roe to make it more festive for the holiday. It's a very refreshing sidedish that goes perfectly with BBQ or sandwiches or can be simply snacked on directly from the jar. My family likes to serve this pickle dumpling-style by taking a slice of daikon and using it as a wrapper for stuffing shredded carrots inside. (I call this a "raw vegan dumpling.") In addition to being fun to eat, it's very easy to make. If you're in a hurry, simply julienne both the carrot and daikon and marinate it in the vinegar sauce and serve as is without assembling them into dumplings as shown.

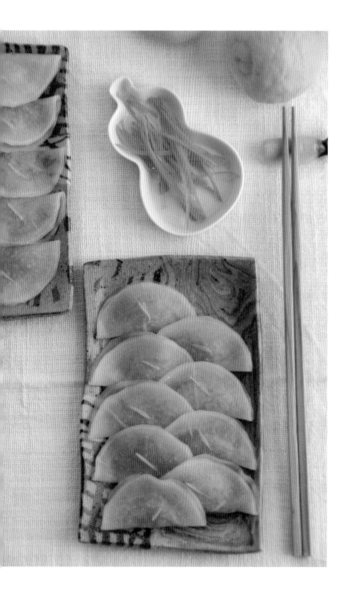

PREPARATION TIME: 15 minutes
COOKING TIME: 15 minutes
SERVES 4

4 in (10 cm) piece of daikon (7 oz/200g)
1 medium carrot (4 oz/100g)
Peel of ¼ yuzu or lemon
1 teaspoon sea salt
¼ cup (65 ml) rice vinegar
1 teaspoon granulated sugar

1. Peel and thinly slice the daikon using a mandoline (or use a sharp knife to cut it into thin slices, about ¹⁄₁₆ in/1.5 mm) and put the slices in a small bowl. Peel and julienne the carrot into thin pieces and put them in a separate bowl.

2. Carefully strip off the topmost layer of yuzu peel using a small sharp knife or vegetable peeler, then julienne the strips into thin slivers.

3. Sprinkle half the salt over the daikon and half over the carrot. Let it sit for 10 minutes to allow the salt to draw out the water. Remove the water either by draining the vegetables in a colander over the sink, or by patting them dry with a paper towel. Squeeze the excess water from the vegetables with your hand.

4. Combine the rice vinegar and sugar in a small bowl. Mix well.

5. Add half of the vinegar sauce to each bowl of vegetables and let them marinate in the refrigerator for 10 minutes.

6. To serve, take about ½ teaspoon carrot and wrap it inside a slice of daikon, folding the daikon in half like a dumpling wrapper. Garnish with yuzu strips on top.

Crunchy Daikon Pickles with Hot Pepper and Kombu

This pickled daikon is highly addictive—a mix of sweet, salty and tangy with a hint of umami from the kombu (which boosts both the flavor and the minerals). Additionally, the dried chili adds a little heat, giving the dish a more balanced flavor. When you pickle fresh daikon, after 30 minutes of pickling, it releases its water, which in turn dilutes the brine, resulting in the flavors being perfectly blended once it's ready. Although the soy sauce might look like too much, the flavors will balance out in the end. Adding sliced celery to the pickling brine along with daikon is one of my favorite variations. This is an easy and delicious pickling recipe that can be adapted for use with other vegetables. Enjoy it as a side dish with steamed rice and soup or as a simple snack with cold beer or sake.

PREPARATION TIME: 10 minutes
COOKING TIME: 10 minutes
MARINATING TIME: 30 minutes to 3 days
SERVES 4

1 lb (450 g) daikon radish
1 small piece of rehydrated kombu, 2 inches
  (5 cm) square
1 whole dried red chili pepper
⅓ cup (80 ml) Kaeshi Sauce (page 40)
⅓ cup (80ml) rice vinegar

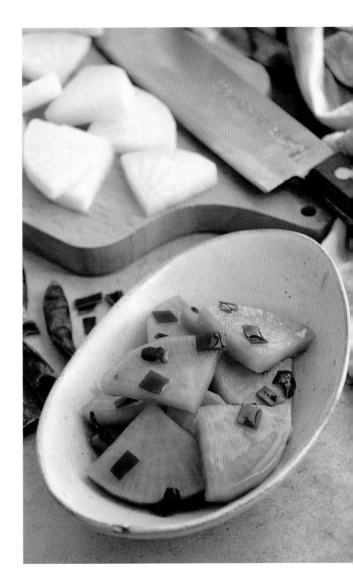

1. Peel and cut the daikon into ¼ in (6 mm) thick quarter moons.

2. Using scissors, cut the kombu into smaller pieces, about ¼ in (6 mm) square.

3. Gently crush the dried chili into small pieces, using your hands, and discard the seeds.

4. Put the daikon, kombu, chili pepper, Kaeshi Sauce and rice vinegar in a resealable plastic bag. Remove the air from the bag and close and seal it tightly. Place the bag in the refrigerator and leave it to pickle for at least 30 minutes. You can let the vegetables pickle for up to 3 days in the refrigerator. The pickles can be stored in the refrigerator for up to 3 weeks.

5. To serve: For a strong flavor, empty the pickles and pickling liquid into a serving bowl, or individual bowls. For a milder flavor, drain the liquid. Serve with steamed rice and miso soup, if you like.

Six Fermented Super Seasonings: Miso, Soy Sauce, Vinegar, Sake, Mirin and Koji

Miso is a fermented soybean paste that has supported a heathy Japanese diet for over 1,300 years. Miso soup is one of the most popular Japanese breakfast items—a mixture of ingredients boiled in dashi stock and seasoned with miso paste. Miso is a great source of essential nutrients (vitamins B12, B2, E and K and dietary fiber) and probiotics that support heathy digestion and slow the effects of aging. Studies show that having a bowl of miso soup every day lowers the risk of breast cancer. Miso also helps to alkalize the body, strengthening the immune system. Made with soybeans, salt and koji, there are many different types of miso. Koji is a fungus (or a mold—Aspergillus oryzae) that contributes a strong, savory flavor to many traditional Japanese foods, such as soy sauce, sake and rice vinegar. The high humidity levels in Japan are conducive to the fermentation process, making miso and other fermented products suitable for the climate. So, how do you know which miso to purchase? Read on!

Miso is classified by its koji content and ingredients as well as by its color. There are 3 basic types of miso based on the type of grain malt used in producing it.

1. Rice Malt Miso—This is the most popular type of miso, accounting for 80% of all miso sold in Japan. It's made from soybeans, rice malt and salt. There are many varieties of rice miso, based on the ratio of ingredients and the length of fermentation, each with slightly different colors and tastes.

2. Barley Malt Miso—This miso, also called "country style" or homestyle, is found in Okinawa and Kyushu. When I make my own miso, I prefer to make this type for its beautiful barley aroma and slightly nutty, sweet flavor. It's made from soybean, barley malt and salt.

3. Soybean Malt Miso—This is produced in the central Tokai region of Japan (mainly Aichi, Mie and Gifu prefectures) and is made from soybeans, soybean malt and salt. This type of miso is called hatcho miso and has the darkest brown color and an intense salty, umami flavor. This type of miso is used to flavor udon noodle soups as well as miso pork cutlets, a well-known local dish from Nagoya.

Miso is also classified by its colors, which fall into three different categories. The color is the result of several factors such as the ratio of ingredients, fermentation time, climate and production location. Together these create the Maillard reaction, in which amino acids in the miso react with the sugar and change color. The longer the fermentation process, the darker the color, and the more antioxidant and anti-aging properties the miso has. Miso also helps the body protect against free radicals and strengthens the immune system.

Here are the three basic miso types based on their colors:

1. Awase miso—Light brownish yellow in color, this is the most versatile and popular miso in Japan. Awase means "combined or blended." This miso has a medium shade, between light and dark. It has a well-balanced flavor that goes well with any type of dish. For this reason, it's the most versatile and commonly used type. If you want to choose just one type of miso, this is the one.

2. Shiro miso—Whitish to light yellow in color, this miso has a sweeter flavor because it isn't fermented as long. It has a shorter shelf life than other misos. It is commonly used for vegetable miso soup, salad dressings and as a pickle seasoning. This variety of miso is popular in the Kansai region of western Japan.

3. Aka miso—Reddish brown in color, this miso has a salty-savory flavor that is a result of its longer fermentation time, which gives it deeper umami flavor and aroma. It's commonly used with seafoods, such as clam miso soup and simmered dishes. Soybean malt miso is included within this group.

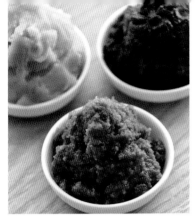
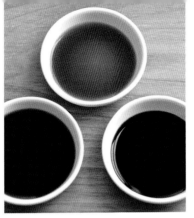
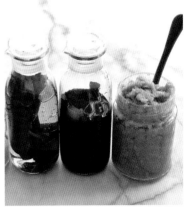

Clockwise from top left: White, red and awase miso

Three shades of shoyu

From left to right: Kombu vinegar, kombu soy sauce and miso

Extra tips about miso

Miso is paired with dashi in Japanese cooking and you often see miso packages labeled "dashi-added." This means that additives such as MSG or other artificial ingredients have been added to the miso. If you want to avoid those, look for a label that lists only three ingredients: soybeans, salt and koji (rice, barley or soybean malts)—preferably also non-GMO products, if that is on your check list. Adding your own vegan or non-vegan dashi is easy to do (see pages 36–39). Also, barley (wheat) koji contains gluten, so make sure to pick other varieties for gluten-free options.

Storage

Be aware that mold can grow on low-salt misos. Keep the miso in a cool, dark place before opening the package, and after opening it store it in the refrigerator. Use a clean, dry spoon when you take miso from the container to prevent mold from forming. After taking miso from the container, flatten the surface and replace the thin white paper that lies directly on the surface of the miso—this prevents the miso from being exposed to air and oxidizing, and prevents it from drying out.

Soy Sauce (Shoyu) is a fermented seasoning liquid made from soybeans, wheat and salt with koji (a fungus called Aspergillus oryzae). It is the most popular condiment in Japanese cuisine and is used in a wide variety of dishes. My first field trip in middle school was to visit the Kikkoman soy sauce factory in Chiba prefecture. Soy sauce was discovered accidentally when the liquid that was accumulated on the surface of the miso was thought so delicious, people started to save it to season their food. I remember when my dad

first made miso at home when I was a child—I saw a big puddle of thick, dark brown liquid in the middle of the miso barrel and I asked him what it was. He explained that it was moisture that appeared on the surface of the miso from the soybeans that were not submerged in liquid. We saved the liquid, called tamari soy sauce, and served it frequently with sashimi. JAS (Japanese Agricultural Standards) divides soy sauce into five different types, depending on the ingredients as well as the length of fermentation.

1. Koikuchi Dark Soy Sauce—Made with an almost equal ratio of soybeans to wheat, koikuchi is the most popular soy sauce in Japan, accounting for 80% of the soy sauce consumed in the country. With a reddish brown color and a great aroma, it's a versatile soy sauce that can be used in any type of dish. In this cookbook, I use koikuchi soy sauce for all my recipes unless noted otherwise.

2. Usukuchi Light Soy Sauce—Made with soybeans and lightly roasted wheat, this light soy sauce is a popular choice in the Kansai region (in western Japan). It has a higher level of sodium than koikuchi, so a little goes a long way. The lighter color is a result of the shorter fermentation period. The light brown color and thinner consistency allows the flavors of the ingredients you're using to shine through.

3. Tamari—Made with soybeans as its primary ingredient, tamari has a thick, syrupy texture and a dark brown color. It's popular in the Tokai region (mainly in Aichi, Mie and Gifu prefectures). The fermentation process is longer than that of other soy sauces, resulting in a darker color and and the highest amount of umami of any soy sauce. Recently, there have been some tamari soy sauces produced that do not contain wheat, making them a popular gluten-free soy sauce outside Japan. This is a great choice for dipping sauces to accompany sashimi and sushi.

4. Saishikomi twice-brewed soy sauce— Saishikomi, which originated in Yamaguchi prefecture, has the darkest brown color of any soy sauce due to the length of the fermentation period. This soy sauce is brewed from another soy sauce, instead of using salted water, which makes it double fermented. This rich, aromatic soy sauce goes well with tofu salad and sashimi as a dipping sauce.

5. Shiro white soy sauce—Made mostly from wheat with a small amount of soybeans, this soy sauce has the lightest brown color and a sweet aroma that results from a shorter fermentation and maturation process. Thus it has less umami flavor than other types of soy sauce. It originated in Aichi prefecture in the Edo period and is popular because it increases the saltiness of a dish without turning the ingredients a dark color. It is often used for steamed egg custards and simmered vegetables.

Kombu Soy Sauce

Kombu soy sauce is simply strips of kombu added to a bottle of soy sauce and allowed to naturally infuse over time. You can start using it after soaking the kombu overnight. It instantly adds another layer of natural umami flavor to an ordinary soy sauce, giving food more flavor without adding anything artificial. You can use this kombu soy sauce as you would any regular soy sauce.

YIELD: approx. 1 cup (250 ml)
SHELF LIFE: Store in an airtight
  container in the refrigerator
  for up to 3 months.

1 cup (250 ml) soy sauce
1 piece, 6-inch (15-cm) kombu

Combine soy sauce and kombu in a container with a lid. Let it brew in the refrigerator at least overnight, or longer, and use up within three months. Leftover kombu can be cut into thin strips and added to soup.

Extra tips about soy sauce and its storage

Soy sauce works well in dishes that are simmered, fried and grilled, and as a dipping sauce. I suggest that you purchase a few different types and taste them to see the wide range of different flavors they have. Natural umami flavor comes from the amino acids created during the fermentation process. The shelf life of soy sauce is generally six months after opening. Some people like to keep it with oil and other condiments near the stove, but it is better to store it in the refrigerator as the flavor does degrade more quickly at room temperature.

Sake The word "sake" literally means "alcoholic drink" in Japanese. Sake is made from rice, water and koji (a fungus called Aspergillus oryzae) and generally has an alcohol content that ranges from 15% to 20%. Here, I am discussing sake that is used as a cooking condiment, a common practice in the Japanese kitchen. Sake not only removes unpleasant odors from ingredients, but it also adds umami flavor, as well as tenderizing meats and fish and enhancing the flavor. It is best to choose a sake for cooking that you would enjoy drinking, the same as with cooking wines. There are many cooking sakes available in the markets, but they usually contain salt, sugar and other additives. Those are not real sake, rather they are a sake-like condiment that has a slightly different flavor from real sake. So when using one of those, be sure to check the flavor of the dish you are cooking as it will tend to get saltier or sweeter than when using regular sake. When you add sake during cooking, make sure to cook off the alcohol completely. If you cannot get sake where you live, you can substitute a sweet marsala wine, white wine, Chinese wine or dry sherry.

Mirin is sweet rice wine that is a staple in every Japanese kitchen. Mirin was enjoyed as a sweet alcoholic beverage in the 16th century. By the late Edo period (19th century), it became a popular condiment and was used to season sauces served on grilled eel and as a dipping sauce for soba noodles. From the Meiji era to the pre-war period, a limited number of people began to use mirin, but it was still a luxury item and was most often used in Japanese restaurants. After a significant tax cut on mirin in the 1950s, it became more affordable for home cooks and is now one of the most popular seasonings in Japanese cuisine. There are three types of mirin available at different price points. While they all say "mirin" on the label, there is only one real mirin on the market—the other two types are mirin-like condiments that have a completely different manufacturing process and ingredients. Let's see what they are.

1. **Hon-mirin (real mirin)**—Golden brown Hon-mirin is the genuine, traditional mirin—the word "hon" means "real" in Japanese. It is made with a mixture of glutinous rice, rice koji and Shochu (alcohol beverage), that is then aged for 40 to 60 days. Hon-mirin adds depth and complexity of flavor to foods, with a natural sweetness that helps eliminate fishiness or gaminess of proteins. To incorporate hon-mirin into a dish, first burn off the alcohol over high heat, as with sake. Sake. Hon-mirin has the highest price point of all mirins and its alcohol content of around 14 percent necessitates that retailers have a liquor license to sell it. Store it in a cool, dark place such as in a cabinet that is away from a heat source and use up within three months after opening. You can purchase hon-mirin at Japanese grocery stores and online. If you can find it, I highly recommend you get Hon-mirin rather than other types of mirin on the market.

2. **Fermented mirin-style seasoning**—This seasoning is similar to hon-mirin in terms of alcohol content (between 8 to 14 percent), but it contains other ingredients—such as salt, glucose syrup, water, alcohol, rice and corn syrup, making

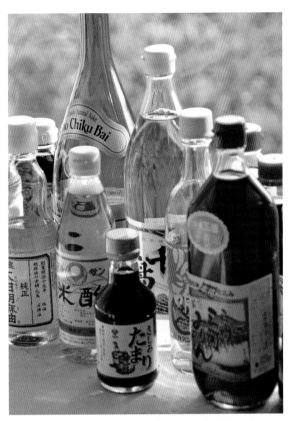

Mighty and mild marinades

it undrinkable. Since salt has already been added, you need to adjust the seasoning of your dish accordingly. To incorporate it into your dish, first burn off the alcohol over high heat, as with sake and hon-mirin. This mirin, which is less expensive than hon-mirin, is available at Asian and Japanese grocery stores and online.

Store it in the refrigerator and use up within three months after opening.

3. **Mirin-style seasoning**—This is not exactly mirin as it only contains a small amount of alcohol (less than 1%), and has sugar or high-fructose corn syrup, salt, vinegar and monosodium glutamate added. This is widely sold in regular supermarkets at a lower price point as an alternative to mirin. Store it in the refrigerator; use within three months after opening.

An Alternative to Mirin
If you are unable to get mirin, you can substitute 1 tablespoon sake or white wine mixed with 1 teaspoon sugar (or ½ teaspoon honey) for 1 tablespoon mirin.

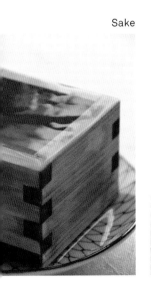

Sake

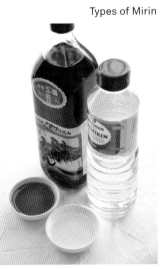

Types of Mirin

Sushi Vinegar

This is a versatile seasoned vinegar that is used not only for making sushi rice, but is also added to many dishes to lend a sweet and sour flavor. You can buy sushi vinegar at almost any grocery store today, but it is easy to make at home and you only need three ingredients, which you might already have in your pantry.

YIELD: approx. 1 cup (250 ml)
SHELF LIFE: Store in an airtight container in the refrigerator for up to 3 months.

1 cup (250 ml) rice vinegar
⅓ cup (80 g) granulated sugar
1 tablespoon salt

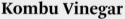

Combine the vinegar, sugar and salt in a container and stir until the sugar and salt have dissolved. Store in the refrigerator.

Kombu Vinegar

This is my everyday vinegar. Simply add a piece of kombu to rice vinegar and let it sit overnight. You will wind up with an aromatic, umami-infused rice vinegar that has a hint of sweetness and is free of additives or artificial flavors. You can start using it after soaking the kombu for overnight.

YIELD: approx. 1 cup (250 ml)
SHELF LIFE: Store in an airtight container in the refrigerator for up to 3 months.

1 cup (250 ml) rice vinegar
1 piece, 6-inch (15-cm) kombu

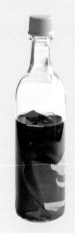

Combine rice vinegar and kombu in a container with a lid. Let it steep in the refrigerator overnight and use it up within three months. Leftover kombu can be cut into thin strips and added to soups, salads or stir-fries.

Rice Vinegar has a sweet, mellow and rich flavor and is widely used in Japanese cooking in such dishes as sushi and pickles. It is made from grains such as rice, wheat or sweet corn, as well as sake, which adds a refreshing note with less acidity. Rice vinegar does not have the intense sourness of most western vinegars. It is used to prevent food—including fish and meat—from changing color, and has also been an important ingredient historically in preventing food spoilage.

Koji is a mold—Aspergillus oryzae—that contributes a strong, savory flavor to so many traditional Japanese foods. It has played a major role in Japanese cuisine since ancient times. All traditional Japanese seasonings are made from koji and thus it is always present on the Japanese table in one form or another. Koji is made from grains or beans such as rice, barley and soybeans. It is impossible to physically see the koji because koji itself is not eaten as it is. Rather, it is used to ferment other ingredients. It is made by breeding a microorganism called koji mold on steamed rice. Seasonings such as miso, soy sauce, mirin, rice vinegar, and sake would not be able to ferment without koji. For example, miso is made by fermenting soybeans with koji and salt. Since miso is not strained (as is soy sauce), if you look carefully, in the case of rice miso, you will see some grains of rice on the surface—these are the rice koji. While there are other types of koji—such as bean koji or barley koji—since rice is a staple of the Japanese diet, rice koji is most widely used.

Other condiments using koji

Koji Vinegar—Combine koji and rice vinegar in a 1:4 ratio in a glass container, cover loosely and let it ferment at room temperature for seven days. Then, store it in an airtight container in the refrigerator for up to three months. The koji infuses natural sweetness into the vinegar without adding any sugar. It is great for pickling and making dressings.

Shoyu Koji—Combine koji and soy sauce in a 1:1 ratio in a glass container, cover loosely and let it ferment at room temperature for seven days. Then, store it in an airtight container in the refrigerator for up to three months. The rich glutamic acid in soybeans gives it a strong umami flavor, which is great for marinating meat, fish and tofu. See the recipe on page 135.

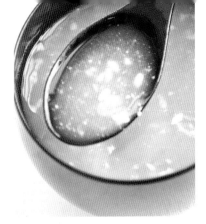

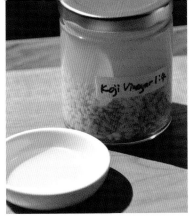

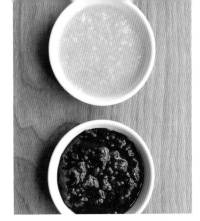

Rice Koji

Koji Vinegar

Top: Shio Koji; **bottom :** Shoyu Koji

Shio Koji

Shio Koji is the most popular salty seasoning in Japan next to miso and soy sauce. You can purchase it in bottles or jars in an Asian grocery store, or you can make your own Shio Koji. All you have to do is mix dried rice koji and salt, add water, and leave at room temperature for seven to 10 days to make an umami-filled seasoning. Though salty, it has a sweet smell, with a creamy texture like rice porridge. When you put it on meat, fish, or vegetables, the moisture in the ingredients is drawn out and the enzymes in the koji break down the proteins. This tenderizes them, while also boosting the flavors and adding umami flavor without a sharp saltiness.

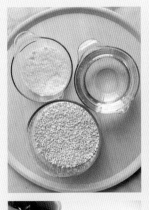

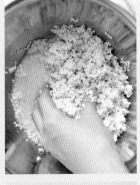

YIELD: approx. 2 cups (500 ml)
SHELF LIFE: Store in an airtight container in the
  refrigerator for up to 3 months.

1¼ cups (7 oz/200 g) dried rice koji
5 tablespoons (⅓ cup/75 g) sea salt
1¼ cups (300 ml) water

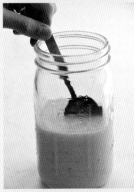

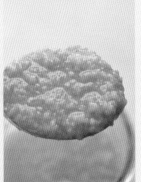

1.   Combine the koji and salt in a medium-size bowl. Using your hands, stir, and occasionally squeeze the Koji and salt tightly in your hands, until well mixed.

2.   Add the water to the koji mixture and mix well, using either your hands or a spatula.

3.   Transfer the mixture to a glass container. (TIP: Using a 1-quart container is recommended as Since carbon dioxide will be released during the ripening process, it is recommended to use a 1-quart container, which will allow enough extra space for the gasses to be released during fermentation. Do not fill the container to the top. Loosen the lid slightly and ferment at room temperature.

4.   Stir at least once a day with a spatula or a spoon to evenly distribute the koji and salted water if they separate. Ferment for one week in the summer, and 2 weeks in the winter. Store in an airtight container in the refrigerator and use it up within 3 months. (TIP: The koji becomes soft, fluffy, and similar in texture to rice porridge texture when it is ready to use. It smells sweet and thick like miso, or ripe bananas and the grains of rice are soft throughout. As the salted koji matures, the koji is broken down and becomes smaller and more watery. The fermenting process continues slightly in the refrigerator as well.)

The Art of Bento

Bento are portable lunch boxes designed to be eaten on the go. These are normally single portions, beautifully designed and arranged. Bento are not only visually appealing and delicious, but also highly nutritious; just a few of the reasons that Japanese bento culture is attracting growing global attention. In Japan, people either make them at home to bring to school or work, or simply purchase them at a local bento shop, convenience store, supermarket, train station kiosk, food court or take-out restaurant. Bento itself has a long history in Japan, dating back to the 5th century. The most popular bento are makunouchi-bento ("intermission bento"), which were first made to be eaten between the acts of kabuki and Noh performances in the late Edo period.

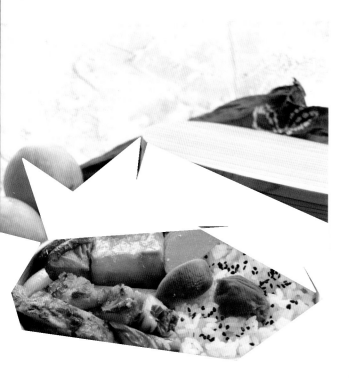

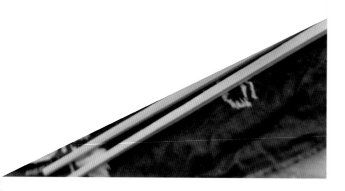

Why bento boxes?

I have loved making bento since I was a little girl. My mom worked outside the home and had a busy schedule, so I made my own bento for school before leaving in the morning. After graduating from college and finding a job, I continued to make my own bentos for the office. The benefits of bento are that I can eat whenever I want, I can be proactive about only including healthy foods in my diet, and I can also save money at the same time! For these reasons, I've made bentos every day of my adult life without fail. Now I have my own family, and I've been making bentos for my son since he was in elementary school. He likes them because they are a varied and fun alternative to school lunches, which are often unhealthy and not very good. I would like to share some of the tips that I've gathered during my long career of making bentos. If you're not familiar with bentos, I hope you will try it out!

Tips for making bento boxes

1. Food safety

Since there are many hours between making and eating your bento, bacteria can grow during that time. To prevent this from happening, here are some important tips.

- Wash your hands frequently before and during the preparation, and use clean cookware and bento boxes.
- Soak a paper towel in a 1:1 combination of water and vinegar and quickly wipe the

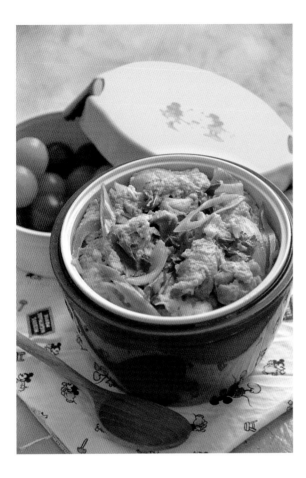

2. Prepare some dishes the night before

Because of the prep work I do the night before, I'm able to make a great bento without spending too much time in the morning. For example, if we have miso-marinated chicken for dinner, I always make a double batch. The chicken, marinated overnight in miso, will be ready to be grilled in the morning, or if that's too much work, you can grill it the night before, while making dinner. Also, some preparations such as boiling the vegetables and cutting the fruit can be done the night before. Deciding on the arrangement of the foods and which bento box you will use is also helpful in saving time in the morning.

3. Choose your bento boxes carefully

There are many different types and sizes of bento boxes available. Choose ones that are easy to handle and made of wood, plastic, aluminum or stainless steel. The size of the bento box should be appropriate to the person who will be eating it and the foods in the box. A two-tiered bento box can hold a lot of noodles and pastas. Deep bento boxes works great as a rice bowl.

4. Tips for assembling your bentos

When you pack a bento, keep in mind that taste, appearance and nutrition are all important elements in creating a great bento lunch.

- Balance the colors. Place darker colors beside lighter colors. Try using five different colors, such as red (tomato, strawberries), yellow (corn, egg), green (broccoli, snow peas), white (rice, noodles) and black (nori, sesame seeds). Using five different colors will also give you five different types of nutrition to create a well-balanced bento.

- Place the rice in the box first, slopping diagonally, so it is at an angle and you can place in the sidedishes at an angle also. The rice should fill about 50% of the bento.

- Place the large, main dish starting at the back and work your way to the front.

- Once you've placed the rice and main dish, you then fill in smaller sidedishes around them. Try to pack the box as tightly as possible, so there are no gaps between the items.

container before packing it to prevent bacteria from growing, especially during the summer when it is hot or if you know that the bento will sit for a long time before being eaten.

- Avoid foods that require refrigeration.
- Except for salads, choose cooked foods.
- Includes seasonings with antibacterial properties (like shiso basil, umeboshi plums and ginger).
- Squeeze excess moisture from the cooked vegetables before packing them in the box.
- Let the contents cool completely before putting the lid on to reduce condensation.
- Use tongs or chopsticks to pack the food, not your bare hands.
- Pack any sauces in a separate container and pour it on just before eating.
- Keep bento in an insulated bag if the weather is very hot.

Homemade Furikake

Furikake is an all-purpose rice topping. Make homemade furikake using katsuobushi flakes leftover from making dashi stock. This is a quick and easy recipe without any artificial flavors, and is great for bentos, breakfast or onigiri rice balls.

MAKES: ½ cup furikake

1 piece rehydrated or leftover kombu, 2 x 5 in (5 x 12 cm)
3 tablespoons leftover katsuobushi flakes
1 teaspoon sesame oil
½ teaspoon sea salt
½ teaspoon brown sugar
2 tablespoons white sesame seeds
1 tablespoon dried aonori flakes

1. Using scissors, cut the kombu into a couple of smaller pieces, put them in a blender and turn them into a powder, about 20 to 30 seconds. Set aside.

2. Cook the leftover katsuobushi in a non-stick skillet over medium heat, stirring constantly with a wooden spoon until completely dried, about 2 to 3 minutes.

3. Add the sesame oil, sea salt and brown sugar to the skillet and cook over medium-low heat for another 1 to 2 minutes, stirring constantly.

4. Add the kombu powder and sesame seeds to the skillet and continue cooking over medium-low heat for another minute. Make sure not to burn the sesame seeds, as they will become bitter.

5. Turn off the heat and add the aonori flakes. Mix until well-combined. Sprinkle on a bowl of steamed rice, onigiri rice balls, noodles, salads as a topping in bentos. Add shichimi hot chili peppers if you prefer it spicy.

6. Store in the airtight jar in a dark, dry place for up to one month.

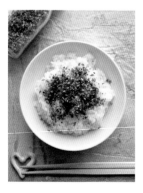
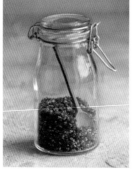

- Instead of laying the sidedishes flat, you can place them tilted upright, to give them a three-dimensional look and make them look more appealing.

- Place shiso leaves or leafy lettuce or other leaves between the dishes to keep them separate, add color and to prevent the flavors from running together.

- Place wet sidedishes (high-moisture content or oily foods) on paper towels to absorb the liquid and prevent it from spreading.

- If you want to make an easy bento, called a nokke-ben, simply place a single main dish on top of the rice.

- Top the rice with furikake rice sprinkles (see recipe at left), sesame seeds or an umeboshi pickled plum to finish.

5. Making simple and quick bentos

If I only have a few minutes to put the bento together in the morning, I suggest making an onigiri rice ball and miso soup bento (the rice is already made in my rice cooker). For quick miso soup, I make tiny miso soup balls called *miso-dama* which are a popular way to create a homemade instant miso soup anytime (see recipe on next page.) You combine miso paste with dashi ingredients including shredded kombu and katsuobushi along with wakame or other ingredients and form them into individual servings balls which are then wrapped in plastic wrap and kept in the freezer. When you want to make a portion of soup, unwrap and place the miso-dama in a cup, add hot water and wait for one minute. Having miso soup in the morning nourishes the body, and makes you feel energized for the rest of the day. And if it's difficult to find the time to have it in the morning, you can have it for lunch instead. I make these miso balls in batches and freeze them so that I can have delicious homemade miso soup whenever I want. I like having soups for lunch and take a thermos to work with me. You can store miso balls in the freezer up to 1 month. Taste the soup, and add more or less miso paste as needed, as the salt varies between different manufacturers.

"Instant" Miso Soup Balls

All the essential ingredients for miso soup can be concentrated in a small miso soup ball that is designed for one individual serving. Make them in batches, then wrap them in plastic and keep them in the freezer so you can have a cup of delicious miso soup anytime you want!

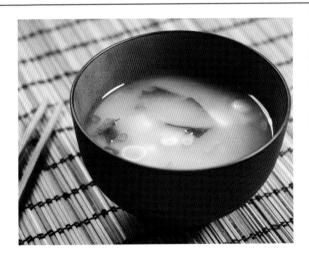

SERVES 4

2 tablespoons miso paste
2 tablespoons shredded dried kombu
2 tablespoons katsuobushi flakes
2 tablespoons dried wakame, nori, tofu, fried tofu or wheat gluten cakes (fu)
2 tablespoons green onions, green part only, thinly sliced

1. Cut a small piece of plastic wrap and place it on your work surface.
2. Place 1 heaping teaspoon of miso paste in the middle of the plastic wrap.
3. Add ¼ of the kombu and katsuobushi to the miso paste, along with the other ingredients.
4. Tightly gather and twist the plastic wrap together to form a ball. Repeat with the remaining ingredients, making 3 more balls. Store them in the freezer in a resealable bag.
5. To serve, add 1 cup (250 ml) of boiling water to a cup with 1 miso soup ball.

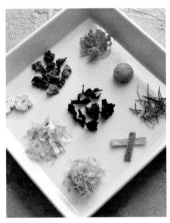
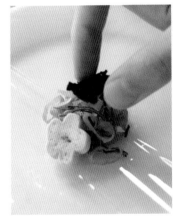
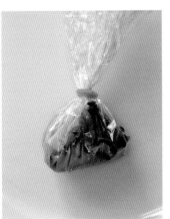
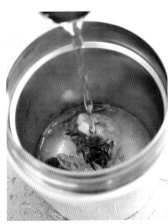
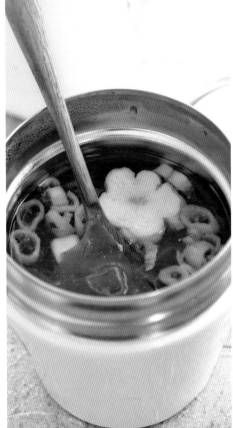

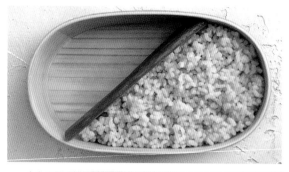

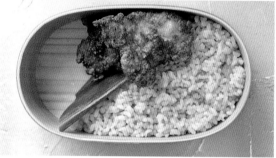

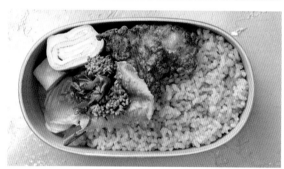

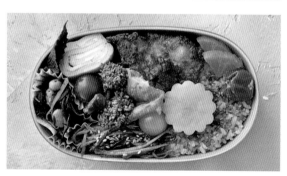

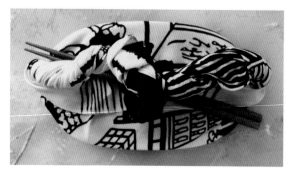

Packing your bento box

Here, I am going to show you the step-by-step process of making an authentic Japanese-style bento box. The only thing you will need to make when you're packing the box is rice. All of the sidedishes can be made the day before and stored in the refrigerator. But if you have time in the morning, you can also prepare the fried chicken. If all the sidedishes are too much to handle, only include the main and one or two sidedishes.

1. Gather all the foods you're going to use to fill the bento box on a table. Fill the bento about 50% full of the rice, placing it diagonally in the box. (I'm using brown rice in the photo.) Use shiso, basil or lettuce leaves to separate the rice and other dishes from one another.

2. Pack the main dish: Japanese Fried Chicken (page 211).

3. Pack a sidedish like rolled omelet (page 177).

4. Pack a salad like Wakame and Broccoli Rabe Salad (page 105). Wrap the salad in a lettuce leaf before placing it in the bento so that the dressing will stay separate from the other dishes.

5. Fill a cupcake liner or silicone cup with 2 tablespoons of rehydrated hijiki and place it into the bento box.

6. Pack the sidedish (2 tablespoons): braised burdock.

7. Pack cherry tomatoes into gaps between the dishes.

8. Place sliced sweet potato on top of the rice. Fill the gaps on the edge of the bento box with shiso leaves or lettuce.

9. Place two thin slices of pickles on top of the rice.

10. Sprinkle furikake or sesame seeds on top of the rice.

11. Place an umeboshi plum on top of rice (optional).

12. Wrap the bento box with a cloth and don't forget the chopsticks or a fork!

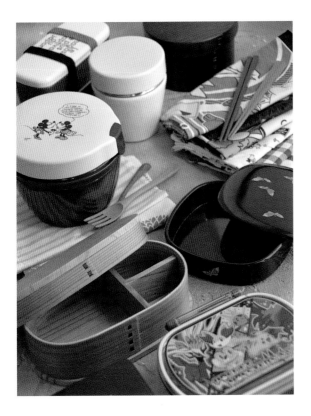

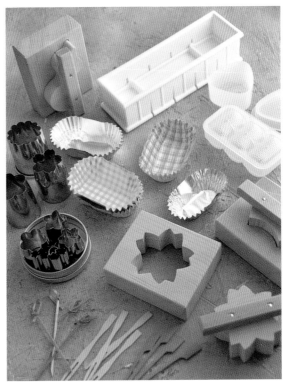

Bento boxes for children vs. adults

When I make bentos for both myself and my son, I make the same dishes for both of us. Try to keep in mind the following basic tips:

- Using cookie cutters to cut boiled carrots, sweet potatoes or daikon interesting shapes can be a fun addition to children's bentos.
- Cut the children's versions into smaller bite-sized pieces than the adult versions, so all the foods are easy to eat without a knife.
- Onigiri rice balls are an easy-to-eat child-friendly dish.
- Creating popular anime or cartoon characters in your child's bento is called kyaraben. (Cut a nori sheet into a character shape by using scissors, for example.)
- Use a fun and colorful bento box, napkin and chopsticks/fork for kids. Be sure the bento box is appropriately sized for them.
- Use colorful cupcake liners to hold smaller, looser ingredients.

Tools for making delicious bentos

There are several items that I always use when making bento.

- Onigiri and sushi molds
- Cupcake liners (waterproof)
- Bamboo toothpicks
- Cookie cutters
- Chopsticks or tongs

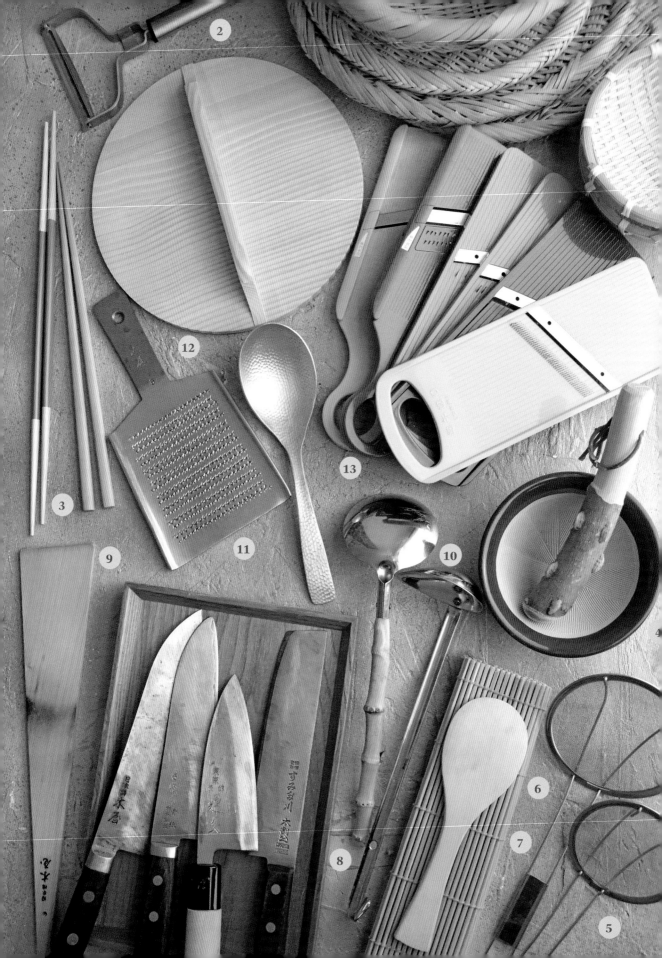

Traditional Japanese Kitchen Utensils

What kind of cooking utensils do you need to create Japanese superfoods at home? Here I've collected all the useful things from my kitchen that you need to know about.

1 Bamboo colanders Used for washing vegetables and draining noodles after being cooked. You can also serve cold noodles in them. Having a range of different sizes from small to large is useful.

2 Vegetable Peeler Used to peel root vegetables such as carrots and radishes. The blade is sharp, so use it with caution.

3 Long kitchen chopsticks These are longer than normal chopsticks and are used for cooking, frying, mixing and serving.

An earthernware nabe hot pot is useful for preparing and serving Japanese hot pots.

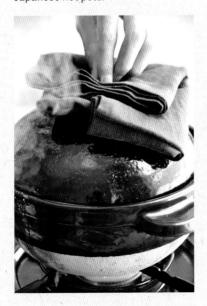

4 Mortar and pestle Used for grinding sesame seeds. Different sizes are available.

5 Mesh ladles A fine strainer or sieve-like device that makes it easier to remove the residue from soups. Also used to remove food from hot oil or from boiling water.

6 Rice paddle Used to serve rice. Soak it in water before using to prevent the rice from sticking to it.

7 Sushi mat Used to roll sushi rice and also to form the shape of an egg omelet.

8 Kitchen knives Used to cut a variety of food. As with all cutlery, exercise propoer precaution.

9 Wooden spatula Used for stir-frying and mashing.

10 Ladles Used for mixing and serving miso soup.

11 Grater Used for grating ginger and wasabi root.

12 Drop lid Placed on top of simmering ingredients, it allows them to absorb flavors more evenly, and also prevents them from falling apart. Wooden, silicone, glass and stainless-steel versions are available.

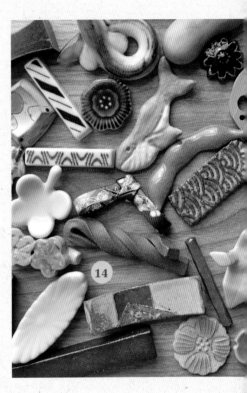

13 Mandolines I have a bit of an obsession with this item. Used to slice any vegetable to the desired thickness. The blade is sharp, so use it with caution.

14 Chopstick rests It prevents the implements from rolling around. They also keep the ends of the chopsticks that touch the food from coming into contact with other objects.

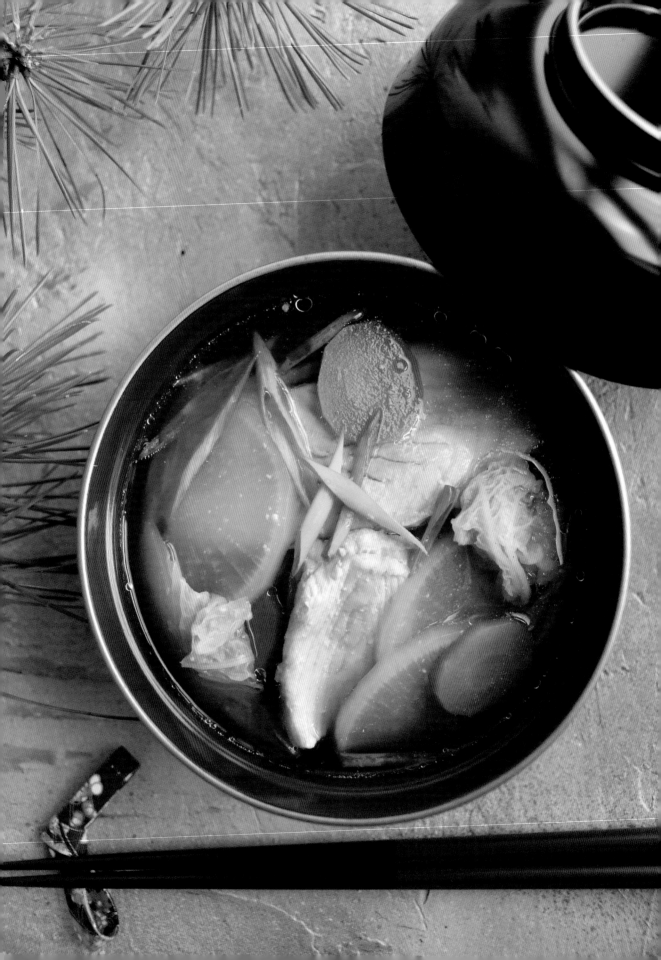

Superfood Soups & Hot Pots

This chapter introduces classic, much-loved miso soups and hot pots using widely available ingredients. Miso soup lies at the heart of Japanese cuisine. A daily staple for many, it serves as a consistent supplier of superfood goodness. This soothing dashi-based treat is primarily made from kombu (kelp), katsuobushi (dried smoked tuna flakes) and miso (fermented soybean paste), three essential Japanese superfoods. Kombu is full of minerals from the sea, while katsuobushi and miso are fermented foods. They provide calcium, necessary for building strong bones, and help to regulate and maintain healthy intestinal function, skin and hair. Incorporating seaweed, which is rich in fiber, into your daily diet also helps in preventing heart disease and cancer.

When the weather turns cold, nabe hot pots are the perfect food. From late October throughout the winter, they're one of the most frequently served dishes in Japanese households. Typically, they're prepared on tabletop gas burners. They warm the body's core, raising metabolism and burning fat. On top of that, they taste so good. Simmer up any of these steaming seasonal soothers and enjoy!

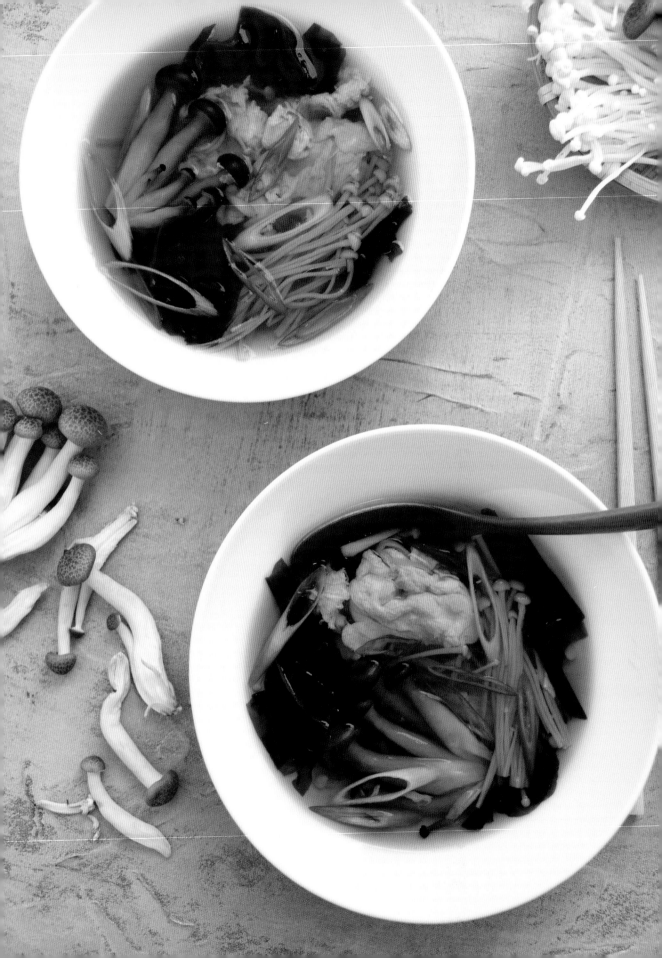

Japanese-style Egg Drop Soup
with Wakame and Mushroom

This light and fluffy Japanese-style egg drop soup is made with Basic Dashi Stock (page 36). Dashi adds a deep savory flavor to so many foods, no wonder it lies at the heart of much of Japanese cooking. This warm and cozy soup is packed with fiber and vitamins from the various mushrooms such as shimeji, shiitake and enoki, as well as minerals from the seaweed in the stock. I prefer to use white soy sauce (see page 49) to keep the soup a light color and to give it a sweeter flavor, but regular (dark) soy sauce will also be fine. You can also add some cooked rice or protein such as chicken or tofu cut into bite-sized pieces, which will turn this soup into a nice hearty meal.

PREPARATION TIME: 10 minutes
COOKING TIME: 15 minutes
SERVES 4

2 cups (150 g) mixed fresh mushrooms, such as shimeji, shiitake, enoki or white mushrooms
1 green onion (scallion), both green and white parts
3 tablespoons fresh or dried wakame
4 cups (1 liter) Basic or Kombu Dashi Stock (pages 36 and 38)
½-in (1.25-cm) piece fresh ginger, peeled and cut into thin strips
2 teaspoons soy sauce (see headnote)
2 teaspoons sake
2 teaspoons mirin sweet rice wine
½ teaspoon sea salt
2 eggs, beaten
1 teaspoon sesame oil

1. Trim the base of the mushrooms, and either separate by hand into individual stalks or slice thinly. Trim the roots off the green onion and cut into thin slices on the bias.

2. Place a strainer in a bowl, add the fresh wakame and fill the bowl with water. Let it sit for a few seconds. Drain and rinse the wakame under running water until the salt is removed and the wakame doubles or triples in size. Squeeze out the excess water and cut into bite-sized pieces. If using dried wakame, follow the instructions on the package, or rehydrate in a bowl of water for 5 minutes, then drain and squeeze out the excess water. Set aside.

3. Put the Basic Dashi Stock, mushrooms and ginger in a medium saucepan and bring to a simmer over medium-high heat. Cook for 5 to 7 minutes, until the mushrooms are tender.

4. Add the soy sauce, sake, mirin and salt to the stock and mushrooms. Let it simmer for a minute over medium-high heat.

5. Holding a fork over the stock, slowly pour the eggs through the tines into the hot dashi stock. Let the stock simmer undisturbed for a minute to allow the eggs to cook.

6. Gently stir the eggs wih the fork and simmer another minute. Add the wakame and sesame oil to the stock.

7. To serve, ladle 1 cup of hot soup into each soup bowl and sprinkle scallions on top.

TIP
You can use Kombu Dashi Stock as a vegan substitute for Basic Dashi Stock.

Chicken Hot Pot
with Mixed Vegetables and Tofu

Nabe hot pots are a very popular one-pot dish eaten with friends and family. They're especially enjoyed during the cold winter months in Japan. A portable gas burner is placed in the center of a table along with a variety of ingredients ready to go into the pot: vegetables, meat, fish, tofu and egg. This is a self-serve dish, which everyone cooks while seated at the table. Serving chopsticks are used to build the customized bowl. If you don't have a portable gas burner, you can make this dish on the stovetop then transfer the pot to the table. The clear broth is made from chicken, kombu, katsuobushi, sake and mirin. It is so rich and savory it will warm you from the inside out. After cooking the tender chicken and vegetable pieces in the stock, dip them into the homemade Ponzu Sauce before popping them into your mouth. I'm sure your guests will love this dish!

PREPARATION TIME: 20 minutes
COOKING TIME: 20 minutes
SERVES 4

2 lbs (900 g) chicken breasts, thighs and wings with skin and bones
5 green onions (scallions), green and white parts, divided
1-in (2.5-cm) piece fresh ginger, divided
4 shiitake mushrooms, rehydrated
1 cup (250 ml) Shiitake Dashi Stock (page 39)
½ head (1 lb/500 g) napa cabbage
One 14-oz (400-g) block medium-firm tofu
3 cups (750 ml) water
2 pieces of dried kombu, 2 x 6 in (5 x 15 cm)
½ cup (125 ml) sake or dry sherry
2 tablespoons mirin (sweet rice wine) or sweet sherry
1 teaspoon sea salt
1 cup (250 ml) Ponzu Sauce (page 40)

1. Cut the chicken into 2-inch (5-cm) pieces. Trim the ends of the green onions, then cut the white parts into 2-in (5-cm) lengths and the green parts into crosswise slices, about ⅛ inch (3 mm) thick. Peel the ginger and cut it into fine strips. Remove the stems from the shiitake mushrooms. Cut the cabbage into about 2-in (5-cm) lengths and separate the white stems from the green leaves. Cut the tofu into 1½-in (4-cm) cubes.

2. Combine the water, shiitake stock, shiitake, kombu, sake, mirin and salt in a large pot or Japanese style donabe hot pot. Heat on a portable stove at the dining table, or on your stovetop, covered, over medium-high heat and bring to a boil.

3. Add the chicken and sliced ginger to the pot and cook over medium heat until the chicken is almost tender, about 3 to 5 minutes. Skim the foam and fat from the surface of the broth using a sieve. Then turn the heat to medium-low and simmer for another 3 to 5 minutes.

4. Add the white stems of the cabbage and the tofu to the pot and simmer, covered, for 3 to 4 minutes over medium-low heat. Skim the foam from the surface again.

5. Add the white parts of the green onions and the leafy green parts of the cabbage to the pot and cook over medium heat for 1 minute, or until all the ingredients are soft and fully cooked. Keep adding more ingredients to the pot as you take out those that are cooked and eat them hot.

6. To serve, divide the Ponzu Sauce, green onions and ginger between four small serving bowls. Each diner can individually dip the cooked ingredients in the sauce before eating.

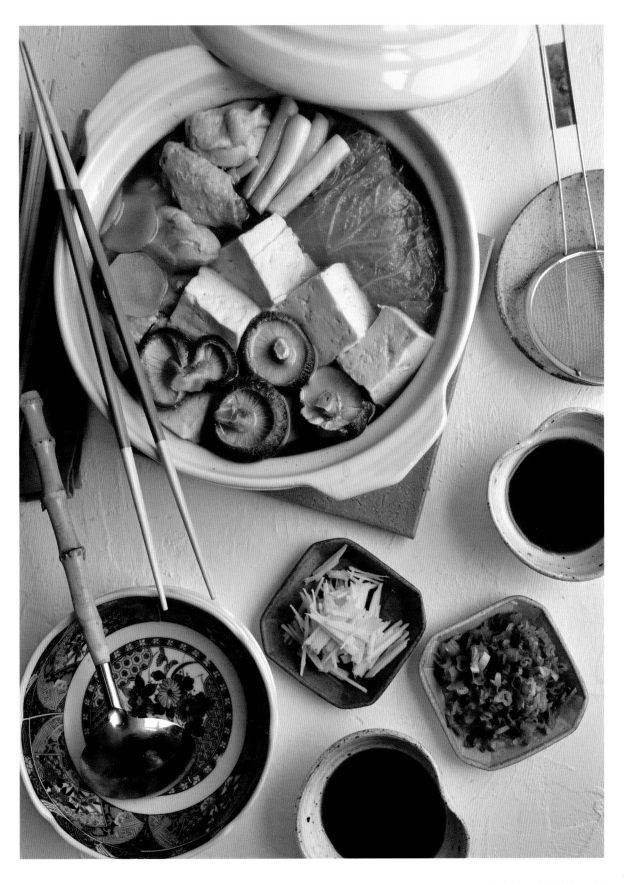

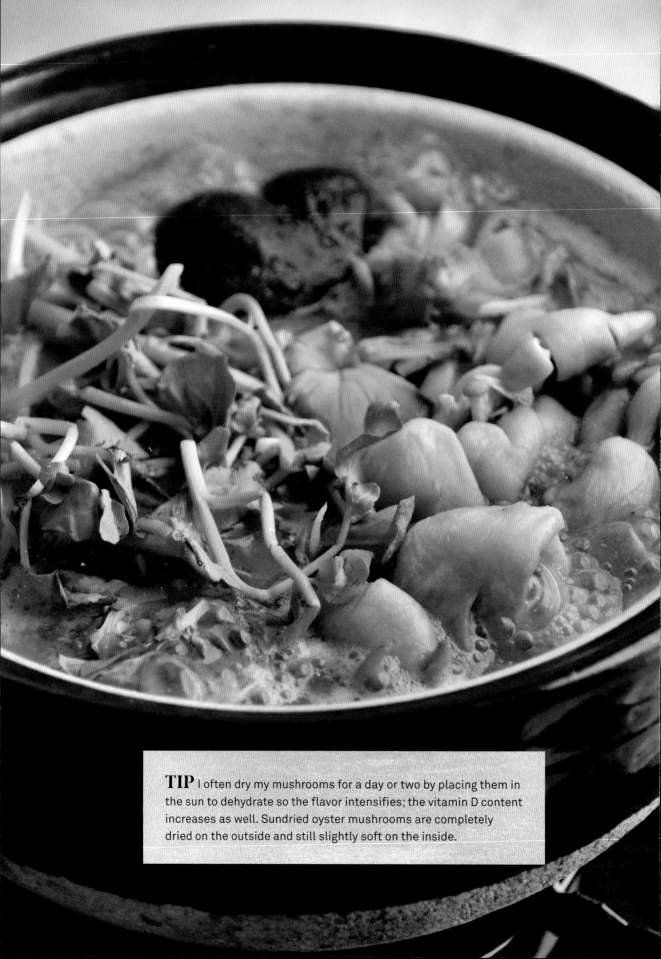

TIP I often dry my mushrooms for a day or two by placing them in the sun to dehydrate so the flavor intensifies; the vitamin D content increases as well. Sundried oyster mushrooms are completely dried on the outside and still slightly soft on the inside.

Mushroom Hot Pot
with Shredded Beef and Watercress

Kombu, which contains the highest levels of glutamate of any food, is a rich source of umami. Katsuobushi contains high levels of inosinate, and dried shiitake mushrooms are packed with guanylate. Cooked together, the amino acids combine to create intense flavor. I also like to add oyster mushrooms, which have a mild flavor and a tender, soft texture that makes them perfect for hot pots. They cook fast and absorb all the delicious flavors from the broth. Enjoy a big bowl of this earthy, hearty homecooked comfort food served over rice or noodles!

PREPARATION TIME: 15 minutes
COOKING TIME: 25 minutes
SERVES 4

10 oz (330 g) mixed mushrooms (such as oyster, shiitake, white, shimeji, maitake, enoki—see pages 20–21)
1 lb (500 g) boneless beef shortribs
1 bunch (4 oz/100 g) watercress
1 in (2.5 cm) fresh ginger
¼ (4 oz/100 g) burdock root
4 cups (1 liter) Basic Dashi Stock (page 36)
4 tablespoons Kaeshi Sauce (page 40)
1 tablespoon tobanjan spicy black bean paste
2 tablespoons nerigoma (Japanese sesame paste), or tahini
Steamed rice or cooked noodles, for serving (optional)

1. Trim the bases of the mushrooms, and either separate them by hand into individual stalks or slice them into bite-sized pieces. If using dried shiitake, soak in hot water for 20 minutes before removing the stems. Cut the shiitake in half.

2. Cut the shortribs into thin strips. Cut the watercress in half lengthwise. Peel the ginger and cut it into fine strips.

3. Peel and slice the burdock root into thin strips, about 2 in (5 cm) in length. Soak the burdock in water for 10 minutes and change the water a couple of times to get rid of the bitterness. Drain well.

4. Combine the stock, Kaeshi Sauce, tobanjan and nerigoma in a large pot and bring to a boil over medium-high heat. Add the shortribs, ginger and burdock and simmer over medium heat for 5 to 7 minutes. Skim the foam and fat from the surface of the pot using a sieve.

5. Add the mushrooms to the pan, reduce the heat to medium and cook for 5 to 7 minutes, until the mushrooms are tender. Add the watercress and cook for one more minute over medium heat. Continue skimming the foam and fat from the surface of the pot using the sieve.

6. To serve, ladle about 1 cup of soup, along with beef and vegetables, into each serving bowl. Serve with a bowl of rice or cooked noodles, if you like.

Mochi Rice Cake Soup
with Chicken and Vegetables

~~~

Ozoni is a traditional Japanese New Year's dish that is filled with mochi rice cake, vegetables and chicken in a flavorful dashi stock. My family has a long-running tradition of celebrating New Year's Day at my grandma's house (now my uncle's and aunt's), where we eat *osechi*, or ceremonial foods. The celebration usually starts at noon with a variety of hot and cold dishes—some traditional, some non-traditional—and the eating continues late into the night. There are two styles of *ozoni*: kanto (a clear stock found in the Tokyo area) and *kansai* (a white miso stock from the Kyoto area). In this Tokyo-style recipe, I use a flower-shaped cutter to prepare the vegetables, to give them some New Year's flair. This is a versatile recipe that can use any vegetables, meat or fish, including leftovers. Sometimes, I make this dish just to clean out my refrigerator!

PREPARATION TIME: 10 minutes
COOKING TIME: 20 minutes
SERVES 4

3-in (7-cm) length daikon
1 carrot
1 cup (2 oz/60 g) spinach
One (8 oz/250 g) chicken thigh
4 cups (1 liter) Basic or Kombu Dashi
  Stock (pages 36, 38)
¼ cup (65 ml) Kaeshi Sauce (page 40)
½ teaspoon sea salt
4 pieces unsweetened mochi rice
  cake 1.5 x 2.5 in (4 x 7 cm) each
1 tablespoon yuzu or lemon peel,
  grated or in strips, optional

1. Peel and slice the daikon and carrot into ⅛-in (3-mm) rounds, then cut them into flower shapes using a cookie or vegetable cutter. Or simply cut them into bite-sized pieces. Trim the roots off the spinach and cut into 1-in (2.5-cm) pieces. Cut the chicken into bite-sized pieces.

2. Combine dashi stock, daikon, carrot and chicken in a pot and bring to a simmer over medium-high heat.

3. Add Kaeshi Sauce and salt to the pot and cook, covered, over low heat for about 8 to 10 minutes.

4. Heat a medium-sized skillet over medium heat; spray or coat lightly with oil if it's not a nonstick surface. Place the mochi in the skillet and cook for about 4 to 5 minutes on each side until the mochi puffs up and turns light brown. Remove the mochi from the skillet.

5. Add the mochi and spinach to the stock and cook over medium heat for 1 to 2 minutes, until the mochi gets a little soft but still retains its shape and the spinach becomes tender. Turn off the heat.

6. To serve, ladle 1 cup of hot soup along with some mochi and vegetables into each soup bowl and top with the yuzu or lemon peel, if using.

TIP
Mochi is sold precut at Asian markets and online. Mochi is also eaten as a dessert, but as this is a savory dish, be sure to buy unsweetened mochi cakes.

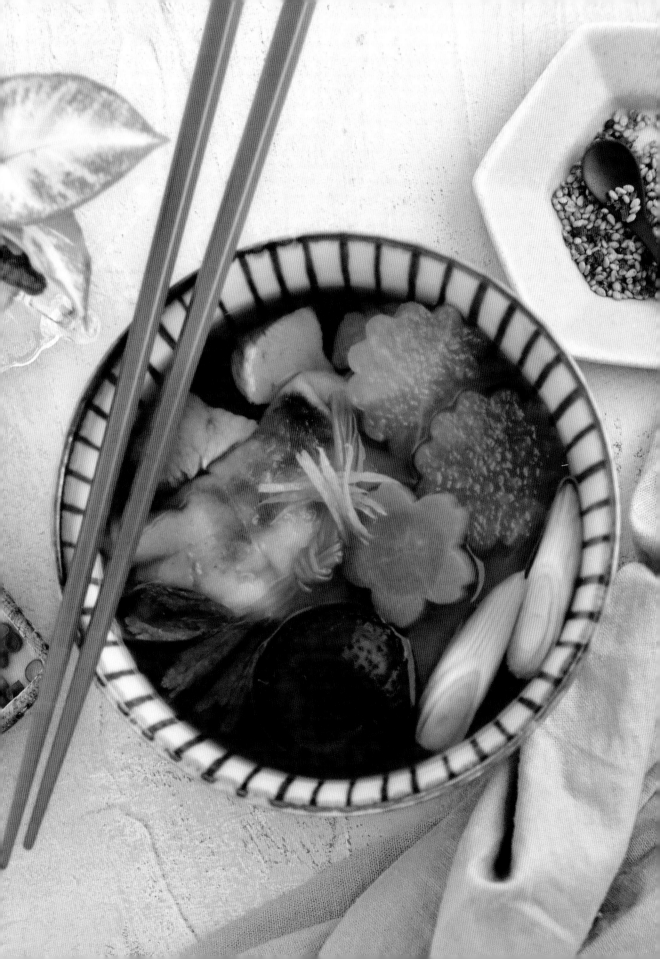

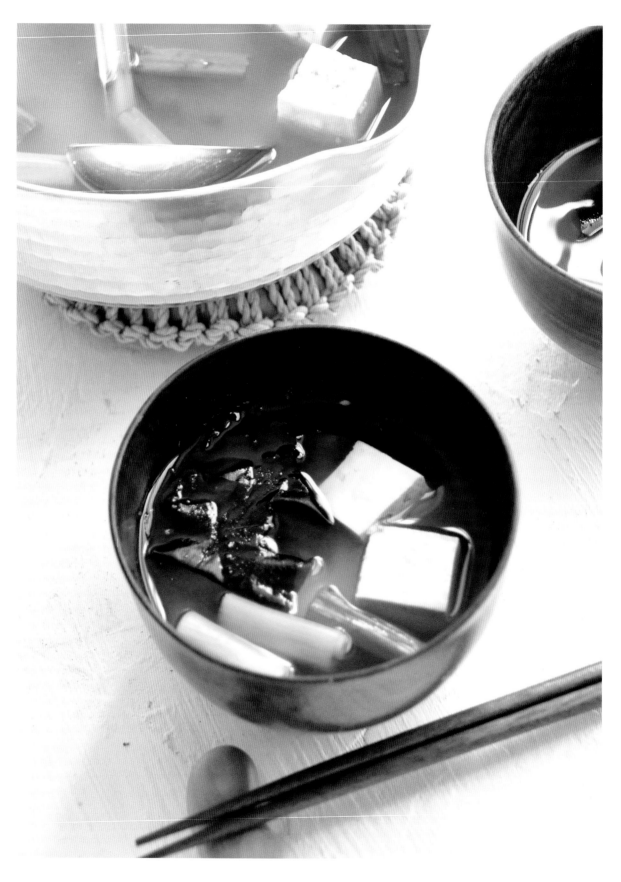

Wakame Miso Soup
with Tofu and Scallions

〜〜〜〜〜

Since my parents ran a seaweed factory when I was growing up, we always had everything we needed to quickly make miso soup at home. The most important ingredient is the dashi. It's the foundation of Japanese cuisine and the backbone of any type of soup. The second most important ingredient is miso. The enzymes found in the koji help break down the rice grains and soybeans into amino acids, creating a sweet and savory flavor. In my family, my dad oversaw making the miso, and we always had plenty of it in a big clay barrel. The final key ingredient is the wakame. It helps reduce high blood pressure and supports healthy heart function. It also provides a lot of dietary fiber, which is why my mom always makes a point of eating seaweed daily. So make a big bowl and enjoy it with steamed rice on the side, or by itself as a light meal.

PREPARATION TIME: 10 minutes
COOKING TIME: 15 minutes
SERVES 4

3 tablespoons fresh or dried wakame
3 cups (750 ml) Basic or Kombu Dashi
 Stock (pages 36, 38)
½ block (7 oz/200 g) medium-firm tofu
2 green onions (scallion)
2½ tablespoons awase miso (page 15)

TIP Miso soup can be stored in the refrigerator for up to 2 days. For a vegan option, use Kombu Dashi or Shiitake Dashi (pages 38–9) instead of Basic Dashi Stock, which has fish in it. For other miso options, see page 15 for basic guidelines on choosing the right miso for your dish. Be sure to add the miso at the end as boiling it kills the beneficial probiotics in the miso.

1. If using fresh wakame, place a strainer in a bowl, add the wakame and fill the bowl with water then let it sit for a few seconds. Drain and rinse the wakame under running water until the salt is removed and the wakame doubles or triples in sized. Squeeze out the excess water and cut into bite-sized pieces. If using dried wakame, follow the instruction on the package, or rehydrate it in a bowl of water for 5 minutes, then drain and squeeze out the excess water. Set aside.

2. Put the dashi stock in a medium saucepan over medium-high heat and bring to a simmer. Cut the tofu into 1-in (2-cm) cubes and add them to the soup. Cook for 2 to 3 minutes over medium-low heat.

3. Cut the green onions in 1-in (2.5-cm) lengths.

4. Add the wakame, green onions and miso to the stock and stir over low heat to dissolve the miso gradually. Remove from the heat just before it boils.

5. To serve, ladle 1 cup of hot soup into each soup bowl.

Salmon Miso Soup

~~~~~~~~~~

This is my favorite fish soup to make when salmon is in season (September to November in Japan). This dish is from Ishikari, a city located on the northern island of Hokkaido, and it uses their local ingredients. It's served as a hot pot called Ishikari nabe, because this is where the best quality salmon is found. The local fisherman prepare this easy, nutritious fish stew with winter vegetables. So, if you need warming up and are looking for a heathy and nutritious dish, this is the perfect choice.

PREPARATION TIME: 15 minutes
COOKING TIME: 20 minutes
SERVES 4

4 skinless salmon fillets (1 lb/500 g)
½ teaspoon salt
2-in (5-cm) piece of daikon
½ carrot
1 potato, any type
2 leaves cabbage or napa cabbage
4 cups (1 liter) Kombu Water or
  Kombu Dashi Stock (page 38)
1 teaspoon fresh grated ginger
4 tablespoons awase miso (page 15)
1 tablespoon unsalted butter, divided
  into 4 pieces
1 tablespoon chopped green onion
  (scallion), white and green parts, to
  garnish

1. Cut each salmon fillet in half crosswise. Sprinkle salt on both sides and let it season for 8 to 10 minutes.

2. Place the fish in a colander set in the sink and slowly pour boiling water over it until the surface turns whiteish in color. Then, rinse it well with cold water.

3. Peel and slice the daikon and carrot into ⅛-in (3-mm) pieces. Peel and cut the potato into 1-in (2.5-cm) pieces and then soak them in a bowl of cool water for 5 minutes and drain. Tear the cabbage leaves in bite-sized pieces and set aside.

4. Combine the Kombu Dashi Stock, daikon, carrot and potato in a medium pot, cover and simmer over medium heat for 7 to 10 minutes.

5. Add the salmon to the pot, reduce the heat to medium-low and cook for about 3 to 5 minutes, covered.

6. Add the ginger, miso and cabbage to the pot, reduce the heat to low, and cook for 2 to 4 minutes or until the cabbage is tender. Taste the broth, adding more miso as needed. Turn off the heat.

7. To serve, ladle 1 cup of hot soup along with some salmon and vegetables into each soup bowl and top with butter and green onions.

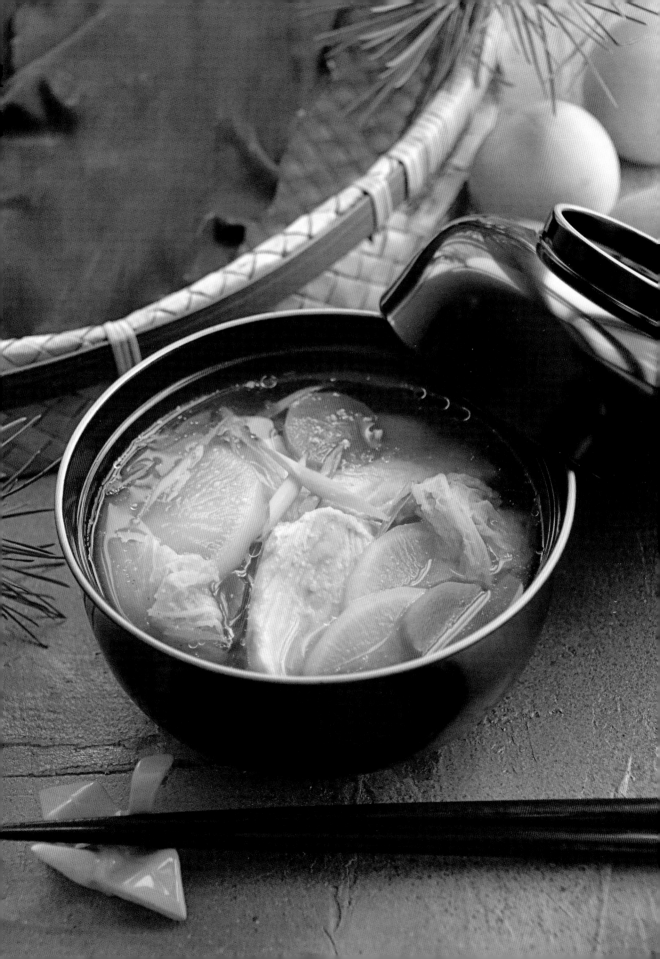

Kabocha Miso Ginger Bisque

Kabocha Japanese pumpkins are denser, starchier and smaller than Western pumpkins, and they have a creamier texture when cooked. They're naturally sweet as well as high in nutrients like beta-carotene and vitamin A. Kabocha lends a subtle, nutty flavor and thickness to the soup. This is a dairy-free (and vegan) recipe with a Japanese twist. Instead of using a cream-based stock, I use Kombu Water seasoned with white miso, which is lighter and sweeter in flavor than regular miso. Enjoy this lighter version of a classic comfort food served hot or cold for breakfast, lunch or dinner.

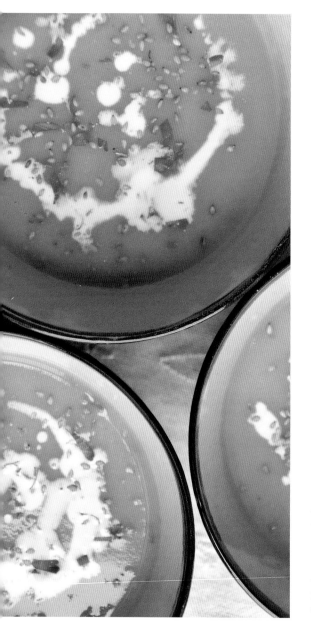

PREPARATION TIME: 15 minutes
COOKING TIME: 30 minutes
SERVES 4 to 5

½ kabocha pumpkin (about 1½ lbs/750 g)
1 medium onion
1 tablespoon extra-virgin olive oil
2½ cups (625 ml) Kombu Water (page 38)
½ cup (125 ml) soy milk or almond milk,
  plus 2–3 tablespoons for drizzling
1½ tablespoons white miso paste (page 15)
½ teaspoon fresh ginger juice
Pinch of sea salt
1 teaspoon white sesame seeds, toasted, to garnish
1 tablespoon finely chopped parsley,
  to garnish (optional)

1. Halve the squash with a sharp knife and scrape out all of the seeds with a spoon. Peel off the skin and cut the flesh into small pieces. Set aside. Peel and thinly slice the onion. Set aside.

2. Heat the oil over medium heat, add the onion and cook for 5 to 7 minutes or until translucent and slightly browned. Add the squash and Kombu Water to the pot and bring to a simmer. Cook for 8 to 10 minutes over medium-low heat, or until the squash is tender when pierced with a fork.

3. Use a food processor or blender to puree the soup in small batches (to avoid accidentally getting splashed with hot liquid, place a kitchen towel over the lid of the food processor or blender). Pour the soup back into the pot.

4. Add the soy or almond milk, miso, ginger juice and salt to the pot and cook over medium-low heat for another 5–7 minutes. Taste for seasoning and adjust as needed.

5. **To serve:** ladle 1½ cups of hot soup into each soup bowl and sprinkle with sesame seeds and parsley. Drizzle the few tablespoons of soy or almond milk on top of each bowl of soup.

Napa Cabbage and Bacon Miso Soup

This is a classic bacon and potato soup with the addition of leafy napa cabbage and savory miso paste, adding a Japanese twist. This recipe is a great example of how miso can elevate the flavor of non-Asian ingredients. A spoonful of miso adds a nice balance and savory flavor to whatever you're cooking. I also appreciate how light this soup is—using Basic, Niboshi or Kombu Dashi Stock not only lends a great umami flavor, but creates a lighter, healthier dish. If you don't have napa cabbage, feel free to substitute green cabbage, kale or spinach.

PREPARATION TIME: 5 minutes
COOKING TIME: 15 minutes
SERVES 4

1 yellow or Yukon gold potato
2 leaves napa cabbage
4 strips of bacon
4 cups (1 liter) Basic, Niboshi or
  Kombu Dashi Stock (pages 36,
  38, 39)
1½ tablespoons awase miso
  (page 15)
1 tablespoon mitsuba Japanese
  parsley or Italian parsley

1. Peel and dice the potato, then soak in a bowl of water. Cut the napa cabbage and bacon into ½-inch (1-cm) pieces.

2. Place a medium pot over medium-high heat. Add the bacon and cook until crispy. Discarded the leftover oil.

3. Add the dashi stock and potato to the bacon and bring to a simmer over medium-high heat. Cook for 3 to 5 minutes, until the potato is tender.

4. Add the napa cabbage to the stock and cook for 3 to 5 minutes over low heat.

5. Add the miso to the stock and stir to combine. Turn of the heat.

6. To serve, ladle 1 cup of hot soup into each soup bowl and sprinkle mitsuba on top.

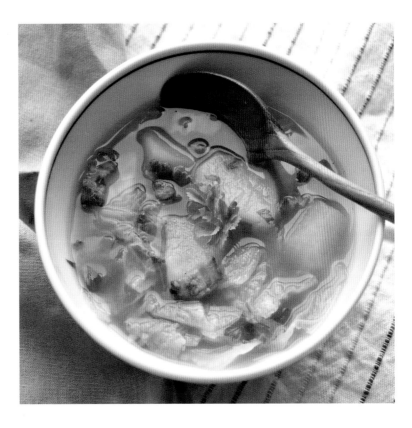

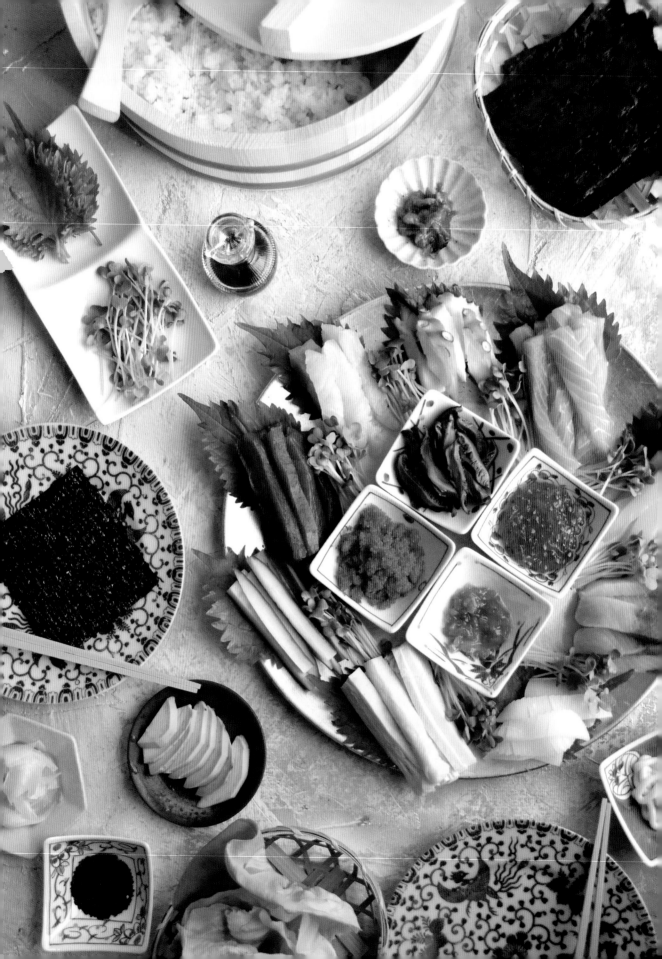

Super-healthy Sushi

During sushi's long culinary history, it has consistently tapped into the superfood fusion of fresh seafood, seaweed and vegetables. The earliest form of sushi dates to around 1000 B.C.E. Called nare-zushi, it was made by sprinkling salt on fish and rice to ferment it, a common form of preservation before refrigeration. Around 1820, vinegar-based Sushi Rice became popular (replacing the time-consuming fermentation process).

Now it's your turn to unlock the one-two power punch of sushi and sashimi. First, you'll make delicious Sushi Rice using homemade Sushi Vinegar. Then I'll introduce you to various styles of sushi including Scattered Sushi, Sushi Rice Stuffed in Tofu Pockets, Ball-shaped Sushi, Hand Rolls, Classic Rolls, Pressed Sushi and Cup Sushi. The recipes are easy to follow and use readily-available ingredients to create beautiful and nutritious sushi at home.

Fatty tuna and salmon, rich in omega-3 acids, often serve as the centerpiece. Hand rolls, with their seaweed wrappers, become small parcels of nutritive power. Finding your favorite flavor combination is up to you, but the healthful benefits are always present.

Colorful Ball-shaped Temari Sushi

These colorful temari-inspired sushi balls are a great dish for a party or gathering. These small bite-sized balls can be topped with any kind of sashimi and vegetables, so they're easy to pull together. For this recipe, I use three popular sushi toppings, salmon, tuna and squid, making eight sushi balls with each topping for a total of 24. I've made this dish for all kinds of occasions: birthday parties, school events and for lunch boxes for hanami, or cherry blossom viewing. This dish is inspired by temari, a traditional Japanese embroidered ball, so each one is decorated to resemble a colorful work of art. Some chefs and home cooks go to extremes in decorating their temarizushi, so you can be as creative with your own unique designs as you like.

PREPARATION TIME: 20
COOKING TIME: 45
YIELDS: 24 pieces

4 cups (660 g) prepared Sushi Rice (page 81)
8 slices of sashimi-grade salmon, 2 in (5 cm) long, 1 in (1.25 cm) wide and ¼ in (6 mm) thick
8 slices of avocado, 2 in (5 cm) long, 1 in (1.25 cm) wide, ¼ in (6 mm) thick
¼ teaspoon fresh dill, chopped, to garnish
4 shiso leaves (Japanese basil), cut in half lengthwise
8 slices of sashimi-grade tuna, 2 in (5 cm) long 1 in (1.25 cm) wide ¼ in (6 mm) thick
¼ teaspoon toasted black sesame seeds
8 slices of sashimi-grade squid, 2 in (5 cm) long 1 in (1.25 cm) wide ¼ in (6 mm) thick
2 tablespoons salmon roe
1 teaspoon lemon peel, thinly sliced into matchsticks
Soy sauce, for dipping
Wasabi (optional)
Pickled sushi ginger (optional)

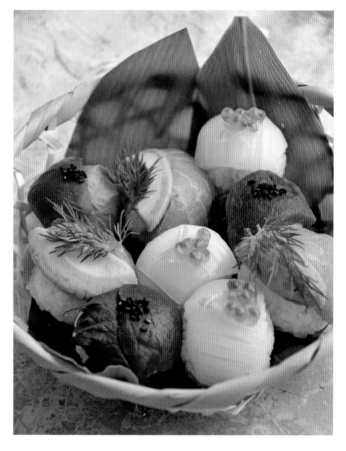

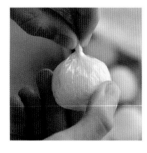
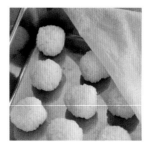
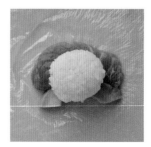
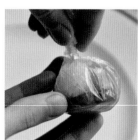

1. Prepare the Sushi Rice.

2. Lay a piece of plastic wrap (8 x 8 inch/20 x 20 cm) on the counter and place 2 tablespoons of Sushi Rice in the center. Make it into a ball shape by gently twisting the plastic wrap. Remove the plastic wrap from the rice and transfer the ball to a large baking pan. Cover the plate with a damp paper towel to keep the balls moist. Continue with the remaining rice, to make a total of 24.

3. Lay the piece of plastic wrap on the counter (reuse the same plastic wrap you used in Step 1) and place one piece of the salmon and one piece of the avocado on it. Then place a rice ball on top. Close the wrap by twisting it gently to make a ball. Remove the plastic wrap from the ball and place it on a serving platter, with the sashimi side facing up, and garnish it with dill. Repeat with the remaining 7 pieces of salmon and avocado. Cover the serving platter with plastic wrap so the rice doesn't dry out.

4. Lay a piece of plastic wrap on the counter, place the shiso basil and tuna on it and then a rice ball on top. Again, close the plastic wrap by twisting it into a ball. Remove the plastic wrap from the ball and place it on the serving platter (from Step 2), with the sashimi side facing up, then garnish with the sesame seeds. Repeat with the remaining 7 pieces of shiso and tuna. Cover with plastic wrap.

5. Lay a piece of plastic wrap on the counter and place the squid on it then a rice ball on top. Twist the plastic wrap into a ball. Remove the wrap and place the ball on the serving platter, with the sashimi side facing up. Garnish with salmon roe and lemon peel. Cover with plastic wrap.

6. Serve with soy sauce, wasabi and pickled sushi ginger on the side, if you like. Dip the balls into the soy sauce and eat immediately.

Sushi Rice

PREPARATION TIME: 10 minutes
SOAKING: 30 minutes
COOKING TIME: 50 minutes
YIELDS: 4 cups (660 g)

1½ cups (340 g) uncooked Japanese short-grain white rice
1½ cups (375 ml) water
1 piece of kombu about 2 x 6 in (5 cm x 15 cm)
4 tablespoons Sushi Vinegar (page 52)

1. Rinse the rice in water to cover in a large bowl by lightly stirring the rice with your hands five to six times, then drain the cloudy water immediately. Do not leave the rice in the cloudy water after the first wash as it will absorb the bran, resulting in an undesirable taste in the rice.

2. Refill the bowl with water to cover the rice. Use the palms of your hands to gently press the rice about 10 times, then drain the cloudy water. Repeat this process three to four times, until the water runs clear.

3. Drain the rice completely in a colander.

4. Combine the rice, 1½ cups (375 ml) water, and kombu in a small (2.5 quarts/2.4 liters) heavy pot or Dutch oven (or in a rice cooker, if using) and soak for 30 minutes.

5. Cover, and cook over medium high heat for 8 to 10 minutes, until the water starts to boil. (TIP: If you are not sure if the water is boiling, you can quickly open the lid to check.) If there is any water remaining above the top of the rice, close the lid and continue cooking for a few more minutes.

6. Turn the heat to low and continue cooking, covered, for 13 to 15 minutes. (TIP: From this point, do not open the lid until the rice is fully cooked.)

7. Remove from the heat and with the pot covered, let steam for another 15 minutes, before removing the lid. If using a rice cooker, follow the manufacturer's instructions.

8. When the rice is done cooking, remove the kombu from the pot with tongs. Transfer the rice to a flat, wooden, medium-size mixing bowl and pour the Sushi Vinegar over the rice while it is still hot. Mix and fluff the rice quickly by using a wet rice paddle so that the rice is seasoned evenly. Cool the rice to room temperature with a handheld fan, then cover the bowl with a damp kitchen towel until you are ready to use it (to prevent it from drying out).

TIP: Store the Sushi Rice in an airtight container in the refrigerator for three days, or in the freezer for up to one month. After defrosting, sprinkle with a little bit of water and use a steamer or microwave for 1 minute to restore its fluffy consistency.

Grandma's Chirashi Scattered Sushi

This is the most popular type of sushi in my family (including my Uncle Yutaka and Aunt Yoshio, whom my grandma left the recipe to). This scattered sushi, chirashizushi, uses vinegar rice mixed with simmered vegetables and topped with thinly cut egg crepes, snow peas and pickled ginger to create a beautiful garnish. My grandma made this dish for all of our birthdays and special occasions, and she always packed the rice in a beautiful "jubako," a traditional lacquered stacking box used for food presentation. My grandma is no longer with us, but now Yoshiko carries on our family traditions by making this on special occasions. Every time I return to Japan to visit my family, Yoshiko brings a box of chirashizushi for me to enjoy. It's a reminder that traditions like there are important ways of honoring beloved family members no longer with us.

PREPARATION TIME: 15 minutes
COOKING TIME: 35 minutes
SERVES 4

3½ cups (600 g) prepared Sushi Rice (page 81)
8 snow peas
1 medium carrot
4 shiitake mushrooms, stems removed
6 oz (170 g) bamboo shoots, or 1 medium zucchini (see Tip)
5 tablespoons Kaeshi Sauce (page 40)
1 tablespoon granulated sugar
1 tablespoon sake
½ cup (125 ml) Basic or Kombu Dashi Stock (pages 36, 38)
2 eggs, beaten
½ teaspoon granulated sugar
Pinch of sea salt
1 teaspoon extra-virgin olive oil
1 tablespoon pickled ginger
1 tablespoon toasted white sesame seed, to garnish (optional)
1 tablespoon shredded nori, to garnish (optional)

TIP To prepare the zucchini, trim off the ends and use a teaspoon to scoop out the spongy, white core and the seeds. Then, cut the zucchini into 2-inch (5-cm) matchsticks.

1. Prepare the Sushi Rice with the recipe on page 81.

2. In a small saucepan, blanch the snow peas in boiling water for 2 minutes. Drain in a colander and rinse with cold water. Trim the ends and thinly cut them on the bias. Set aside.

3. Cut the carrots into thin matchsticks. Cut the shiitake mushrooms and bamboo shoots into thin strips. Along with the Kaeshi Sauce, sugar, sake and stock, cook, covered, over medium heat for 12 to 15 minutes or until the liquid has been absorbed by the vegetables. If using zucchini, add it toward the end and cook it for only about 1 minute so it retains a crunchy texture.

4. In a small bowl, whisk together the eggs, sugar and salt until smooth.

5. Place a nonstick skillet over medium heat and add the oil. Pour half of the egg mixture into the middle of the skillet and swirl the pan until it evenly coats the bottom. Cook until the egg is golden and the edges begin to lift from the pan, about 1 to 2 minutes, then flip the egg with a spatula and cook on the other side for 30 seconds. Place the egg on a cutting board on top of a paper towel. Repeat the process with the remainder of the egg mixture.

6. Stack the two egg crepes on top of each, roll them up and cut them into thin strips.

7. In a medium bowl, combine the Sushi Rice and the vegetable mixture. Use a spatula to mix them until well combined.

8. Scoop the rice onto serving plates. Garnish with the thin egg strips, snow peas and pickled ginger along with sesame seeds and shredded nori, if you like.

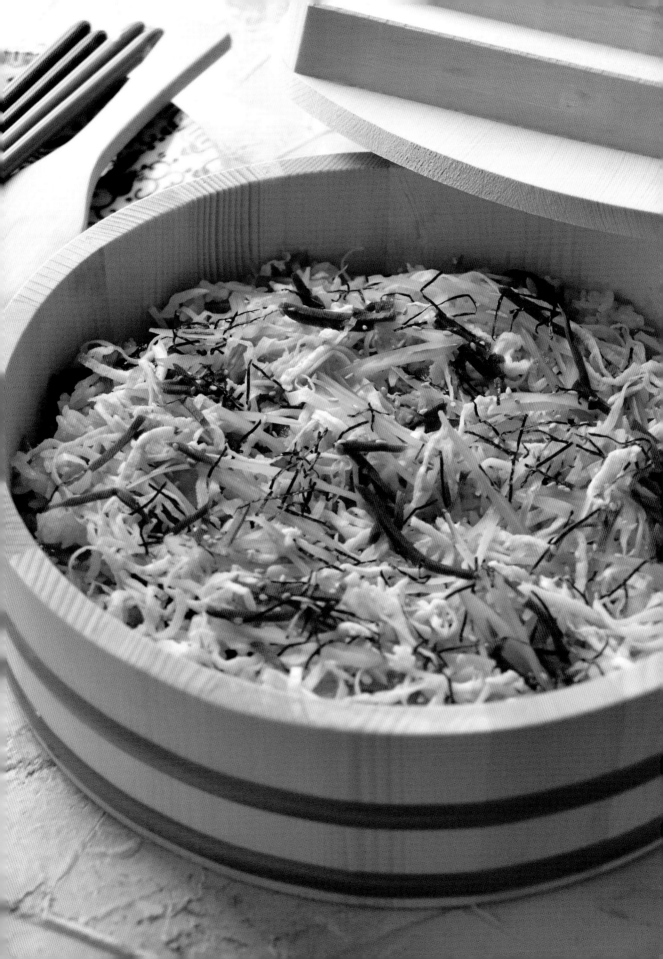

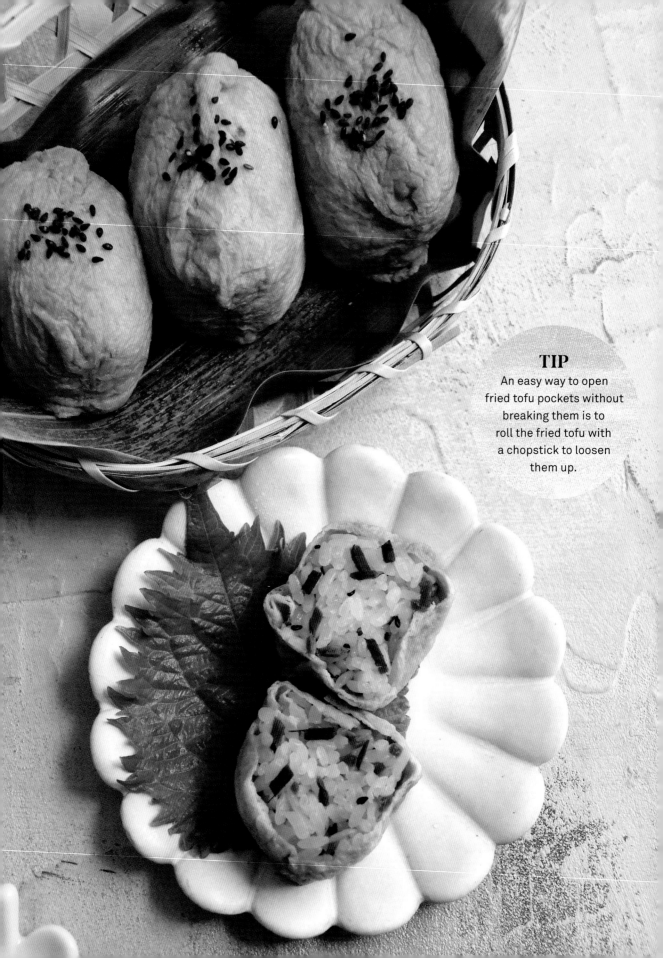

TIP
An easy way to open
fried tofu pockets without
breaking them is to
roll the fried tofu with
a chopstick to loosen
them up.

Tofu Pocket Inari Sushi

Here's another family favorite we would all share during lunch breaks at the seaweed factory. Known as Inarizushi, it's made with a sweet and savory Sushi Rice stuffed into fried, seasoned tofu pockets. They're easy to eat and travel well, so they're often packed in school lunches and for field trips. If you've never used fried tofu before, this will be your introduction to a great ingredient. Called aburaage, it's a light, puffy, flat rectangle approximately 2.5 by 5 inches (6 by 12 cm). It comes in both plain and seasoned varieties, and you can find it in the refrigerated or frozen section of any Asian grocery store. A versatile ingredient, I always keep it on hand in the freezer so it's there when I need it.

PREPARATION TIME: 15
COOKING TIME: 30
YIELDS: 10 pieces

3½ cups (600 g) prepared Sushi Rice (page 81)
5 sheets of fried tofu (2.5 x 5 in/6 x 12 cm)
1 cup (250 ml) Kombu, Basic or Second-Brew Dashi Stock (pages 36–8)
4 tablespoons Kaeshi Sauce (page 40)
1½ tablespoons granulated sugar
3 tablespoons minced pickled ginger
1 tablespoon toasted black sesame seeds

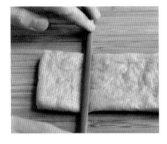

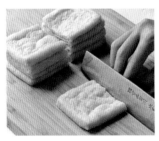

1.   Prepare the Sushi Rice with the recipe on page 81.

2.   Place one piece of the fried tofu on a cutting board. Roll a chopstick back and forth over it a couple of times to loosen it. Cut the fried tofu crosswise to form two halves, each with a pocket. Repeat with the remaining four pieces of tofu, for a total of 10 small pockets.

3.   Place the fried tofu in a colander and slowly pour about 2 cups (500 ml) of boiling water over it. Gently rinse it under cold running water, then squeeze out the excess water.

4.   Combine the Kombu Dashi (or the version you prefer), Kaeshi Sauce and sugar in a pot and bring to a boil over medium-high heat. Add the fried tofu pockets and cover with a drop lid (if you don't have a drop lid, cut a piece of parchment paper to fit inside the pot and use it to cover the surface). Cook for about 8 to 12 minutes over medium heat or until most of the liquid is absorbed into the fried tofu. Transfer the tofu to a plate and let it cool to room temperature, about 5 to 10 minutes. If the tofu pockets are too wet, gently squeeze out the sauce, being careful not to break them.

5.   In a medium-sized bowl, combine the rice, ginger and the black sesame seeds and mix well. Divide into 10 equal portions.

6.   Set a small bowl with water on the table. Wet your hands and form the rice into a small oval that will fit into the tofu pocket. Then, stuff the rice into the pocket and close the end by folding it over.

7.   To serve, place the stuffed pockets with their seams facing down and the smooth side facing up. Sprinkle on additional black sesame seeds for garnish, if you like.

Futomaki Thick Rolls

Futomaki thick rolls are a casual type of sushi roll eaten in Japan as an everyday treat or as a party staple. They're also a popular portable meal that can be found at train stations throughout Japan. They're perfect for the home cook as they can be assembled with several different fillings, including premade, rolled omelet pieces and simmered shiitake mushrooms, to make a thick roll, as big as 2 inches (5 cm) wide. When I make this dish to serve guests, I tend to add even more fillings, such as simmered gourd strips, boiled leafy green vegetables and codfish flakes for a heartier, more substantial result. Here, I've created an easy at-home version of the dish, so I narrowed the fillings down to four basic accessible options. If you can't find sashimi-grade tuna, you can always use smoked salmon instead.

PREPARATION TIME: 15 minutes
COOKING TIME: 30 minutes
YIELDS: 4 thick rolls

3½ cups (600 g) prepared Sushi Rice (page 81)
2 eggs, beaten
½ teaspoon granulated sugar
Pinch of sea salt
1 teaspoon extra-virgin olive oil
2 Japanese or baby cucumbers
7 oz (200 g) sashimi-grade salmon or tuna
8 shiitake mushrooms, simmered
7 oz (200 g) yellow pickled daikon (optional)
½ oz (15 g) kaiware sprouts or microgreens (optional)
4 sheets, 8 x 7-in (20 x 18-cm) nori
Pickled sushi ginger, to garnish (optional)
4 shiso leaves, to garnish (optional)
Soy sauce, for dipping (optional)

TIP When you place the nori on the bamboo mat, put the shiny side face down and the rough side face up. You can easily see the difference between the two sides.

1. Prepare the Sushi Rice with the recipe on page 81.

2. In a small bowl, whisk together the eggs, sugar and salt until smooth. Place a nonstick skillet over medium heat and lightly coat with oil. Pour half of the egg mixture into the middle of the skillet and swirl the pan so it evenly coats the bottom. Cook for about 1 to 2 minutes, until the egg is golden and the edges begin to lift from the pan, then flip the egg with a spatula and cook on the other side for 30 seconds to 1 minute. Place the egg on a paper-towel-lined cutting board. Repeat the process with the remaining egg mixture. Cut the egg crepes in half and set aside.

3. Trim the ends off the cucumber and cut into 8 lengthwise strips, about ½ in (1.3 cm) thick.

4. Cut the salmon lengthwise into 8 strips about ½ in (1.3-cm) thick.

5. Thinly slice the shiitake mushrooms.

6. Cut the yellow pickled daikon into 8 lengthwise strips, about ½-in (1.3 cm) thick. Cut the roots off the kaiware sprouts (if you're using them).

7. On a cutting board, place a bamboo mat and put the nori on top. Spread a thin layer of rice on top of the nori and gently flatten it with a rice paddle or your wet hands. Lay a half piece of egg crepe on top of the rice. Then place the cucumber, salmon, shiitake mushrooms, pickled daikon and kaiware sprouts in a line down the center of the rice. Lift the end of the mat with the rice and roll everything together with your hands, gently pressing it to form a roll. Continue making three more rolls with the remaining ingredients.

8. Cut each roll into 8 slices, wiping the knife blade with a wet paper towel after each cut. Serve the rolls with pickled sushi ginger and soy sauce on the side, if you like.

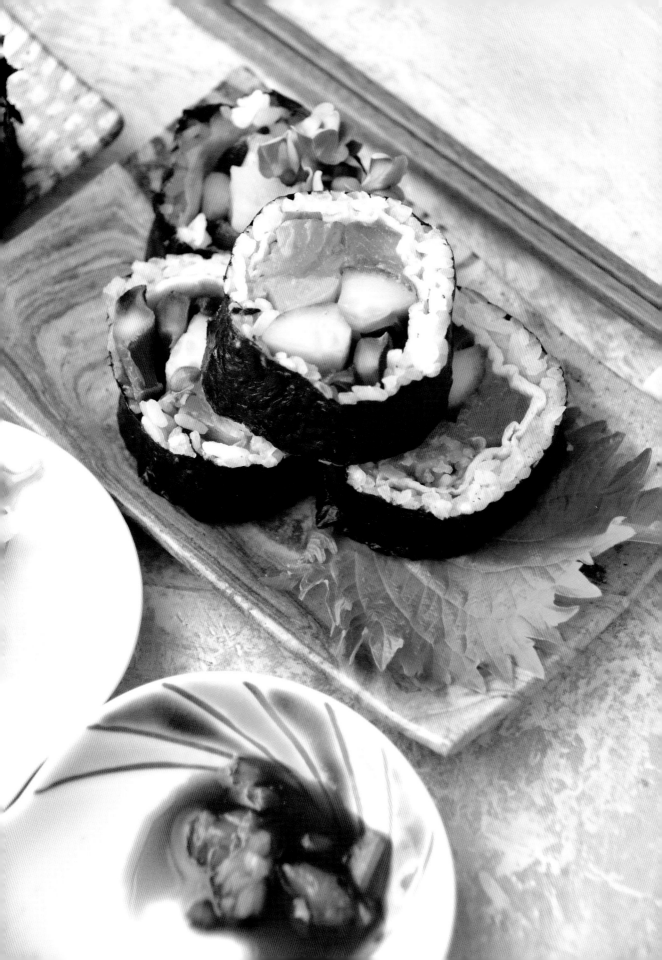

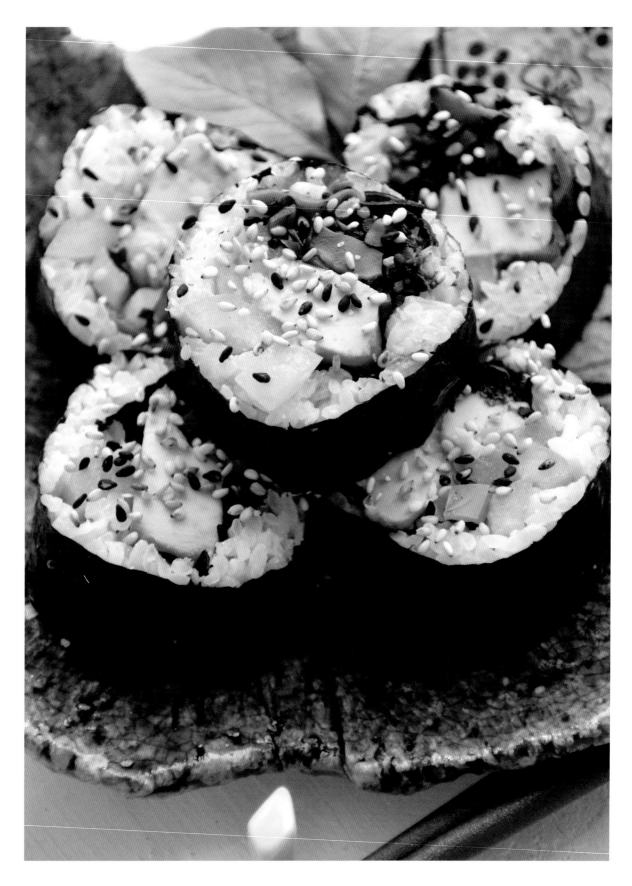

Avocado Hijiki Sushi Rolls

When I make Hijiki Stir Fry (page 95), I always make a big batch so I can enjoy it several different ways, not just with steamed rice, the traditional way. This dish came about a few years ago when I transformed leftovers into my son's lunch. With only a little bit of cooked rice on hand for his lunch box, I wanted to try something new that would be fun and easy to eat without chopsticks. To make up for the shortage of rice, I substituted a few slices of avocado. These rolls have a nice contrast between the creamy avocado and the crunch of the cucumber, radish or asparagus. I've added yellow bell peppers, but you can use whichever vegetables you like. This is similar to the Hijiki Stir Fry recipe used for making Hijiki Hot Dogs (page 112), or you can sprinkle it on top of streamed rice, salads or noodles. It keeps in the refrigerator for up to 5 days or in the freezer for a month, stored in a resealable plastic bag.

PREPARATION TIME: 10 minutes
COOKING TIME: 30 minutes
YIELDS: 4 rolls

3½ cups (600 g) prepared Sushi Rice
  (page 81)
4 dried shiitake mushrooms
4 tablespoons dried hijiki seaweed
1 carrot
1 avocado
½ bell pepper (yellow, red or green)
  or cucumber
1 tablespoon extra-virgin olive oil
½ tablespoon brown sugar
3 tablespoons Kaeshi Sauce (page 40)
1 teaspoon sesame oil
4 sheets nori
1 tablespoon toasted mixed sesame
  seeds, white and black

1. Prepare the Sushi Rice by following the recipe on page 81.

2. Soak the shiitake in 1 cup (250 ml) cold water for 30 minutes or in hot water for 10 minutes or until tender. Squeeze out the liquid and remove the stems, then thinly slice. Set aside.

3. Soak the hijiki in 4 cups of cool or hot water. Then, drain and rinse in fresh water five to six times, in the sink with a strainer and a bowl, until the water runs clear. Set aside.

4. Cut the carrot into 1½-inch (4-cm) matchsticks. Set aside.

5. Peel, pit and cut the avocado in half lengthwise and then into ½-in (1.25-cm) slices. Remove the stem and seeds from the bell pepper, then cut into thin strips and set aside.

6. In a skillet set over medium heat, add the oil and fry the shiitake mushrooms and carrots for 2 to 3 minutes. Add the hijiki to the skillet, lower the heat to medium and fry for 2 to 3 minutes.

7. Add the brown sugar and Kaeshi Sauce and continue frying until all the ingredients are soft, about 3 to 4 minutes. Right before turning the heat off, drizzle the sesame oil over the skillet and cook for an additional 30 seconds. Turn off the heat. Set aside.

8. Place a bamboo mat, covered with plastic wrap or parchment paper, on a cutting board and put a piece of nori on top. Spread a thin layer of rice on the nori and gently flatten it with a rice paddle or your wet hands. Place ¼ of the hijiki stir fry and 2 to 3 slices each of avocado and bell pepper in a line down the center of the rice. Lift the end of the mat with the rice and roll everything together with your hands, gently pressing to form a roll. Continue making rolls with the remaining ingredients.

9. Cut each roll into 8 slices, wiping the knife with a wet paper towel after each slice.

10. To serve, sprinkle sesame seeds on top of the rolls.

Pressed Sushi with Grilled Mackerel

∼∼∼∼∼∼∼∼

If you think sushi is just rolls and nigiri, think again! Oshizushi means "pressed sushi," the rice molded into a wooden or plastic box then topped with a variety of ingredients. Despite the festive look, it's a versatile dish made year-round for both daily consumption and seasonal parties and celebrations. Here, I make it without using a traditional box mold. All you need is a piece of plastic wrap or parchment paper and your clean, dry hands! This might be rather rustic-looking sushi, but the layers of Sushi Rice combine with the shiso, pickled ginger and salty grilled mackerel on top to create some satisfying bites. Pressed sushi can be found in bento boxes sold at train stations and airports throughout Japan. Each region has its own version, highlighting local specialties.

PREPARATION TIME: 15 minutes
COOKING TIME: 45 minutes
SERVES 4

3½ cups (600 g) prepared Sushi Rice (page 81)
2 mackerel fillets, about 10 oz (330 g) total
Pinch of sea salt
2½ tablespoons toasted white sesame seeds, divided
6 shiso leaves or 2 tablespoons fresh cilantro/coriander leaves
3 tablespoons pickled ginger, excess vinegar squeezed out
2 radishes, thinly sliced
1 tablespoon Sushi Vinegar (page 52)

1. Prepare the Sushi Rice by following the recipe on page 81.

2. Sprinkle salt on both sides of the mackerel and let it season for 10 minutes, then pat it dry with a paper towel.

3. Cut a piece of parchment paper to fit inside a medium-sized skillet. Turn the heat to medium-low and place the fish in the skillet on top of the parchment with the skin side down.

4. Cook for 4 to 6 minutes, covered, until the skin turns crispy and golden brown.

5. Gently flip the fish over with a spatula and cook the other side for 2 to 4 minutes or until it's golden brown and thoroughly cooked. The color of the fish changes from transparent to white and has a firmer texture, when it's done cooking.

6. Remove the fish from the skillet and let it cool on a plate at room temperature. Remove the excess oil from the fish with a paper towel. Combine the Sushi Rice and 2 tablespoons of the sesame seeds in a medium bowl and divide the mixture in half.

7. Place a piece of plastic wrap or parchment paper that's slightly longer than the fish (about 13 in/33 cm or so) on the counter. Place half of the Sushi Rice in the middle of the plastic wrap and form it into a log the same size as the fish. Enfold the rice tightly with the plastic wrap and form the shape into a rectangle with your hands so that the fish can sit on top of the rice.

8. Place the block of Sushi Rice on the kitchen counter. Gently open the plastic wrap and layer 1½ tablespoons of pickled ginger slices over the rice. Then place 3 shiso leaves on top of the ginger.

9. Place the fish on the rice with the skin side facing up. Replace the plastic wrap, wrapping it tightly around the rice while forming it into a rectangular shape with your hands. Repeat with the second half of the rice and the remaining ingredients. Put the two wrapped rectangles in the refrigerator for 30 minutes to set.

10. In a small bowl, combine the radish and the Sushi Vinegar and mix well. Let it sit for about 5 minutes in the refrigerator.

11. To serve, cut each Sushi Rice brick through the plastic wrap (so it will hold its shape) into 5 to 6 pieces. Wipe the knife with a wet paper towel after each slice. Then unwrap and serve. Sprinkle the remaining sesame seeds on top and garnish with pickled red radishes on the side.

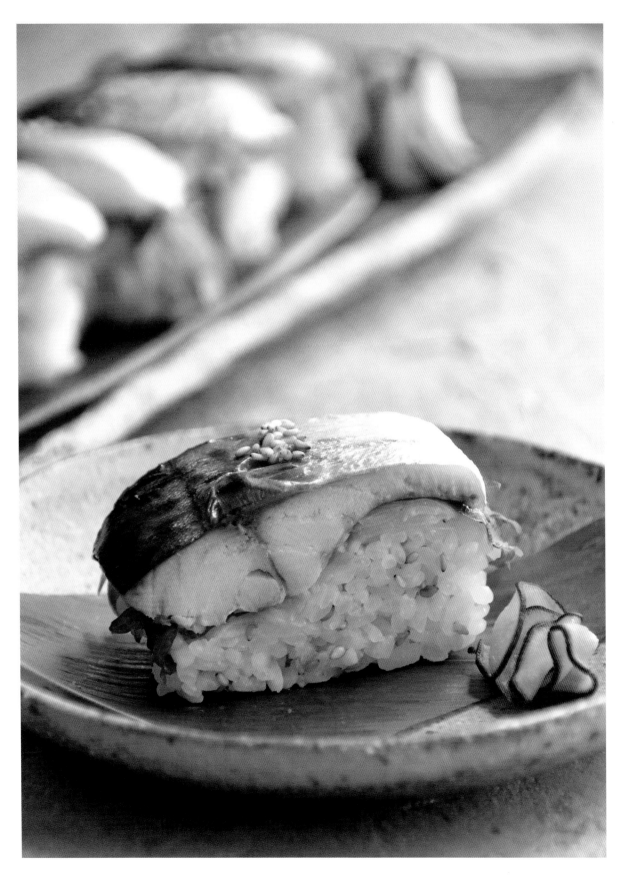

Cup Sushi

This is my favorite type of sushi not found in roll form. It's great for birthday parties, picnics and family gatherings. You can use any type of small cups, about 10 ounces (280–300 ml) should do the trick. My vessel of choice is a short, clear glass so you can see the beautiful layers of colorful ingredients before digging in. You can use any type of sashimi-grade fish, and if you want to transform this into Western-style sushi (which is also delicious), you can use prosciutto instead of fish and add sliced olives and a sprinkle of Parmesan cheese on top.

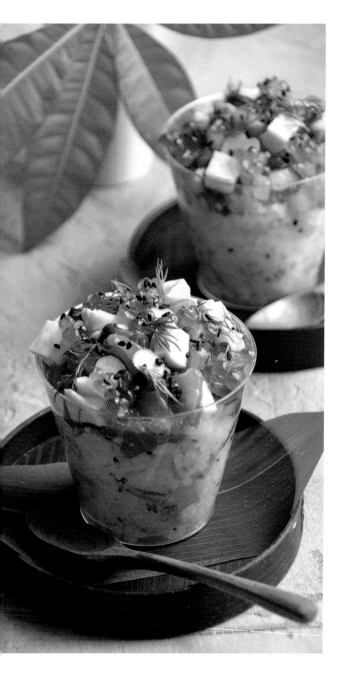

PREPARATION TIME: 15 minutes
COOKING TIME: 30 minutes
SERVES 4

3½ cups (600 g) prepared Sushi Rice (page 81)
7 oz (200 g) sashimi-grade salmon
1 Japanese or baby cucumber (5 oz/150 g), peeled and seeded
½ rolled omelet
4 radishes
Pinch of sea salt
10 shiso leaves
1 tablespoon Kaeshi Sauce (page 40)
¼ teaspoon garlic, grated
1 teaspoon Shio Koji (page 53)
2 teaspoons sesame oil
1 teaspoon toasted black sesame seeds
4 tablespoons salmon roe
1 tablespoon dill, to garnish (optional)

1. Prepare the Sushi Rice by following the recipe on page 81.

2. Cut the salmon, cucumber and rolled omelet into ½-in (1.25-cm) cubes.

3. Thinly slice the radishes.

4. Sprinkle the salt over the cucumber and radish slices and let sit for 5 minutes. Pat dry with a paper towel.

5. Cut the shiso leaves into thin strips.

6. In a medium bowl, combine the salmon, cucumber, radishes, half the shiso leaves, the Kaeshi Sauce, garlic, Shio Koji and sesame oil. Mix well. Let marinate for 5 to 10 minutes in the refrigerator.

7. In a medium-sized bowl, combine the Sushi Rice, ½ teaspoon sesame seeds and the remaining shiso. Use a spatula to mix well.

8. Fill the cups about three-quarters full of the rice, then top with the sashimi filling and the omelet. Garnish with the salmon roe and sesame seeds. Add some dill and drizzle the leftover Kaeshi Sauce on top, if you like.

Hand-rolled Party Sushi

Hand-rolled sushi is my go-to dish for last-minute gatherings or when you're short on time but can't arrive empty-handed. Cut the fish into thin strips, then add the sliced vegetables of your choice. This is a DIY sushi roll: you provide all the components and then let your guests do the work! Fun and easy, right? You can use any sashimi-grade fish such as salmon, squid, shrimp, yellowtail, tuna, red snapper, scallops, sea urchin or salmon roe. If you're vegan, swap out the sashimi and use koji-cured tofu instead.

PREPARATION TIME: 20 minutes
COOKING TIME: 20 minutes
YIELDS: 14 to 16 hand-rolled sushi

4 cups (660 g) prepared Sushi Rice (page 81)
10 oz (300 g) sashimi-grade fish (see above)
¾ cup (75 g) vegetables, such as cucumber,
  avocado and pickled daikon
¼ cup (25 g) kaiware sprouts or microgreens
½ rolled omelet
4 simmered shiitake mushrooms
4 sheets nori
Pickled sushi ginger, to garnish (optional)
Condiments such as wasabi, mayonnaise, black
  sesame seeds or ume plum paste (optional)
Soy sauce, for dipping

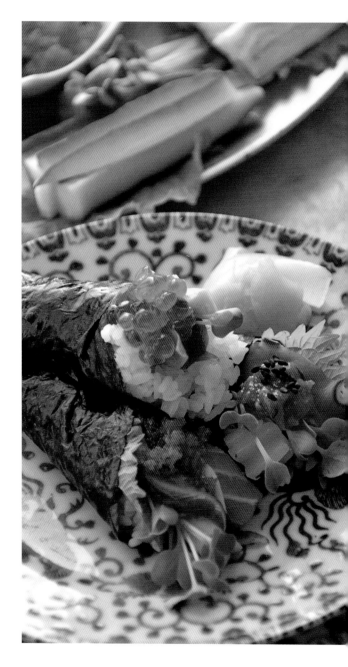

1. Prepare the Sushi Rice by following the recipe on page 81.

2. Cut the fish into strips that are about 3 in (7.5 cm) long and ½ inch (1.25 cm) wide.

3. Cut the vegetables into pieces that are 3 in (7.5-cm) long by ¼ inch (6 mm) wide. Remove the roots from the kaiware sprouts or the microgreens you're using.

4. Cut the rolled omelet into pieces that are the same size as the vegetables.

5. Cut the shiitake mushrooms into thin strips and the nori into quarters.

6. Place the Sushi Rice in a large serving bowl with a spatula. Arrange the sashimi, fresh vegetables, rolled omelet and shiitake on a serving platter. Put the nori on a separate plate and all the condiments together also on their own plate.

7. To make a roll: put a piece of nori, with the rough side facing up, on your plate. Put 1½ tablespoons of Sushi Rice on the nori, then add the sashimi and the vegetables. Add whichever condiments you like on top of the rice. Roll all the ingredients together into a small cone. Dip the roll in soy sauce and eat immediately.

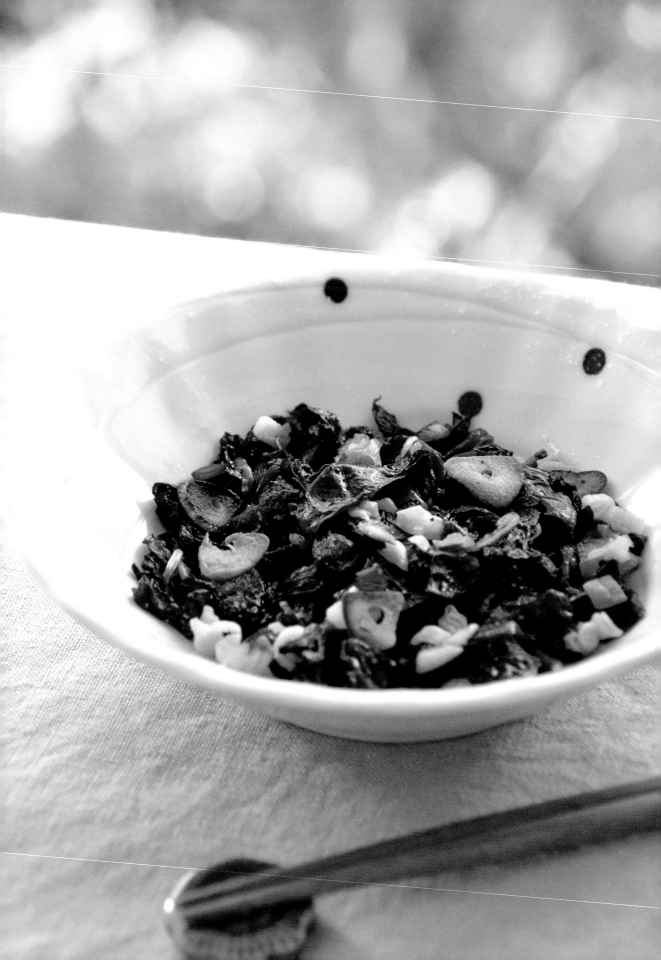

My Go-to Superfood Seaweed Recipes

Seaweed is the ocean's superfood secret. Rich in minerals not only from the ocean but also from the rivers running into it, ocean vegetables occupy a prime position in the superfood pantheon. Seaweed is rich in iodine and alginic acid. Iodine activates the metabolism and boosts energy and focus. Alginic acid is a soluble dietary fiber found in the slimy components of wakame. It binds to the salt in other foods and helps remove it from the body. Alginate also aids in cholesterol reduction and helps regulate the body's balance of gut bacteria.

In order to prevent diseases caused by arteriosclerosis and to slow the effects of aging, seaweed is a recommended part of your daily diet. This section highlights three of Japan's most popular offerings: wakame, kombu and hijiki, with recipes ranging from the traditional (Wakame Rice Ball) to more modern takes (Hijiki Hot Dogs). I've also included recipes for repurposing kombu left over from making dashi stock. Unlocking all the goodness in these healthful ingredients is a defining element of Japanese cooking and one of the keys to unleashing the power of superfoods.

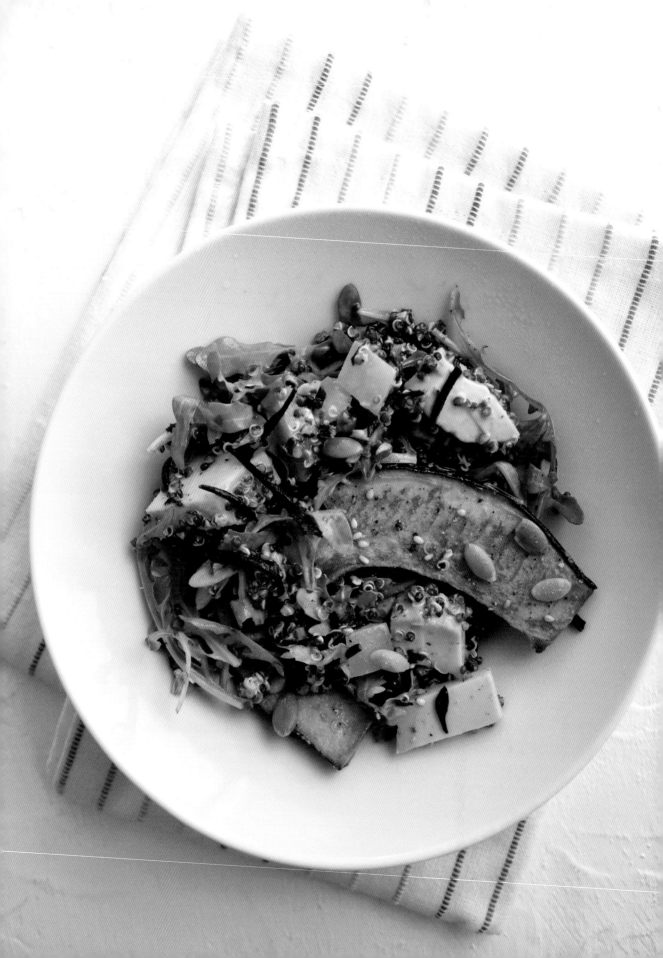

Red Quinoa Salad with Hijiki and Kabocha Pumpkin

~~~

This isn't a typical Japanese dish, but it's packed with authentic Japanese flavors you might be familiar with. I boil the quinoa in the kombu stock so that the savory umami notes infuse the plain quinoa with a depth of flavor. Hijiki is something the Japanese have been eating as part of a healthy diet for centuries. It's a versatile dried seaweed that's not only delicious but also highly nutritious, packed with iron, magnesium and calcium. It's also rich in dietary fiber. With its smoky, savory flavor and a pleasant crunchy texture, it can be adapted in numerous ways. Hijiki needs to be rehydrated before cooking, and you need to eat it within a day or two. Store it in a cool, dry place for up to a year. This salad will keep in the refrigerator for up to 3 days.

PREPARATION TIME: 15 minutes
COOKING TIME: 30 minutes
SERVES 4

8 oz (250 g) kabocha pumpkin
4 tablespoons extra-virgin olive oil, divided
½ teaspoon sea salt
2 tablespoons dried hijiki strands
½ cup (85 g) red quinoa
1 cup (250 ml) Kombu Dashi Stock (page 38)
1 ripe avocado
½ yellow bell pepper
2 cups (50 g) arugula or any leafy greens
4 tablespoons Sushi Vinegar (page 52)
1 tablespoon Japanese mayonnaise or regular mayonnaise
2 tablespoons fresh lemon juice
1 tablespoon toasted pumpkin seeds, to garnish (optional)
½ tablespoon toasted white sesame seeds, to garnish (optional)
½ tablespoon crushed red pepper corns, to garnish (optional)

1. Line a baking sheet with a silicone liner or parchment paper. Preheat the oven to 325ºF (160ºC).

2. Scoop out the seeds from the kabocha and thinly slice it vertically into ⅛-in (3-mm) pieces, placing the pieces on the baking sheet. Drizzle 1 tablespoon of the olive oil over the kabocha and sprinkle with the salt. Bake the kabocha for 7 to 10 minutes or until golden brown and tender when pierced with a fork. Remove it from the oven and transfer it from the baking sheet to a wire rack. Let cool for 10 minutes.

3. Place the hijiki in a bowl and fill with plenty of water. Let it sit until it's softened, about 15 to 20 minutes, or in hot water for 4 to 5 minutes or follow the manufacturer's instruction on the package. The water will turn brown at first. Drain the water in a colander and rinse in fresh water 5 to 6 times in the sink with a strainer until the water runs clear. Squeeze out the excess then set aside.

4. Place a fine mesh strainer in a bowl, add the quinoa and rinse it under running water for 30 seconds. Transfer the quinoa to a small saucepan, add the stock and cook over medium heat until tender and almost all the stock has been absorbed, about 10 to 12 minutes.

5. Cut the avocado into bite-sized pieces. Dice the pepper into ½-in (1.25-cm) pieces. Wash the arugula, pat it dry with a paper towel and chop it into bite-sized pieces. Set aside.

6. In a small bowl, combine the remaining 3 tablespoons of olive oil, Sushi Vinegar, mayonnaise, lemon juice and sea salt. Mix well.

7. In a large bowl, combine the kabocha pumpkin, hijiki, quinoa, avocado, peppers, arugula and the dressing and toss all together. Taste and add a pinch more salt if necessary.

8. To serve, plate the salad and sprinkle pumpkin seeds, sesame seeds and crushed red pepper on top, if using.

Smashed Cucumber Salad with Wakame and Ginger

You can make this great side dish in less than 10 minutes, marinating the vegetables, typically cucumbers, in a sweet vinegar sauce. My grandmother always made this for me when I spent summers at her house, though she always used silky wakame. She had a farm and grew a ton of cucumbers in the summer. She'd sit on the wood floor in her kitchen and use a mandoline to carefully slice the cucumbers into a big gold bowl. As an adult, whenever I make this cool and crunchy treat for my family, it makes me smile, thinking of her.

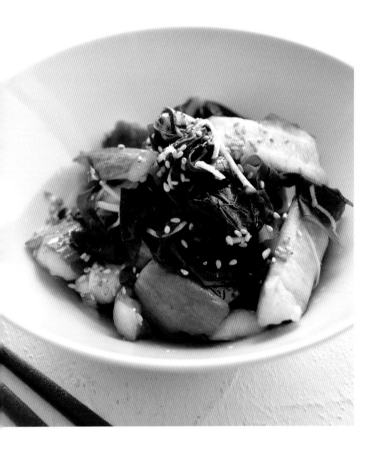

PREPARATION TIME: 10 minutes
COOKING TIME: 10 minutes
SERVES 2

¼ cup (45 g) fresh or dried wakame
2 Japanese or 1 medium cucumber
¼ teaspoon sea salt
3 tablespoons Sushi Vinegar (page 52)
½-in (1-cm) piece ginger, peeled and cut into thin strips
¼ teaspoon toasted white sesame seeds, to garnish

1. Place a strainer in a bowl. Add the fresh wakame and fill the bowl with water, letting it sit for a few seconds. Drain and rinse the wakame under running water until the salt is removed and the wakame doubles or triples in size. Squeeze out the excess water and cut into bite-sized pieces. If using dried wakame, follow the instruction on the package or rehydrate in a bowl of water for 5 minutes, draining then squeezing out the excess water. Set aside.

2. Put the cucumber on the counter, breaking it down with a rolling pin or a meat mallet. "Smash" it into bite-sized pieces then place them in a small bowl. Sprinkle with the sea salt and set aside for 5 minutes.

3. Wipe the salt and excess water from the cucumbers with a paper towel. Combine the Sushi Vinegar, cucumber, wakame and ginger in a medium-sized serving bowl. Toss all the ingredients well and serve with sesame seeds sprinkled on top.

Hijiki Stir Fry with Bacon, Bell Pepper and Edamame

There are two different types of hijiki: me hijiki (sprouts), which looks like black tea and has a tender texture, and naga hijiki (long), which is the stem part of the plant and has a crispy texture. I make my version of hijiki stir fry with me hijiki, bacon, edamame and red bell peppers as a side dish. It has a nice smoky and savory flavor with a pleasantly crunchy texture. So watch out: it's pretty addictive! This is a versatile dish that can be adapted in any number of ways. Try adding avocado and tofu, using it as a sandwich filling or serving it with noodles.

PREPARATION TIME: 15 minutes
COOKING TIME: 15 minutes
SERVES 4

4 tablespoons dried me hijiki seaweed
½ red bell pepper
4 strips bacon
4 tablespoons frozen edamame soybeans (without pods), defrosted
1 tablespoon Kaeshi Sauce (page 40)
1 teaspoon brown sugar
½ teaspoon toasted white sesame seeds, divided
Steamed rice, for serving (optional)

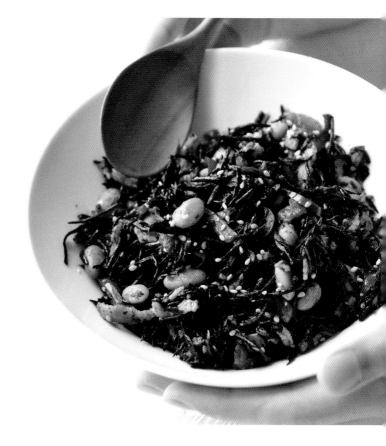

1. Soak the hijiki in cool or hot water. Then, drain and rinse it in fresh water 5 to 6 times in the sink with a strainer and a bowl, until the water runs clear. Set aside.

2. Cut the red pepper into 1-in (2.5-cm) matchsticks. Set aside.

3. Cut the bacon into ½-in (1.25-cm) pieces and fry in a skillet over medium-high heat until crispy, about 1 to 2 minutes. Add the red peppers, edamame and hijiki and fry for 2 to 3 minutes.

4. Add the Kaeshi Sauce, brown sugar and half of white sesame seeds and continue frying over medium-low heat until the liquid is almost evaporated, about 2 to 3 minutes. To serve, sprinkle the remaining sesame seeds on top and serve with steamed rice, if you like.

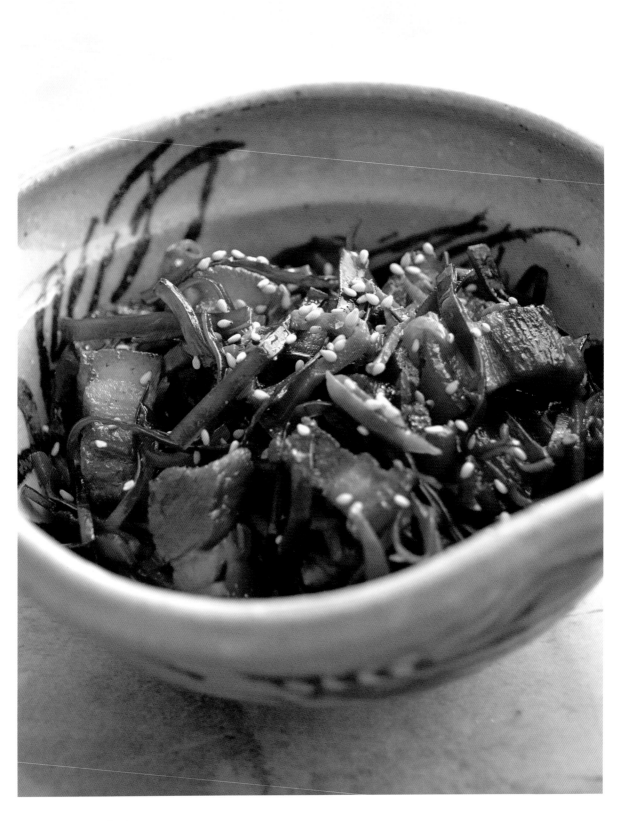

Okinawa-style Braised Kombu with Pork

Called kubu irichii in Japanese, this is one of the classic dishes found in Okinawa, the southernmost island of Japan. Okinawans are famous for being centenarians. Not only do they live longer, they have low rates of chronic illness. What's the secret to these long and healthy lives? Many theories have been posited, but one thing for certain is that Okinawans eat a lot of fresh seafood and sea vegetables. Here, you can use dried kombu and soak it in water before cooking it. Another option is using kombu left over from making the dashi. This is a great way to repurpose, storing your leftover kombu in the freezer until you're ready to use it. For a vegan option, use Kombu Dashi (page 38) instead of the Basic Dashi Stock (page 36) and substitute medium-firm tofu, zucchini or eggplant for the pork belly.

PREPARATION TIME: 15 minutes
COOKING TIME: 60 minutes
SERVES 4

14 oz (400 g) pork belly or pork shoulder
3–4 sheets (6 oz/175 g) kombu, left over
   from making dashi stock
1 tablespoon neutral-flavored oil
2 carrots, cut into matchsticks
2 cups (500 ml) Basic or Kombu Dashi
   Stock (pages 36, 38)
2 teaspoons brown sugar
2 tablespoons Kaeshi Sauce (page 40)
2 teaspoons sesame oil
2 teaspoons toasted white sesame seeds
Steamed rice, for serving (optional)

1. Put the pork belly in a medium-sized pot and add just enough water to cover it. Boil the pork belly for 8 to 10 minutes until a toothpick comes out clean. Let it cool for 10 minutes and then cut it into ½-in (1.3 cm) pieces.

2. Cut the kombu into thin strips.

3. Heat the oil in a medium-sized pot and cook the pork over medium-high heat. Once the pork turns light brown, add the kombu and carrots and cook for another 6 to 8 minutes.

4. Add the dashi stock you're using and the brown sugar to the pot, cover then bring to a boil over medium-high heat. Reduce the heat to low and add the Kaeshi Sauce. Simmer for 25 to 30 minutes over low heat, slowly reducing the broth.

5. Add the sesame oil and mix well.

6. When the broth has been absorbed and all the ingredients have softened, turn off the heat.

7. Serve in bowls, sprinkled with sesame seeds or over steamed rice.

Kabocha Pumpkin Hijiki Croquettes

Kabocha pumpkin is loaded with beta-carotene and vitamin A, a powerful source of antioxidants that help boost your immune system. These kabocha croquettes with hijiki were my favorite food growing up. Velvety and creamy mashed kabocha is filled with iron-packed hijiki and sweet onions, then formed into bite-sized balls. They're briefly deep-fried until crispy, then served with a sweet and tangy tama miso sauce on top. This is everybody's favorite dish when I host lunch or dinner events. The croquettes disappear quickly and leave everyone wanting more. Enjoy serving these little bites as a main dish with steamed rice or as an appetizer paired with your favorite cocktail.

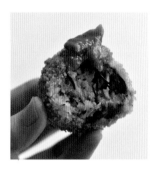

PREPARATION TIME: 20 minutes
COOKING TIME: 40 minutes
YIELDS: 16 to 18 croquettes

Half (1½ lbs/750 g) kabocha pumpkin
2 tablespoons dried hijiki strands
2 onions, minced
2 tablespoons salted butter
⅓ cup (40 g) potato starch or cornstarch
2 eggs, beaten
1½ cups (200 g) panko breadcrumbs
Neutral-flavored oil, for deep-frying
¼ teaspoon sea salt
3 tablespoons Tama Miso (page 205)
3 tablespoons ketchup
2 cups (200 g) shredded cabbage, for serving (optional)
1 tomato, cut into 8 pieces, for serving (optional)
Steamed rice, for serving (optional)

1. Fill a large pot halfway with water and place a steamer on top. Scoop out the seeds from the kabocha, cut it into 2-in (5-cm) pieces and place them in the steamer. Turn the heat to high, cover the pot and steam the kabocha for about 15 to 20 minutes or until it's tender when pierced with a fork. Turn off the heat, remove the kabocha from the steamer and discard the water. Put the kabocha pieces on a plate and let them cool for 10 minutes.

2. Place the hijiki in a bowl and fill it with cool water. Let it sit until softened about 15 to 20 minutes or in hot water for 4 to 5 minutes. The water will turn brown at first. Drain the hijiki in a colander and then rinse it in fresh water 5 to 6 times in the sink in a strainer until the water runs clear. Squeeze out the excess water and set aside.

3. In a pot, heat the butter over medium heat. Add the onions and cook for 4 to 6 minutes, until light brown and translucent.

4. Peel the kabocha skin with your hands or a knife and put the pieces into the steamer (the bottom part of the pot). Mash the kabocha with a potato masher until smooth and creamy. If the kabocha is too wet, turn the heat to medium-low and allow the moisture to evaporate for 2 to 3 minutes while mixing well with a spatula.

5. Add the hijiki and the onions to the kabocha mixture and combine.

6. Using a tablespoon, scoop out the kabocha mixture and roll it into a golf-ball-sized bite in your hands. Place it on a baking sheet, then repeat the process with the remaining kabocha mixture. Cover the baking sheet with plastic wrap and chill it in the refrigerator for 10 to 15 minutes.

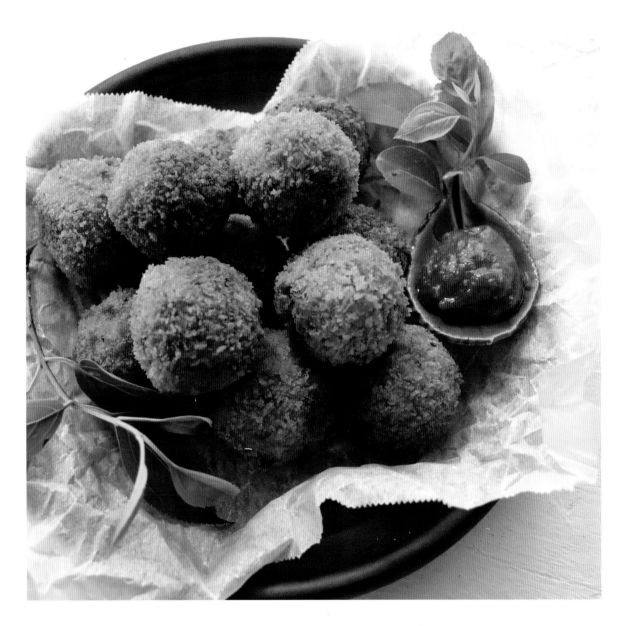

7. In a small bowl, combine the eggs and potato starch and mix well. In another small bowl, add the panko.

8. Remove the kabocha balls from the refrigerator. Dip one in the egg mixture and then coat it with the breadcrumbs. Repeat with all the kabocha balls, setting them on a plate as they're completed.

9. Fill a large heavy-bottomed pot with about 1 in (2.5 cm) of oil and bring it to 325º F (160º C) over medium heat. Gently drop each croquette into the oil and cook for a total of 2 to 3 minutes or until golden brown and crispy on all sides. Don't overcrowd the pot—if all the pieces don't fit at one time, fry them in batches. Give each ball at least 1½ in (4 cm) of space. Drain the croquettes on a wire rack with a paper-towel-lined tray beneath it and sprinkle them generously with sea salt. Combine the Tama Miso and the ketchup in a small bowl and mix well.

10. Plate the croquettes with some of the miso ketchup sauce on top and serve with the cabbage and tomatoes on the side, along with a bowl of steamed rice, if you like.

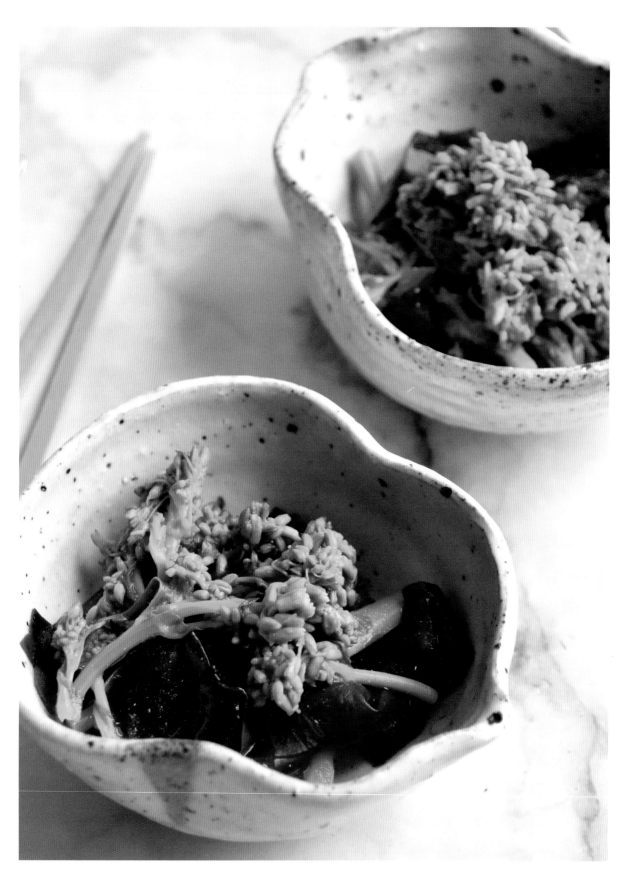

Wakame and Broccoli Rabe Salad
with Sesame Mustard Vinaigrette

When I think of spring, I always crave *this* salad. It's traditionally made from nanohana, which is similar to broccoli but is a lighter shade of green with vivid yellow flowers. When I was in high school, I commuted by bicycle, my route taking me past nanohana fields, like a beautiful, bright yellow carpet. I often stopped at the farm stand to pick up freshly cut young sprouts so my mom could make them into a salad. This dish introduced me to the idea of eating flowers as a vegetable. When I moved to the United States, I couldn't find nanohana but discovered that broccoli rabe served as the perfect substitute. The mustard dressing gives an extra kick of flavor. If you're looking for a new vegetable dish for your next meal, try making this instead of your usual choices.

PREPARATION TIME: 5 minutes
COOKING TIME: 10 minutes
SERVES 4

3 tablespoons fresh or dried wakame
½ medium bunch (5 oz/150 g)
    broccoli rabe
½ teaspoon Dijon mustard
2 teaspoons Kaeshi Sauce (page 40)
1 tablespoon Kombu or Basic Dashi
    Stock (pages 36, 38)
1 teaspoon maple syrup
⅛ teaspoon salt
2 teaspoons rice vinegar
1 teaspoon sesame oil

1. Place a strainer in a bowl, add the fresh wakame and fill the bowl with water, letting it sit for a few seconds. Drain and rinse the wakame under running water until the salt is removed and the wakame doubles or triples in size. Squeeze out the excess water and cut it into bite-sized pieces. If you're using dried wakame, follow the instructions on the package or rehydrate it in a bowl of water for 5 minutes. Then drain and squeeze out the excess water and set aside.

2. Cut and discard 1 in (2.5 cm) from the bottom of the broccoli rabe, then cut it into 2-in (5-cm) pieces. Fill a medium-sized pot halfway with water and bring it to a boil. Add the broccoli rabe and cook the pieces over high heat, about 1 to 2 minutes or until just tender. Drain well in a colander and place under cold running water for 30 seconds to shock the pieces and stop the cooking. Gently squeeze out the excess water.

3. Combine the mustard, Kaeshi Sauce, dashi stock, maple syrup, salt, rice vinegar and sesame oil in a bowl large enough to hold the broccoli rabe. Mix well.

4. Add the wakame and broccoli rabe to the bowl with the mustard dressing. Gently mix the salad so that the broccoli rabe is coated in dressing, being careful not to break up the florets. Serve as is or in small individual bowls.

Wakame Rice Balls

Rice balls are pure Japanese soul food. Steamed, short-grain rice made into a triangle or a ball and often wrapped in black nori—onigiri are cheap, easy to eat and the perfect choice for a meal on the go. There are no rules as to fillings, so be creative. Popular options include grilled salmon, umeboshi, salted kombu, mentaiko spicy cod roe, tuna salad and furikake sprinkles. These popular treats are not only quick and easy to make, they're also healthy and delicious. There are three ways to form the onigiri—using your bare, wet hands, plastic wrap or using special onigiri molds. Keep the ingredients at room temperature and be sure to finish them up within a day. About a half cup of rice (85 g) for each onigiri works best. Always use freshly cooked or warm rice, as cold rice won't stick together. Place the rice ball on one hand to start. The other hand is used to hold the rice as you clamp down, bending your fingers into a V to make the triangular shape. Use the pictures below to guide you along. You'll get it down soon enough.

PREPARATION TIME: 10 minutes
COOKING TIME: 60 minutes
SERVES 4

1½ cups (340 g) uncooked Japanese short-grain white rice
1¼ cups (300 ml) water
1 piece of dried kombu (3 in/7.5 cm square)
2½ tablespoons mirin
2½ tablespoons sake
2 teaspoons sea salt, divided
1 teaspoon peeled and minced fresh ginger
2 tablespoons fresh or dried wakame
2 teaspoons toasted white sesame seeds

1. In a large bowl, cover the rice with water, rinsing it by lightly stirring it with your hands 5 to 6 times then draining the cloudy water immediately. Don't leave the rice in the cloudy water after the first wash as it'll absorb the bran and give the rice an unpleasant flavor.

2. Refill the bowl with water, covering the rice. Use the palms of your hands to gently press the rice about 10 times, then drain the cloudy water. Repeat this process 3 to 4 times, until the water runs clear. Refill the bowl with the washed rice and 1½ cups of water and soak for 30 minutes.

3. While soaking the rice, prepare the seasoning stock by combining 1¼ cups of water (10 oz or 300 ml), the kombu, mirin, sake, 1 teaspoon of the sea salt and the ginger in a small (2.5-quart/2.4-liter) saucepan or Dutch oven and soak for 30 minutes also.

4. Place a strainer in a bowl, add the fresh wakame and fill the bowl with water, letting it sit for a few seconds. Drain

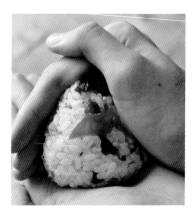 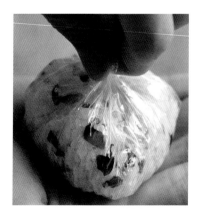 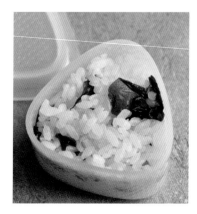

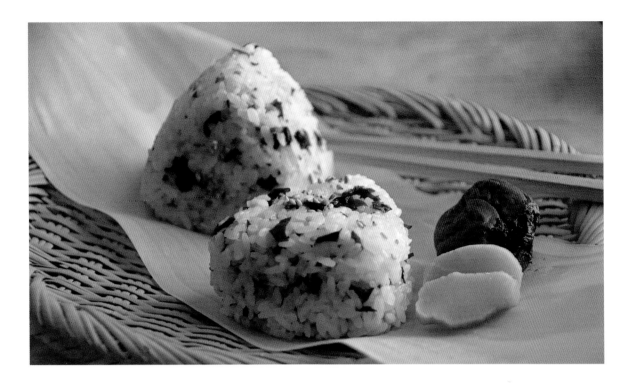

and rinse the wakame under running water until the salt is removed and the wakame doubles or triples in size. Squeeze out the excess water and cut the wakame into bite-sized pieces. If you're using dried wakame, follow the instructions on the package or rehydrate it in a bowl of water for 5 minutes. Drain and squeeze out the excess water. Set aside.

5. Drain the rice completely in a colander.

6. Combine the seasoning stock, kombu and rice in the saucepan or Dutch oven and mix well.

7. Cook covered over medium-high heat for 8 to 10 minutes until the water starts to boil. (You can lift the lid quickly to check.) If there's some water left, replace the lid and continue cooking for a few more minutes.

8. Turn the heat to low and cook, covered, for 13 to 15 minutes. (TIP: From this point on, don't lift the lid until the rice is fully cooked.)

9. Turn off the heat and with the pot covered, let the rice steam for another 15 minutes before removing the lid. If you're using a rice cooker, follow the manufacturer's instructions.

10. Transfer the rice to a large bowl. Combine the rice, wakame and the sesame seeds, using a spatula to mix it well.

11. Using your hands: Set a bowl of water and a plate containing 1 teaspoon of the sea salt on your work surface. To prevent the rice from sticking to your hands, wet them in the bowl and rub your palms with the salt before working with the rice. Place a clump of rice in one hand and gently mold it into a round shape. Use your thumb, index finger, middle finger and third fingers to form a triangle. Keep rotating and pressing the rice with your fingers a couple of times until you're happy with the shape. Don't squeeze the rice too hard, as you want to keep it soft and fluffy.

12. Using plastic wrap: Spread a piece of plastic wrap (10 x 10 in or 25 x 25 cm) over a bowl and add the rice. Lift the corners of the wrap and twist it twice to form a ball shape first. Then make a triangle with your fingers as previously described.

13. Using a mold: Rinse the mold then fill it with rice almost to the rim (about 90 percent full) and put on the top. Don't overstuff the mold. Remove the lid and flip it over on the plate. There should be a release button to press so that the rice comes out easily.

14. To serve, place the onigiri on a plate and sprinkle on the remaining salt and sesame seeds, if you like.

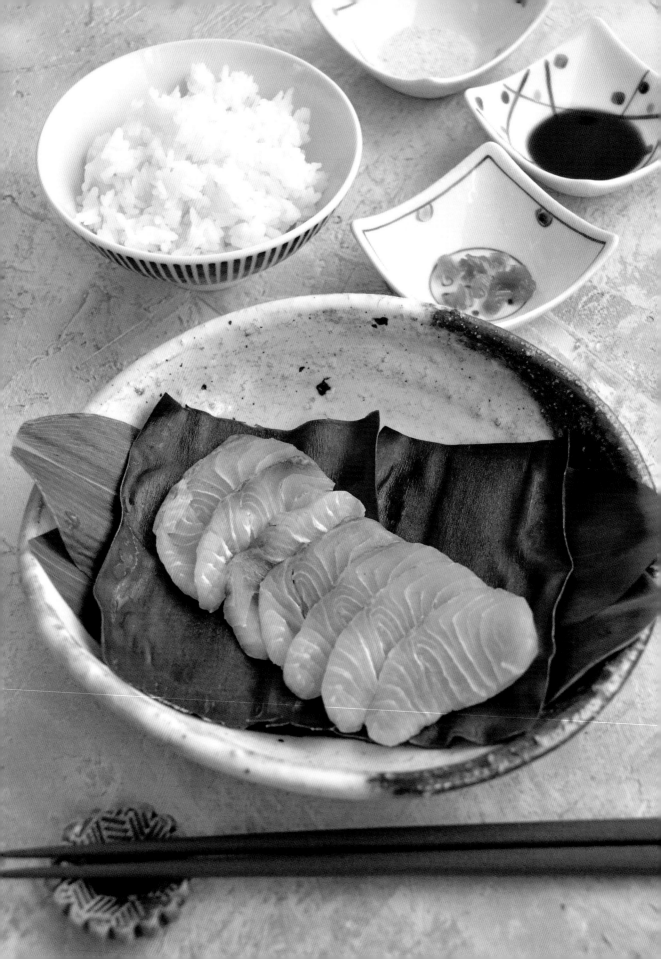

Kombu-cured Sashimi

What a genius idea to wrap fish in kombu and infuse it with umami flavor! This amazing preparation couldn't be easier. Simply lay sashimi-grade fish on a sheet of kombu, cover it with another sheet of kombu and let it cure overnight. The result is remarkable, as the natural saltiness of the kombu adds an extra layer of flavor to the fish. This light, no-fuss dish is a perfect appetizer or an ideal main dish when served with steamed rice. When you handle the kombu, you might find a white, powder-like crystallized substance on the surface. Include it in the dish. It's mannit, a natural glutamic acid and a source of the dish's savory, delicious umami flavor. Serve kombu-cured fish as is or with wasabi, sea salt and/or soy sauce.

PREPARATION TIME: 10 minutes
COOKING TIME: 3 hours, up to 1 day (including curing time)
SERVES 4

8 pieces dried kombu (3 x 8 in/7.5 x 20 cm)
2 tablespoons sake
12 oz (350 g) sashimi-grade fish such as amberjack, sea bream, fluke, red snapper, sea bass or tilefish
½ teaspoon wasabi (optional)
Pinch of sea salt (optional)
½ tablespoon soy sauce (optional)
Steamed rice, for serving (optional)

1. Gently wipe the surface of the kombu with a paper towel, leaving the white powder (see the headnote).

2. Moisten both sides of the kombu with the sake, using a brush or a paper towel.

3. Slice the fish into ⅛-inch (3-mm) pieces.

4. Cover a medium-sized tray with a piece of plastic wrap, then layer on the kombu and fish by placing one sheet of kombu on the bottom, then topping it with a slice of the fish (see the first picture below). Then, place another sheet of kombu on top of the fish as if you're making a sandwich (see the second picture below). Make sure that the kombu and fish are stacked on top of each other and that the pieces of fish don't touch each other.

5. Tightly wrap the kombu and fish together with plastic wrap (see the third picture below) and place a flat plate or another medium-sized tray onto the kombu. Let it cure in the refrigerator for at least 3 hours or up to a day.

6. Cut each piece of kombu widthwise into two pieces.

7. To serve, place the cut kombu sheets on a plate and add the slices of fish on top. Serve with the wasabi, sea salt and/or the soy sauce on the side and rice, if you like.

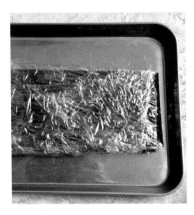
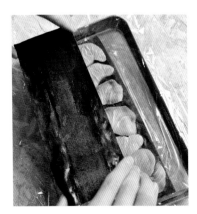
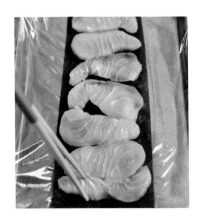

Swordfish-stuffed Kombu Rolls

Kombu rolls, or kobumaki, are a signature New Year's dish. Made with fish and root vegetables, such as carrots and burdock root, they're tightly rolled and beautifully tied with kanpyo dried gourd before being simmered in a flavorful dashi soy sauce. At the turn of the year, we enjoy a special dish called osechi ryori, a Japanese tradition of serving a variety of small dishes, each having a special meaning for the coming year. If you're lucky enough to receive an invitation to a Japanese-style New Year's feast, you'll definitely find kombu rolls on the table. Here, for an easier preparation, I don't use the kanpyo dried gourd, as it can be difficult to tie the rolls with the thin strips. Using toothpicks works just as well. Kombu sheets come in different sizes, but as long as you keep the kombu and the fish the same width, the rolls will be easy to handle and will cook evenly. If you're using long hidaka kombu, simply soak it in water to rehydrate it and then cut it in half, a perfect size for this recipe. You can store the kombu rolls for up to 5 days in the refrigerator, and they're a great addition to a bento box.

PREPARATION TIME: 15 minutes
COOKING TIME: 1 hour, 40 minutes
SERVES 4

Three 6-in (15-cm) squares of dried
  kombu
4 cups (1 liter) water
10 oz (330 g) swordfish fillets,
  skin removed
12 toothpicks
1-in (2.5-cm) piece fresh ginger,
  peeled and sliced
3 tablespoons Kaeshi Sauce (page 40)
1 tablespoon brown sugar
Steamed rice and miso soup,
  for serving (optional)

1. Clean the surface of the kombu with a dry towel. Soak and rehydrate the kombu in 4 cups of water in a large bowl for 15 to 20 minutes. Cut the kombu squares in half so you have 6 pieces. Reserve the soaking water.

2. Cut the swordfish fillets into strips about 4 by 1 in (10 x 2.5 cm) long. The widths of fish and kombu should be closely matched when rolling them up together.

3. Lay out a piece of kombu on a cutting board with the longest side facing you. Place a strip of swordfish across the lower edge and tightly roll the kombu up over the swordfish. Use 2 toothpicks per roll to hold the kombu and swordfish together by putting each toothpick about 1 in (2.5 cm) from the edges. Repeat with the remaining ingredients.

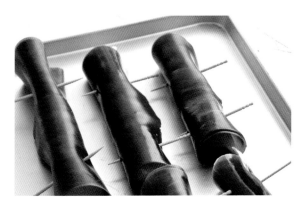
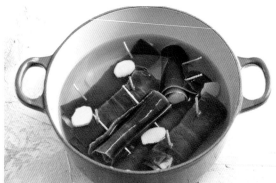

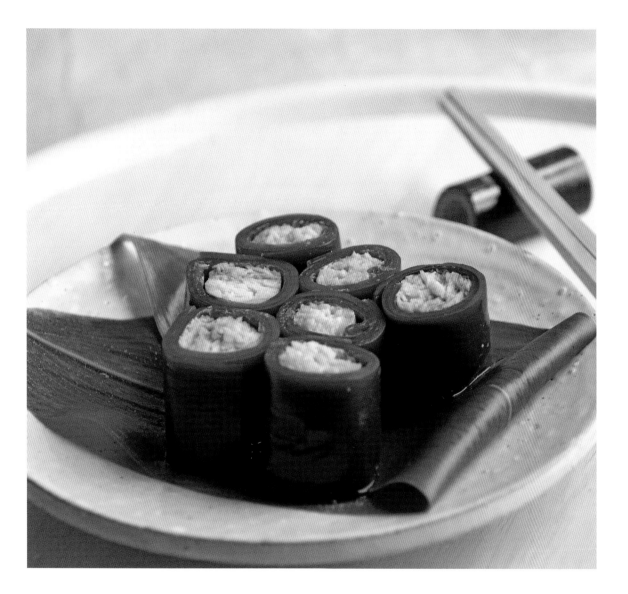

4. Place the reserved kombu water, the kombu rolls and the ginger in a medium-sized pot. Cover and bring to a boil. Skim the foam from the surface using a sieve.

5. Reduce the heat to medium-low, cover with a drop lid, in addition to the pot's lid and simmer for 30 minutes. If you don't have a drop lid, cut a piece of parchment paper to fit the diameter of the pot.

6. Add the Kaeshi Sauce and the brown sugar and continue simmering over medium-low heat for about an hour or until tender. Turn off the heat and let the kombu rolls cool in the pot for 30 minutes.

7. To serve, remove the toothpicks and cut each kombu roll into three bite-sized pieces and serve with steamed rice and miso soup, if you desire.

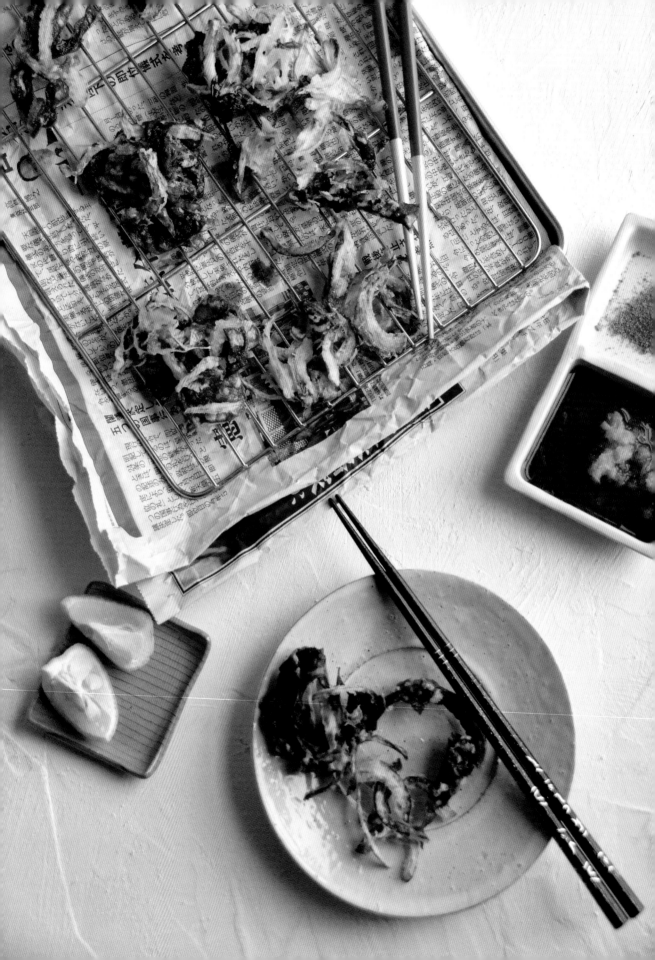

Wakame and Onion Tempura

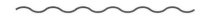

Whenever my mother made this dish, the house turned into a tempura party. She would fry so many different ingredients—squid, shrimp, sweet potato, kabocha, lotus root, green peppers, mushrooms and eggplant—and in such large quantities that we had leftovers to use as noodle soup toppings the next day. She always said that since she was making a mess in the kitchen deep-frying, why not make a lot? So what's the secret to tempura's crispy exterior? Some people say that using seltzer or adding eggs makes the ideal batter, but my mother first lightly dusted the ingredients with homemade tempura flour (made with flour and potato starch), then coated each piece with tempura batter made with ice water, flour and potato starch. The key is to add ice cubes to the batter to make sure it stays very cold. This lets you achieve a feather-light batter and crispy crusts every time!

PREPARATION TIME: 15 minutes
COOKING TIME: 30 minutes
SERVES 4

½ cup (75 g) fresh or dried wakame
1 onion
2 tablespoons grated daikon
4 tablespoons Ponzu Sauce (page 40)
¼ teaspoon matcha green tea powder
½ teaspoon salt
6 tablespoons flour, divided
6 tablespoons potato starch or cornstarch, divided
½ cup (125 ml) cold water
Neutral-flavored oil

1. Place a strainer in a bowl, add the fresh wakame and fill the bowl with water, letting it sit for a few seconds. Drain and rinse the wakame under running water until the salt is removed and the wakame doubles or triples in sized. Squeeze out the excess water and cut into bite-sized pieces. If using dried wakame, follow the instructions on the package or rehydrate it in a bowl of water for 5 minutes. Drain and squeeze out the excess water, then set aside.

2. Combine the grated daikon and the Ponzu Sauce in a small bowl and mix well. In a separate bowl, combine the matcha green tea powder and the salt and mix well. Set aside.

3. Combine 3 tablespoons of the flour and 3 tablespoons of the potato starch in a medium bowl. Toss to coat the wakame and the nion in the flour, shaking off any excess. Set aside.

4. In a deep fryer or heavy pot, heat the oil to 325°F (160°C) over medium-high. Lay paper towels beneath a rack.

5. Add the water to the remaining flour and the potato starch in the bowl and mix well. It's O.K. to leave some lumps in the batter.

6. Coat the wakame and onion lightly with the batter. Use a spoon to scoop the battered pieces of wakame and onion out of the bowl and drop them into the oil. Fry them until they float to the top, have turned light brown in color and are crispy, about 1 to 2 minutes. Transfer them to a rack to drain. Serve them with the Ponzu Sauce and the matcha salt on the side.

Simmered Mushrooms with Kombu, Chicken and Bok Choy

White beech are the mushrooooms I prefer for this tempting concoction. They're ivory colored with a smooth, silky skin, a sweet, mild flavor and a great texture and mouthfeel. They pair well with just about any type of ingredient. You first cut off the bottom root and then break the bunch into pieces with your hands. Served as an appetizer or as a side dish for a main meal, it's also great for lunch and can be stored for up to 2 days in the refrigerator. You can add protein to this dish, such as chicken thighs, or you can use firm tofu for a vegetarian option. I also use doubanjiang, a popular Chinese ingredient, to season the dish. The spicy and salted fermented bean paste adds a deeply savory kick.

PREPARATION TIME: 15 minutes
COOKING TIME: 20 minutes
SERVES 4

3–4 sheets (about 6 oz/175 g) rehydrated or leftover kombu from making dashi stock

5 oz (150 g) white beech, enoki or any other kind of mushrooms

1 boneless chicken thigh (5 oz/ 150 g) or the equivalent amount of firm tofu

1 large bok choy (5½ oz/160 g)

2 cups (500 ml) Basic, Niboshi or Kombu Dashi Stock (pages 36, 38, 39)

4 tablespoons Kaeshi Sauce (page 40)

1 tablespoon rice vinegar

1 tablespoon doubanjiang (spicy black bean paste)

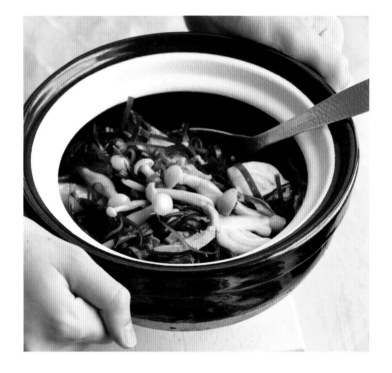

1. Cut the kombu into thin strips. Cut the root off the white beech mushrooms and break the bunch into pieces with your hand. Cut the chicken into thin strips. Cut the bok choy leaves into 2-in (5-cm) pieces and the stems lengthwise and then into quarters.

2. Combine the kombu, mushrooms, chicken and stock in a medium-sized pot, cover and cook over medium-high heat for 6 to 8 minutes.

3. Add the bok choy, Kaeshi Sauce, vinegar and doubanjiang, cover, reduce the heat to medium-low and cook for another 5 to 7 minutes, until the kombu and mushrooms become tender and the liquid is almost gone.

4. Serve as an appetizer or with steamed rice as a main meal.

Spicy Wakame Pepperoncino

I really like using wakame for this dish, as it retains its chewy texture even after being fried with garlic. It's a hybrid recipe, a fusion of Italian and Korean to which I also add a small amount of Kaeshi Sauce for a hint of umami. If you really want to make it in the Italian style, add some freshly grated Parmesan cheese. No matter what flavor direction you take, using fresh wakame rather than dried will make a difference in terms of both the flavor and texture. When you fry fresh wakame in oil, it turns into a silky but "meaty" vegetable, the perfect vehicle for the minerals and superfood goodness it delivers.

PREPARATION TIME: 5 minutes
COOKING TIME: 10 minutes
SERVES 4

½ cup (75 g) fresh or dried wakame
1 tablespoon extra-virgin olive oil
2 gloves garlic, sliced
1 small dried chili pepper, thinly
  sliced
½ tablespoon Kaeshi Sauce
  (page 40)
½ tablespoon unsalted butter

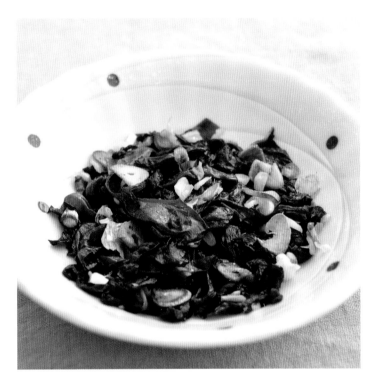

1. Place a strainer in a bowl, add the fresh wakame and fill the bowl with water, letting it sit for a few seconds. Drain and rinse the wakame under running water until the salt is removed and the wakame doubles or triples in size. Squeeze out the excess water and cut it into bite-sized pieces. If you're using dried wakame, follow the instruction on the package or rehydrate it in a bowl of water for 5 minutes, draining and squeeze out excess water. Set aside.

2. Add the oil, garlic and the chili pepper to a skillet. Turn the heat to medium-low and sauté the garlic and chili. Just before the garlic starts to turn light brown, add the wakame and cook over medium-low heat for 1 to 2 minutes.

3. Add the Kaeshi Sauce and the butter to the pan and cook for 30 seconds to 1 minute. Taste and add a pinch of salt as needed.

Hijiki Hot Dogs

My mom has always made hijiki stir-fry using whatever vegetables she finds in the refrigerator, but always adds carrot and dried shiitake. In my family, we double (or triple!) the recipe, making a batch in a big pan that lasts for 3 to 4 days as a quick snack. As tasty as it is, you can still get tired of just eating it the traditional way, with a bowl of rice. One day we tried putting it in a bun as a hot dog topping, and a new tradition was born! This is my "East meets West" mashup, marrying two popular and iconic dishes from Japan and the United States. Sounds weird but tastes great!

PREPARATION TIME: 10 minutes
COOKING TIME: 25 minutes
SERVES 4

4 shiitake mushrooms, rehydrated
4 tablespoons hijiki
1 medium carrot
1 tablespoon extra-virgin olive oil
½ tablespoon brown sugar
3 tablespoons Kaeshi Sauce (page 40)
1 teaspoon sesame oil
8 beef hot dogs
8 hot dog buns
Yellow mustard, to taste
4 tablespoons chopped scallions, the green part only, to garnish
1 teaspoon toasted sesame seed, to garnish

1. Remove the stems from the shiitake mushrooms, thinly slice them, then set aside.

2. Soak the hijiki in 4 cups of cool or hot water (see Tip). Drain and rinse it in fresh water 5 to 6 times in the sink with a strainer and a bowl, until the water runs clear. Set aside.

3. Cut the carrots into 2-in (5-cm) matchsticks.

4. In a skillet set over medium heat, add the oil and fry the shiitake and the carrots for 2 to 3 minutes. Add the hijiki to the pan and fry 2 to 3 minutes more.

5. Add the brown sugar and the Kaeshi Sauce and continue frying until all the ingredients are soft, about 3 to 4 minutes. Right before turning the heat off, drizzle the sesame oil into the skillet and cook for an additional 30 seconds. Turn off the heat and set it aside.

6. Fill a pot with water and boil the hot dogs for 5 minutes.

7. Put each hot dog in a bun and top with 2 tablespoons of the hijiki. Drizzle with the yellow mustard and top with the green onions and the sesame seeds, if desired. Store the leftover hijiki in the refrigerator for up to 4 days. It can be eaten on top of steamed rice, noodles or salads or packed in your lunch box.

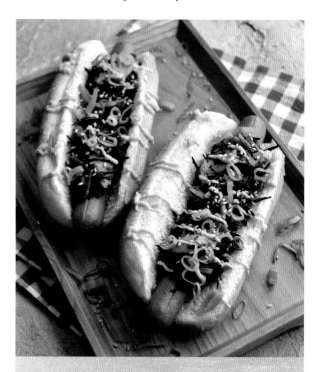

TIP Hijiki will expand five to eight times in volume after being soaked in cool water for 15 to 20 minutes or in hot water for 4 to 5 minutes. When you soak hijiki, the water will turn brown at first, but as you keep rinsing and replacing the water (at least 5 to 6 times) it will run clear. At that point, it's ready to be cooked and savored!

Kombu Water Blueberry Smoothies
with Lemon Yogurt and Maple Syrup

Because the kombu here is soaked in water and is uncooked, the water has a smooth, clear taste similar to coconut water. My mom encouraged me to drink a glass of refreshing mineral-rich, plant-based kombu water every day before breakfast, as a way to give her growing children the healthy nutrients they needed. To be honest, it wasn't a favorite of mine, as I always thought of kombu as an ingredient in warm, savory miso soups rather than cold beverages. However, the concept of a healthier alternative to sodas and juices has grown on me through the years. The hint of savory umami flavor makes my morning Blueberry Smoothie an instant mineral booster, and it's a new favorite of mine!

PREPARATION TIME: 10 minutes
COOKING TIME: 5 minutes
SERVES 4

2 cups (500 ml) Kombu Water (page 38)
1 tablespoon freshly squeezed lemon juice
1 cup (100 g) fresh or frozen blueberries
1 cup (250 ml) plain Greek yogurt
2 tablespoons maple syrup
Fresh mint leaves, for garnish (optional)

Place the Kombu Water, lemon juice, blueberries, yogurt and maple syrup in a blender and process until smooth. If the smoothie seems too thick, add more about ¼ cup more Kombu Water. To serve, pour the beverage into glasses and garnish with mint leaves, if desired.

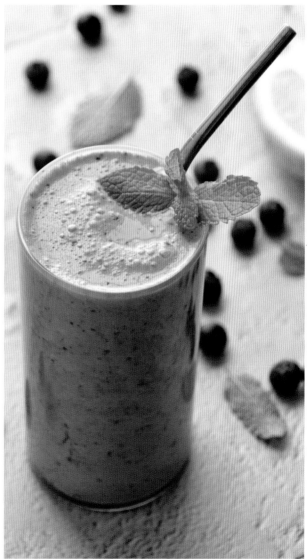

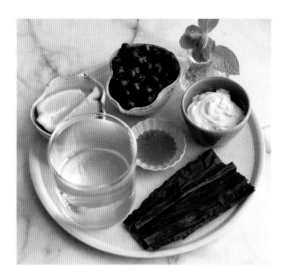

Avocado Toast with Wakame and Radish

~~~~~~~~

Over the past few years, avocado toast has become one of my favorite breakfasts. And I'm not alone. I had my first avocado toast during brunch with a friend at a tiny café in New York a few years back. I wasn't sure what to expect, but I was immediately hooked after my first bite. This simple combination quickly became my favorite dish to make whenever I have the two main components on hand. It's so simple, healthy and delicious. Best of all, it's a versatile base: I can add anything I want on top. Fried eggs, feta cheese and leafy greens are my favorite toppings, but I always come back to my Japanese roots by adding a bit of wakame for an extra boost of minerals. The inspiration actually comes from an appetizer my mom makes. She lightly mashes avocado and mixes it with seaweed and a touch of soy sauce, then sprinkles some shredded radish on top. We sometimes add umeboshi pickled plums for an extra kick of tart, pungent flavor, having the dish with a bowl of steamed rice. Back home, I never imagined eating my mom's preparation on a slice of bread, but I now realize that the toast serves as a perfect substitute for the rice. So here's my take on Japanese-style avocado toast. I hope it will become your favorite breakfast (or lunch or snack) too.

PREPARATION TIME: 10 minutes
COOKING TIME: 10 minutes
SERVES 4

2 tablespoons fresh or dried wakame
2 ripe large avocados
1 tablespoon freshly squeezed lime
  juice
1 teaspoon sesame oil
½ tablespoon Kaeshi Sauce
  (page 40)
4 slices sourdough bread
1 tablespoon Japanese mayonnaise or
  regular mayonnaise
2 radishes, shredded
1 teaspoon toasted white sesame
  seeds, to garnish
Shichimi togarashi chili pepper
  or cayenne pepper, to sprinkle
  (optional)
8 lettuce leaves, to garnish (optional)
12 cherry tomatoes, to garnish
  (optional)

1. Place a strainer in a bowl, add the fresh wakame and fill the bowl with water, letting it sit for a few seconds. Drain and rinse the wakame under running water until the salt is removed and the wakame doubles or triples in size. Squeeze out the excess water and cut it into ¼-in (6-mm) pieces. If you're using dried wakame, follow the instruction on the package or rehydrate it in a bowl of water for 5 minutes. Drain and squeeze out the excess water, then set aside.

2. Cut the peeled, seeded avocados in half. In a bowl, lightly mash them with a fork, keeping some of it chunky. Add the wakame, lime juice, sesame oil and Kaeshi Sauce to the bowl and mix well.

3. Toast the bread, let it cool slightly, then spread it with the mayonnaise.

4. Put the avocado mixture on top of the toast. If you want to make a crisscross pattern, press down on the avocado mixture with the back of a fork. Sprinkle the radishes, sesame seeds and shichimi togarashi chili pepper (if you like spice) on top, served with lettuce and tomatoes on the side, if using.

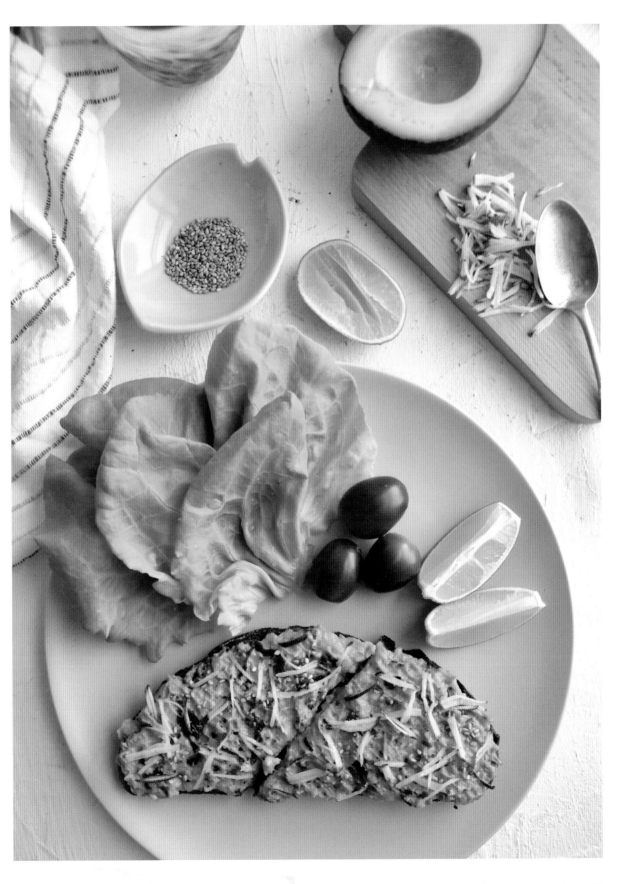

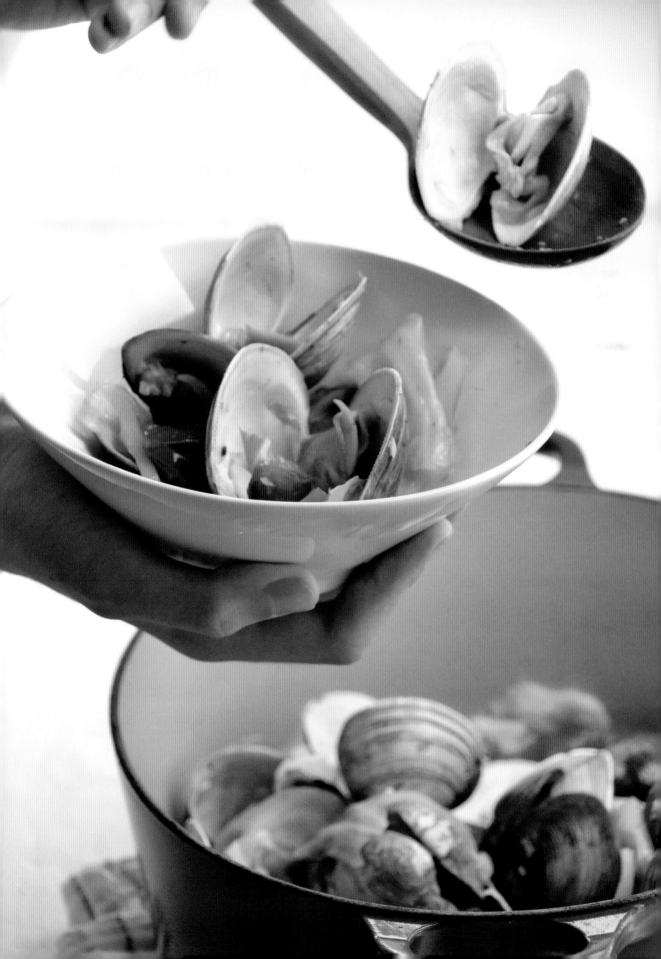

Super Seafood Dishes

Japan is known for its abundance of seafood as well as its wealth
of methods of preparing it. Beyond being a source of protein,
fish is rich in vitamins D and B-12, iodine, calcium and selenium.
With its low saturated fat, fatty acids and numerous healthful
compounds, eating seafood can help stave off high blood
pressure, macular degenation, osteoporosis and diabetes. The
risk of heart attack and stroke is also signficantly reduced just by
adding a couple servings of seafood to your diet each week.

Properly preparing fish is very important. In Japanese cuisine,
the first step after buying fish is to sprinkle it with salt.
This draws out excess water and boosts its umami flavor.
Next, a two-part washing of the fish—first with boiling,
then with cold water—allows seasonings to better penetrate
the flesh, resulting in a more delicious dish. These traditional
cooking methods will give you restaurant-quality fish at home,
harvesting the healthful benefits of the sea for yourself.

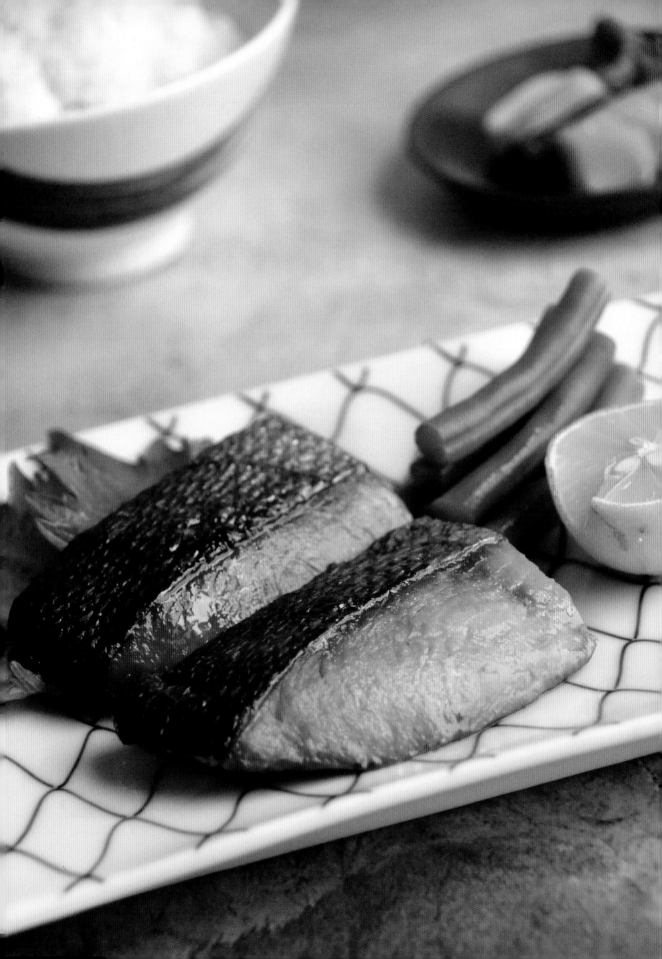

Koji-cured Grilled Salmon

Koji is a fungus (a mold—Aspergillus oryzae) that contributes a strong, savory flavor to many traditional Japanese foods. Today, many professional chefs and home cooks are being recognized for using this magical ingredient, but it's been a key component in Japanese cooking for centuries. Naturally packed with probiotic properties, koji helps strengthen the immune system. Here, I use Shio Koji (salted koji) to marinate salmon. As a salt substitute, it not only lends the necessary seasoning, it also adds maximum umami flavor and a natural sweetness. You'll achieve a pleasing depth of flavor after marinating with Shio Koji for a day. You can cook the salmon after 8 hours, but I highly recommend at least 12 hours of marination, and up to three days in the refrigerator for optimal flavor. Cutting the salmon fillets in half crosswise will allow them to tenderize more quickly. Be sure to remove the excess Shio Koji from the salmon before cooking, to prevent it from burning.

PREPARATION TIME: 10 minutes
MARINATING TIME: 3 hours to 3 day
COOKING TIME: 20 minutes
SERVES 4

4 salmon fillets with skin, about 1 lb (500 g)
4 tablespoons Shio Koji (page 53)
20 green beans
Pinch sea salt
2 limes (optional)
8 shiso leaves (Japanese basil) (optional)
Steamed rice, for serving (optional)

1. Cut each salmon fillet in half crosswise.

2. Put the salmon and the Shio Koji in a medium-sized freezer-safe resealable bag. Press the air out and seal it tightly. Press the Shio Koji into the salmon so that the entire surface is coated. Put in the refrigerator to marinate for at least 8 hours and up to 3 days.

3. Trim both ends of the green beans and cut them in half. Boil them in a small pot of water for about 2 to 4 minutes, until tender. Drain and sprinkle with a pinch of salt. Cut the limes in half and set aside.

4. Wipe the excess Shio Koji off the salmon with a paper towel and discard.

5. Line a medium-sized skillet with parchment paper, cutting it to fit. Put the salmon, skin side down, on top of the parchment paper and cook, covered, on medium-low for 5 to 7 minutes. When the bottom is cooked, as the skin turns light brown, flip the salmon with a spatula and cook the other side for about 3 to 5 minutes, over low heat, until it starts to brown. Or broil the salmon at 350°F (180°C) for 15 to 20 minutes.

6. Serve the salmon on the shiso basil with the green beans and lime on the side and over steamed, rice if desired.

TIP
You can adapt this recipe by switching the salmon to chicken, pork chops or spareribs for your next BBQ. Shio Koji is a fermented rice condiment (see page 53). You can purchase Shio Koji at any Japanese supermarket or online. It's available in two forms: either as a white paste that looks similar to rice porridge or as a clear bottled liquid. Or create your own at home with my recipe. You can also continue marinating uncooked salmon for up to one month in the freezer, but reduce the amount of Shio Koji from 1 tablespoon to ½ tablespoon per fillet instead.

Crispy Tuna with Green Onion Sauce

~~~~~~~~

Tatsuta-age is a popular Japanese method of cooking either fish or chicken by first marinating the food in soy sauce and sweet rice wine, dusting it with potato starch and frying it until crispy. It's then all served with a pungent green onion sauce, at room temperature, accompanied by vegetables. While chicken is commonly used, here I use tuna and add ginger and garlic to the marinade. The sweet and savory green onion vinaigrette is served over the fish to soak up all the delicious flavors. The name refers to the Tatsuta River, which flows through the northwestern part of Nara prefecture, a famous spot for viewing the vivid colors of maple leaves during the fall season. You can store the fish in the refrigerator for up to 2 days and serve it in your bento box—just make sure to drain the excess liquid before you pack it.

PREPARATION TIME: 10 minutes
COOKING TIME: 20 minutes
SERVES 3 to 4

2 tuna steaks, about 14 oz (400 g)
Pinch of sea salt
1 teaspoon grated garlic
1 teaspoon peeled and grated fresh ginger
3 tablespoons Kaeshi Sauce, divided (page 40)
2 tablespoons finely minced green onions, both the green and white parts
1 tablespoon Sushi Vinegar (page 52)
1 tablespoon Basic Dashi Stock (page 36) or water
⅓ cup (40 g) potato starch or cornstarch
Neutral-flavored oil, for deep frying
5 lettuce leaves
½ teaspoon toasted sesame seeds
Pinch of shichimi togarashi Japanese seven spice or cayenne pepper (optional)

1. Line a plate with paper towel. Cut the tuna into 2-in (5-cm) pieces and lay them on a plate. Sprinkle them with salt on both sides. Cover the plate with plastic wrap and chill in the refrigerator for 10 minutes.

2. Combine the garlic, ginger and 2 tablespoons of the Kaeshi Sauce in a medium-sized bowl and mix well. Add the tuna to the bowl and return everything to the refrigerator for 10 to 15 minutes to marinate.

3. In a small bowl, combine the remaining 1 tablespoon of the Kaeshi Sauce, the green onions, vinegar and dashi stock and mix well. Set aside.

4. Preheat the oil in a skillet over medium-high heat to about 350°F (175°C).

5. Pat the tuna pieces with a paper towel. Put the potato starch on a plate and dip the tuna on both sides to lightly coat the pieces. When the oil is preheated, use tongs to lower the pieces of tuna into the pot, allowing space around them. Fry them in batches, if necessary, for about 2 to 3 minutes per side, until golden brown. When each side has reached its desired degree of doneness, remove the pieces from the skillet and drain on a paper-towel-lined rack. Then, transfer the fried tuna to a serving bowl lined with the lettuce leaves. Pour the green onion sauce over the tuna while it's still hot.

6. Serve the tuna garnished with sesame seeds and a pinch of shichimi togarashi (Japanese seven spice) on top, if desired.

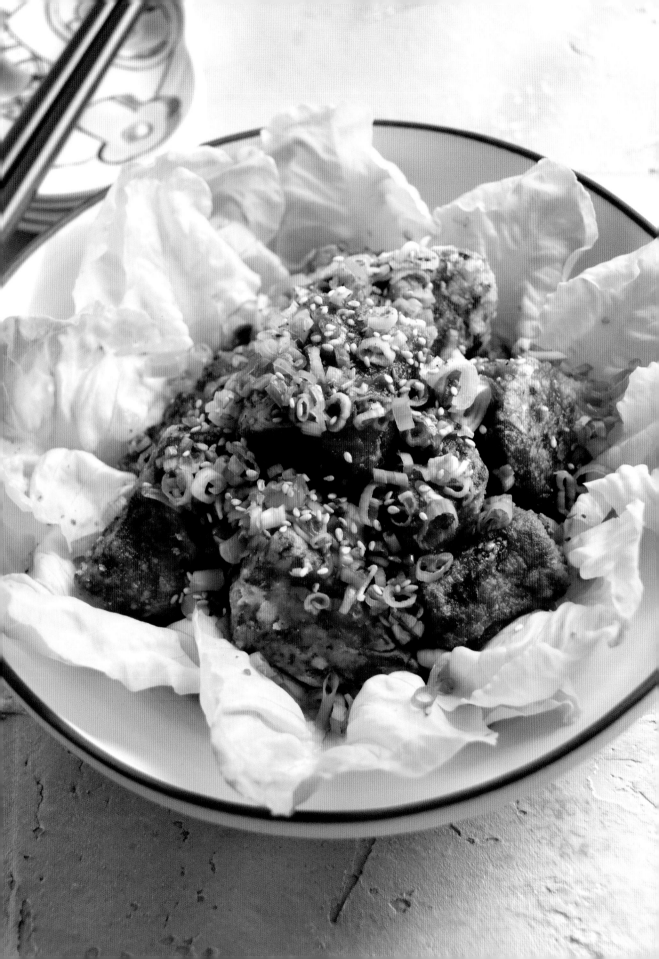

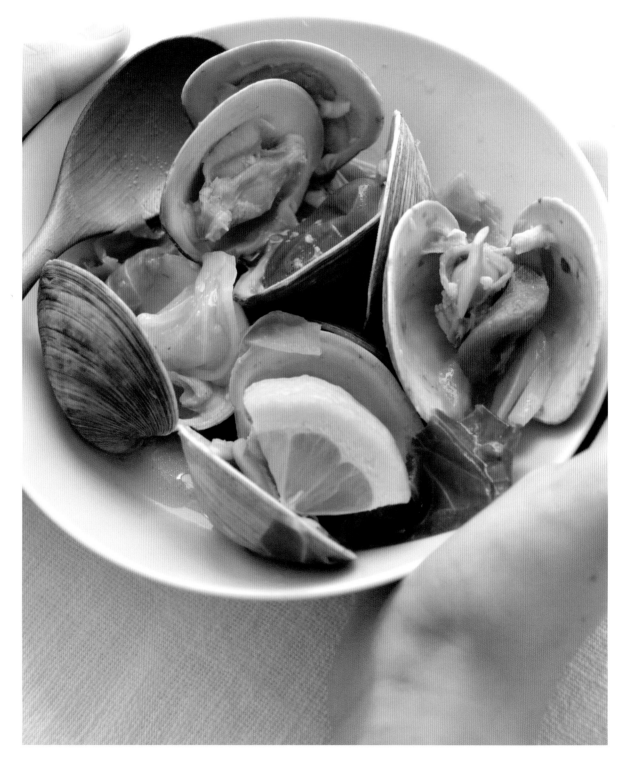

Clams Steamed in Sake with Ginger and Shio Koji

~~~~~~

Clam digging is a popular tradition in Japan between April and June. Growing up, I visited the nearby beaches of Chiba prefecture every year with both my family and on school field trips. It's said that if you find one clam, you'll end up finding 30 more in the same spot. If you can't find a single clam, it's time to move to another part of the beach for a fresh start. When you're finished, you pay by weight when you check out. Once we got home, my mom soaked the clams in warm water. Here I've put my own spin on this family recipe by adding sake and Shio Koji, a popular seasoning for Japanese home cooking that is made with koji fermented rice, salt and water. Shio Koji, which looks like rice porridge, tastes slightly sweet and salty, with a mild fermented smell like sweet miso paste. You can easily make Shio Koji at home (see page 53). Enjoy the flavor of fresh clams over rice or pasta or serve with crusty bread.

PREPARATION TIME: 15 minutes
COOKING TIME: 15 minutes
SERVES 4

2¼ lbs (1 kg) fresh medium-sized clams in their shells
3 green cabbage leaves (5 oz/150 g)
1 tablespoon extra-virgin olive oil
1 tablespoon peeled and minced fresh ginger
1 tablespoon minced garlic
1 cup (250 ml) sake
½ cup (125 ml) Kombu Water (page 38)
2 tablespoons Shio Koji (page 53)
8 cherry tomatoes, cut in half
2 tablespoons unsalted butter
½ lemon, cut into 4 wedges

1. Fill a large bowl with warm water, about 120°F (50°C). Add the clams and wash them with your hands for 1 to 2 minutes to remove dirt and sand. Leave in the water for 10 minutes, then wash the clams under running water to remove any remaining dirt and sand then drain well.

2. Tear the cabbage into 2-in (5-cm) pieces.

3. In a large pot over medium heat, add the olive oil, ginger and garlic and cook for 30 seconds. Add the sake, Kombu Water and Shio Koji and boil until the liquid has reduced to two-thirds its original volume.

4. Add the clams to the pot and cook, covered, over medium heat until the shells have opened, about 4 to 6 minutes. Discard any unopened ones.

5. Add the cabbage, cherry tomatoes and butter to the pot, give everything a gentle shake and cook over medium-low heat for another 2 to 3 minutes.

6. Serve the clams in bowls with the broth spooned over them. Garnish with the lemon wedges.

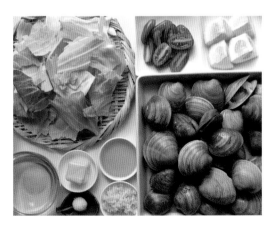

Sashimi and Wakame Salad
with Crispy Wonton Chips

〜〜〜〜〜〜

This sashimi salad is one of my favorite summertime dishes that I've been making for years. I prefer to use yellowtail, but you can use any firm white fish such as red snapper, fluke, black sea bass, tilefish or sea bream. A white-fish-based sashimi goes beautifully with this creamy wasabi vinaigrette made with homemade Sushi Vinegar, extra-virgin olive oil, Japanese mayonnaise and a touch of wasabi. This dressing is delicious, so make extra—it can be stored in the refrigerator for up to 2 weeks—as it's also good to use on other dishes, such as simple green salads, grilled fish and meats or noodles. There's no cooking involved, except for the crispy wonton chips, which are an optional garnish. The wonton chips are my take on Japanese-style croutons, and they give the salad a great texture and crunchiness. If you don't want to use fried wantons, you can substitute rice crackers or corn chips. If you're craving sushi but want to stay on a low-carb diet, this makes a satisfying, healthy and light meal.

PREPARATION TIME: 10 minutes
COOKING TIME: 10 minutes
SERVES 4

12 oz (350 g) sashimi-grade yellowtail or other sashimi-grade firm white fish (see the headnote)
3 tablespoons fresh or dried wakame
8 wonton wrappers (about 3 x 3 in/ 8 x 8 cm)
Neutral-flavored oil, for deep frying
3 tablespoons Sushi Vinegar (page 52)
3 tablespoons sesame oil
3 tablespoon Japanese mayonnaise
Wasabi, to taste
Pinch of sea salt
4 cups (120 g) mixed salad greens
¼ piece red onion, thinly sliced
1 teaspoon toasted white sesame seeds, to garnish

1. Slice the sashimi into bite-sized pieces.

2. Place a strainer in a bowl, add the fresh wakame and fill the bowl with water, letting it sit for a few seconds. Drain and rinse the wakame under running water until the salt is removed and the wakame doubles or triples in size. Squeeze out the excess water and cut it into bite-sized pieces. If you're using dried wakame, follow the instructions on the package or rehydrate it in a bowl of water for 5 minutes. Drain it, squeeze out the excess water, then set aside.

3. Cut the wonton wrappers into ½-in (1-cm) strips. Heat the oil to 325°F (160°C) over medium-high in a small deep fryer or a heavy pot. Lay out a paper towel under a rack.

4. Cook the wontons in the oil until light brown in color, about 1 to 2 minutes. Scoop them out of the oil with a metal sieve, allowing the oil to drain off before transferring them to the rack.

5. Combine the vinegar, oil, mayonnaise and wasabi in a small bowl and mix well. Taste, adding a pinch of salt if needed. Combine the mixed greens, onion, fluke and wakame in a medium-sized bowl. Slowly drizzle ⅔ of the dressing over the salad and toss well. Taste the salad and add more dressing, if necessary.

6. To serve, place the salad on a serving platter, on individual plates or simply use the same bowl you tossed the salad in. Sprinkle with the sesame seeds and lay the crispy wonton strips on top, if using.

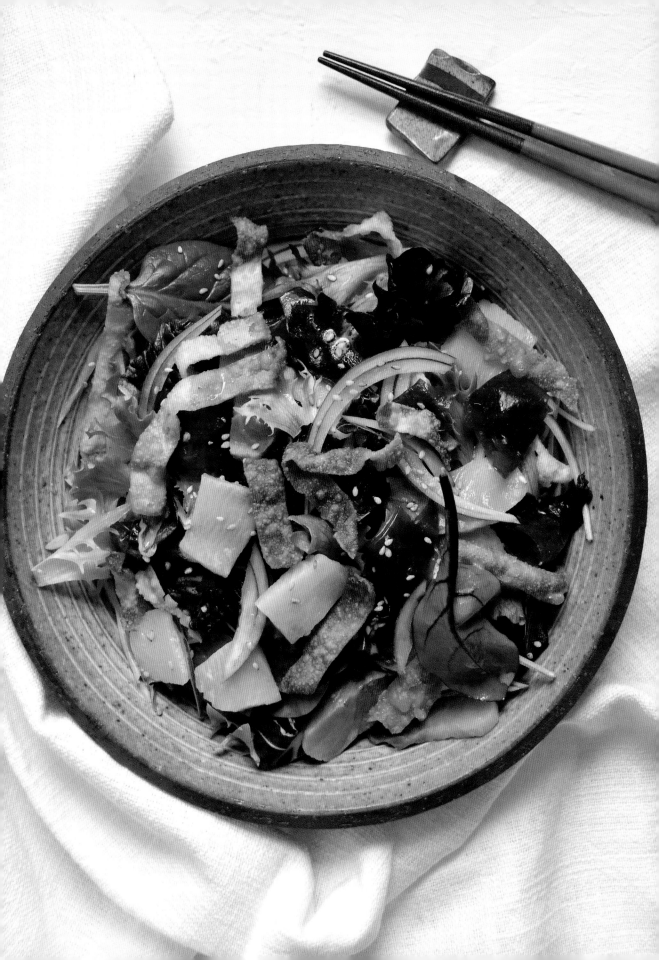

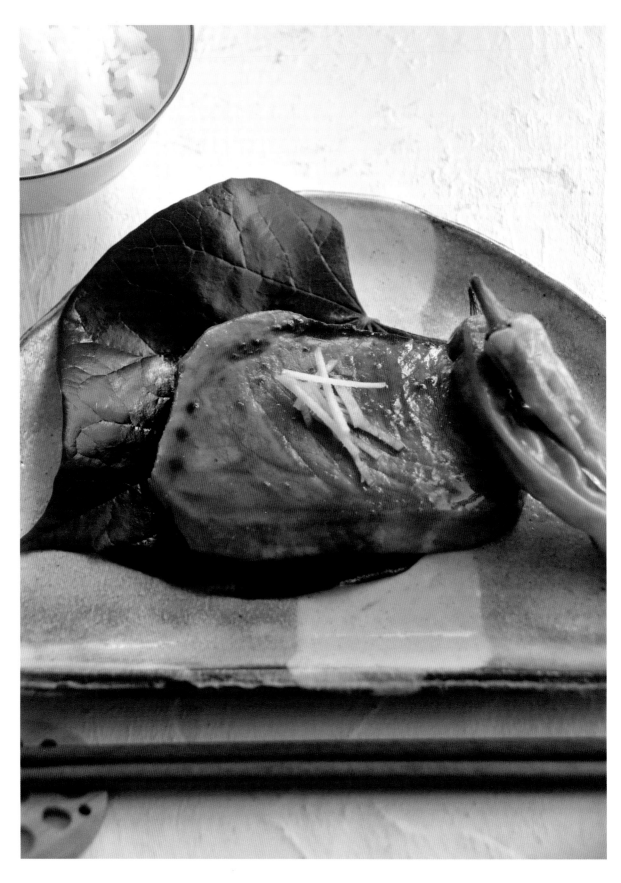

Swordfish Steaks Simmered with Sweet Ginger Soy and Shishito Peppers

I grew up in a large family where not only my parents but my grandmother, aunts and uncles all worked at the seaweed factory since its founding in the 1960s. Through the decades, there have been many meals shared while sitting around a big table. This recipe is one of my favorite fish dishes made by my aunt Keiko. She always helped feed us kids when my mom was too busy to cook. As an adult, I still crave her simmered swordfish and ask her to make it for me every chance I get. The mild, rich fish carefully simmered with dashi stock and Kaeshi Sauce (page 40) always comes out perfect. Aunt Keiko uses a drop lid while cooking so the sauce slightly thickens and the fish becomes tender and flaky. If you don't have one, you can easily make your own by cutting parchment paper or aluminum foil to fit inside the pan.

PREPARATION TIME: 10 minutes
COOKING TIME: 25 minutes
SERVES 4

4 swordfish fillets, about 1½ lbs (680 g) and ¾ in (2 cm) thick
½ teaspoon sea salt
1 in (2.5 cm) piece fresh ginger
¾ cup (185 ml) Kombu Water (page 38)
¼ cup (65 ml) Kaeshi Sauce (page 40)
1 tablespoon brown sugar
8 shishito or banana peppers
Steamed rice, for serving (optional)

TIP
It is important to salt the fish before cooking so that the moisture is drawn out, bringing out the natural umami flavor. Pouring boiling water over the fish is also an important step, as it will get rid of excess fat and the fishy aroma, helping to refine the flavors.

1. Remove the skin from the fish and sprinkle salt on both sides. Let it season for 10 minutes.

2. Place a colander in the sink, put the fish in it, and slowly pour boiling water (about 2 cups/500 ml) over it, turning the fish halfway through. The surface of the fish will turn slightly whitish in color. Rinse it well with cold water, then set aside.

3. Peel the ginger, cutting half of it into fine strips, to be set aside for garnish. The other half should be sliced thinly to be simmered with the fish.

4. Combine the fish, Kombu Water, Kaeshi Sauce, sugar and sliced ginger in a medium-sized pot and cover it with a drop lid. Bring to a boil and cook for about 3 to 5 minutes. Reduce the heat to medium and cook for an additional 3 to 5 minutes, until the fish is almost done (it'll continue to cook for a minute after it comes off the heat) and the sauce has been reduced by half.

5. Just before the fish is done, add the shishito peppers and cook for about 1 minute. When the swordfish feels firm when pressed, it's done. Use a spatula to lift the fish out of the pot without breaking it and transfer it to individual plates.

6. Serve the fish with the ginger strips on top, the shishito peppers on the side and some of the sauce drizzled over. Serve over steamed rice, if desired.

Pan-fried Salmon Fillets
in a Spicy Sweet Soy Vinaigrette

Nanbanzuke is fried fish that's marinated in vinegar and a dashi soy sauce then served with seasonal vegetables. It's a popular summertime dish in Japan, easy to prepare using accessible ingredients, which also makes it a great weeknight dinner. The dish was first introduced by Spanish and Portuguese missionaries in the 16th century and is similar to escabeche. You can also use chicken or shrimp. This is a great make-ahead dish for your next dinner party. You can prepare it and keep it in the refrigerator for a couple of days while it absorbs all the delicious flavors. Use a thermometer to determine when the oil is the correct temperature, which is about 350ºF (175ºC).

PREPARATION TIME: 15 minutes
COOKING TIME: 25 minutes
SERVES 4

4 skinless salmon fillets, 1 lb (500 g)
Pinch of sea salt
½ red bell pepper
½ green bell pepper
¼ red onion
1 lemon
3 tablespoons Basic or Second-Brew
  Dashi Stock (pages 36–7)
1 tablespoon rice vinegar
⅛ teaspoon dried red chili flakes
  (optional)
4 tablespoons Kaeshi Sauce
  (page 40)
1 tablespoon maple syrup
Neutral-flavored oil, for deep frying
⅓ cup (40 g) potato starch or
  cornstarch
1 tablespoon fresh coriander leaves
  (cilantro), to garnish (optional)

1. Cut the salmon into ½-in (1-cm) pieces. Put them on a plate lined with a paper towel and sprinkle the pieces with salt on both sides. Cover with plastic wrap and set in the refrigerator for 10 minutes.

2. Cut the red and green peppers into 2-in (5-cm matchsticks and thinly slice the onion. Thinly slice half the lemon into 6 to 8 slices and squeeze the remaining half. You'll need about 1 tablespoon of lemon juice.

3. In a medium-sized bowl, combine the lemon juice, dashi stock, vinegar, chili flakes, Kaeshi Sauce and maple syrup. Mix well and add the cut vegetables to the bowl. Set aside.

4. Preheat the oil in a pan over medium-high heat to about 350ºF (175ºC).

5. Pat the salmon dry with a paper towel and lightly coat the pieces with the potato starch in a bowl or on a plate. When the oil reaches the correct temperature, drop in the fish using tongs. Deep-fry the salmon in batches for about 2 to 3 minutes per side over medium-low heat. When the salmon gets golden brown, remove it from the pan and drain it on a paper-towel-lined rack. Then transfer the fried salmon to the bowl of cut vegetables and dashi vinegar sauce. Gently stir to combine, cover and let marinate in the refrigerator for at least 15 to 20 minutes and up to two days before serving.

6. Serve the salmon garnished with the sliced lemon and the fresh cilantro/coriander leaves on top, if using.

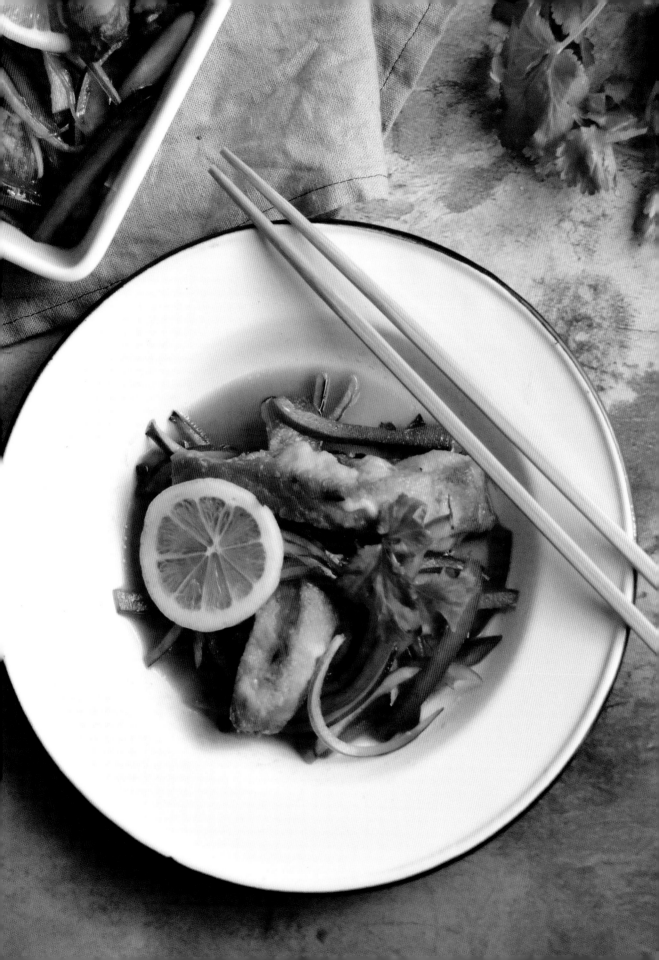

Turnips with Shrimp and Wakame
in Shoyu Koji Gravy

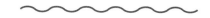

For as long as I can remember, my mom has taught me the importance of eating seasonally. That's the best way of drawing the deepest flavors from the best ingredients. Turnips are one of the most popular winter staples in Japan, and when I see them arrive at local markets—big and round with gorgeous green leaves—I realize that winter has arrived. Turnips look like radishes, but they're sweeter, with an earthy flavor and a soft, tender texture when cooked. This dish is prepared in the ankake style—turnips, shrimp and leafy wakame are briefly cooked in a rich dashi stock and seasoned with Shoyu Koji, which lends a beautiful amber color. It's then thickened with potato starch. It's a filling but delicate dish that is perfect for cold winter nights.

PREPARATION TIME: 10 minutes
COOKING TIME: 15 minutes
SERVES 4

14 oz (400 g) turnips, preferably with
  the leaves attached
24 medium fresh shrimp, about 10 oz
  (300 g), when peeled and deveined
2 cups (500 ml) Basic Dashi Stock
  (page 36)
3 tablespoons fresh or dried wakame
2 tablespoons Shoyu Koji (see the
  next page)
¼ teaspoon sea salt
1 tablespoon sake
2 teaspoons potato starch or
  cornstarch
2 teaspoons water
½ teaspoon ginger, peeled and grated

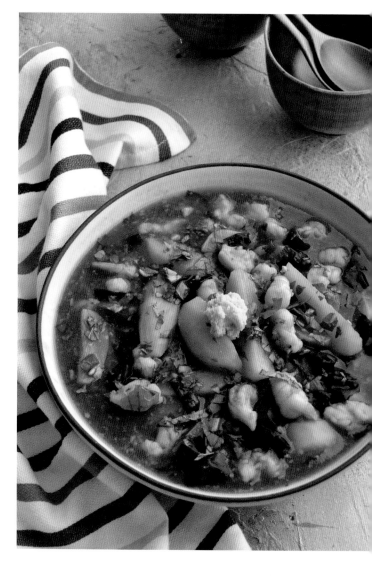

How to Make Shoyu Koji

Combining the taste of shoyu with the superfood power of koji, this simple combination can be used in place of regular soy sauce for an extra depth of savory flavor. But Shoyu Koji truly shines in its role as a marinade. Overnight in the fridge, it infuses carbohydrates with a subtle sweetness, breaking down proteins into amino acids and tenderizing meat.

1¼ cups (7 oz/200 g) dried rice koji
1¼ cups (300 ml) soy sauce, plus 1 to 2 tablespoons for adding later

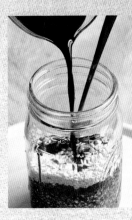
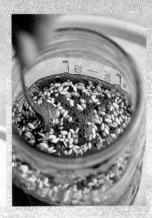

1. Combine the koji and soy sauce in a glass jar and stir it with a spoon until well mixed. (TIP: Since carbon dioxide will be released during the fermentation process, it's important to use a container large enough to hold the ingredients along with a little extra space. A 1-quart container

is recommended. Loosen the lid slightly to allow the gas to escape and let it ferment at room temperature.

2. Stir it at least once a day with a spoon to evenly distribute the koji and soy sauce. The koji will have absorbed quite a lot of soy sauce by the next day, so you'll need to add more soy sauce—just enough to cover the koji. Ferment for one week in the summer and two weeks in the winter. Store in an airtight container in the refrigerator. (TIP: The koji becomes soft, fluffy and similar in texture to rice porridge when it's ready to use. It's thick, smells sweet like miso and the grains of rice have no core.)

3. As the Shoyu Koji matures, the koji is broken down and becomes smaller and more watery. Store the finished product in the refrigerator and use it up within three months. Use it for pickles, stir fries, marinades, dipping sauces, dressings, seasoning rice, noodles and soups.

1. Trim off the turnip leaves. Chop 2 leaves into ½-in (1-cm) pieces and set aside. Reserve the remaining leaves for another use such as stir fries and soups. Trim and discard the root ends. Peel and cut the turnips lengthwise in 6 wedges.

2. Cut the shrimp into bite-sized pieces.

3. Combine the Basic Dashi Stock and the turnips in a saucepan over medium-high heat and bring to a simmer. Cook for 10 to 13 minutes until the turnips are tender.

4. Place a strainer in a bowl, add the fresh wakame and fill the bowl with water, letting it sit for a few seconds. Drain and rinse the wakame under running water until the salt is removed and the wakame doubles in size. Squeeze out the excess water and cut

into bite-sized pieces. If you're using dried wakame, follow the instructions on the package or rehydrate it in a bowl of water for 5 minutes. Drain it, squeeze out the excess water, then set aside.

5. Add the shrimp, Shoyu Koji, salt and sake to the stock and simmer for 2 to 4 minutes over medium-low.

6. Combine potato starch and water in a small cup and mix until smooth. Add it to the pan, reduce the heat to low and stir until the sauce is smooth and thickens, about 2 to 3 minutes. Add the wakame, then turn off the heat.

7. Serve in a medium-sized bowl or in four individual bowls and garnish with the grated ginger and sliced turnip greens on top.

Octopus Salad with Wakame and Okra

Octopus salad is a popular dish on any izakaya (Japanese pub) menu. The octopus is always sold pre-boiled, so you simply cut and plate the ingredients, then drizzle a savory miso vinaigrette over the top. It's a light and refreshing appetizer for summer that's great served with cold beer or sake. The octopus is translucent when it's raw but turns pure white with a bit of dark purple after it's cooked. Don't peel the skin, that's what lends this dish its appealing contrast of colors.

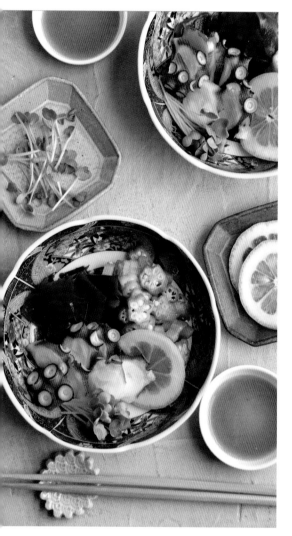

PREPARATION TIME: 5 minutes
COOKING TIME: 15 minutes
SERVES 4

3 tablespoons fresh or dried wakame
10 oz (330 g) octopus
8 okra
Pinch of salt
3 tablespoons Tama Miso (page 205)
1 tablespoon Sushi Vinegar (page 52)
2 tablespoons Basic Dashi Stock (page 36)
1 teaspoon maple syrup
1 teaspoon fresh lemon juice
4 slices of lemon, to garnish
Radish sprouts, to garnish (optional)

1. Place a strainer in a bowl, add the fresh wakame and fill the bowl with water, letting it sit for a few seconds. Drain and rinse the wakame under running water until the salt is removed and the wakame doubles or triples in size. Squeeze out the excess water and cut it into bite-sized pieces. If you're using dried wakame, follow the instruction on the package or rehydrate it in a bowl of water for 5 minutes. Drain it, squeeze out the excess water, then set aside.

2. Thinly slice the octopus.

3. Lay the okra flat on a cutting board and sprinkle them with the salt. Rinse them off under running water in the sink.

4. Fill a small saucepan halfway with water, cover and bring to a boil. Add the okra and cook over medium-high heat for about 2 to 3 minutes or until soft. Drain and rinse in cold water. Cut the stems off and slice thinly crosswise.

5. In a small bowl, combine the miso, vinegar, stock and maple syrup and mix well.

6. Place the wakame, octopus, and okra in a serving bowl or on four individual plates and drizzle the miso vinaigrette over. Garnish with the sliced lemon and the radish sprouts, if using.

Mackerel Braised in Miso

This is one of the most popular fish dishes in all of Japanese cooking. When I think of this dish, I always think about my grandmother. She loved fish, and simmering was her favorite way to prepare it. When my sisters and I slept over at her house, she often made this for us. There are two quick tips for making this dish even more delicious. First, salt the fish before cooking it, letting it sit for about 10 minutes. This not only helps to draw the moisture from the fish but also to get rid of any fishy smell. Second, place the fish in a colander and pour hot water over it until the surface turns white. Then, rinse it with cold water. This helps the seasoning infuse the fish and yields a richer flavor.

PREPARATION TIME: 10 minutes
COOKING TIME: 20 minutes
SERVES 2

2 mackerel fillets, about 10 oz (330 g)
¼ teaspoon salt
½ zucchini or 8 sugar snap peas
½ cup (125 ml) Kombu Water (page 38)
¼ cup (65 ml) Tama Miso (page 205)
1 teaspoon brown sugar
1-in (2.5-cm) piece fresh ginger, peeled and thinly sliced
¼ onion, thinly sliced and soaked in water
4 shiso leaves, to garnish (optional)
Steamed rice, for serving (optional)

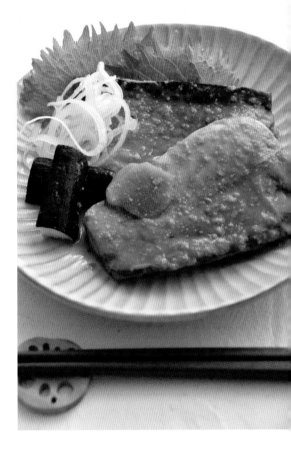

1. Cut each fillet in half crosswise to make four pieces about 4 in (10 cm) each. Sprinkle salt on both sides and let the pieces sit for 10 minutes.

2. If you're using zucchini, cut it into pieces that are ½ x 1½ in (1.25 x 3.75 cm). If you're using sugar snap peas, remove and discard the stem ends and strings from the pods.

3. Place the fish in a colander and slowly pour boiling water, about 2 cups (500 ml), over the fish until the surface turns whitish in color. Then rinse the fish well with cold water.

4. Combine the fish, Kombu Water, miso, sugar and ginger in a medium pot and bring it to a boil over medium-high heat, about 3 to 4 minutes. Use a drop lid or parchment paper cut to fit the size of the pan. Turn the heat down to medium-low and cook for an additional 3 to 4 minutes until the fish is almost done, as it'll continue to cook for a minute when it's off the heat.

5. Just before the fish is done, add the zucchini or peas to the pot and cook for about 1 minute. Drain the onion.

6. Serve the fish with the shiso, sliced onions, zucchini and ginger and drizzle some of the sauce over the fish. You can also serve this over steamed rice.

Scallop Sashimi and Wakame Salad
with Yuzu Vinaigrette

There's no cooking involved in this delicous treat. You simply prep the ingredients and assemble them on a platter. This dish is quick to make and is a great appetizer, as well as a beautiful party dish. I love the naturally sweet flavor of sashimi scallops and their melt-in-your-mouth texture, which is quite different from when they're cooked. You're not curing the scallops in the yuzu juice, as you want to retain the sweet, soft texture of their fresh, raw flavor.

PREPARATION TIME: 15 minutes
COOKING TIME: 10 minutes
SERVES 4

14 sashimi-grade scallops, about
   12 oz (350 g)
3 tablespoons fresh or dried
   wakame
½ cup (50 g) radishes
1 tablespoons Sushi Vinegar
   (page 52)
1 tablespoon fresh yuzu or lemon
   juice
2 tablespoons extra-virgin olive oil
1 tablespoon maple syrup
1 tablespoon Kaeshi Sauce
   (page 40)
Pinch sea salt
2 tablespoons kaiware radish
   sprouts or microgreens, to
   garnish
¼ teaspoon toasted white sesame
   seeds

1. Slice each scallop crosswise into two pieces and chill in the refrigerator.

2. Place a strainer in a bowl, add the fresh wakame and fill the bowl with water, letting the wakame sit for a few seconds. Drain and rinse it under running water until the salt is removed and the wakame doubles or triples in size. Squeeze out the excess water and cut into bite-sized pieces. If you're using dried wakame, follow the instructions on the package or rehydrate it in a bowl of water for 5 minutes, then drain and squeeze out the excess water. Set aside.

3. Thinly slice the radishes with a mandoline or a sharp knife.

4. In a small bowl, combine the vinegar, yuzu juice, olive oil, maple syrup, Kaeshi Sauce and salt. Mix well.

5. Lay the scallops, wakame and radishes on a serving platter and pour the dressing over. Garnish with the radish sprouts and the sesame seeds.

TIP
You can use any type of radish for this dish, such as daikon, French breakfast, watermelon or traditional red radishes. Otherwise, use any crunchy vegetable you prefer, such as Japanese cucumber or fennel, thinly slicing them.

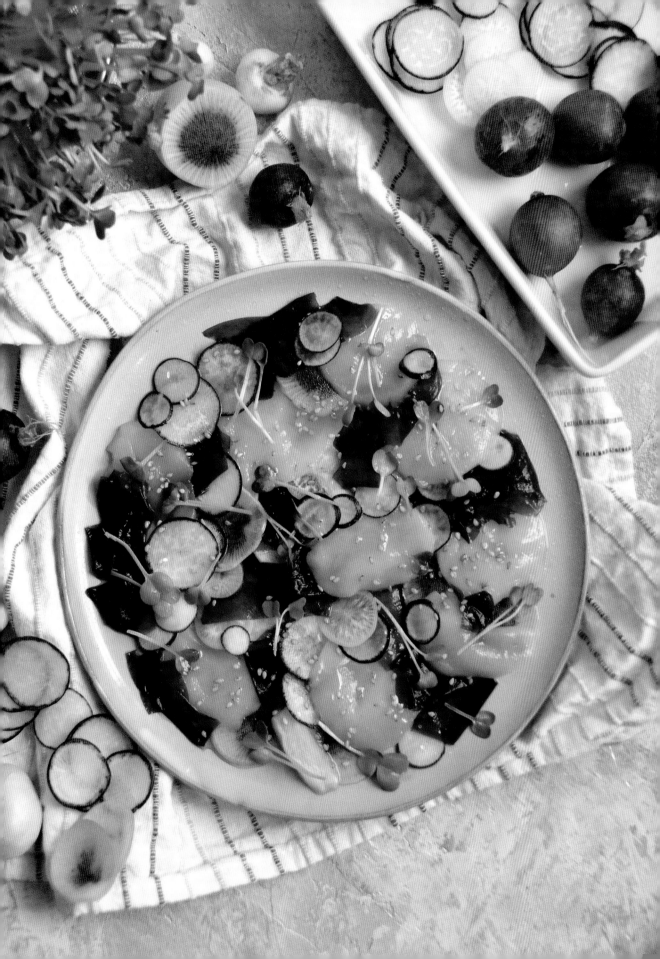

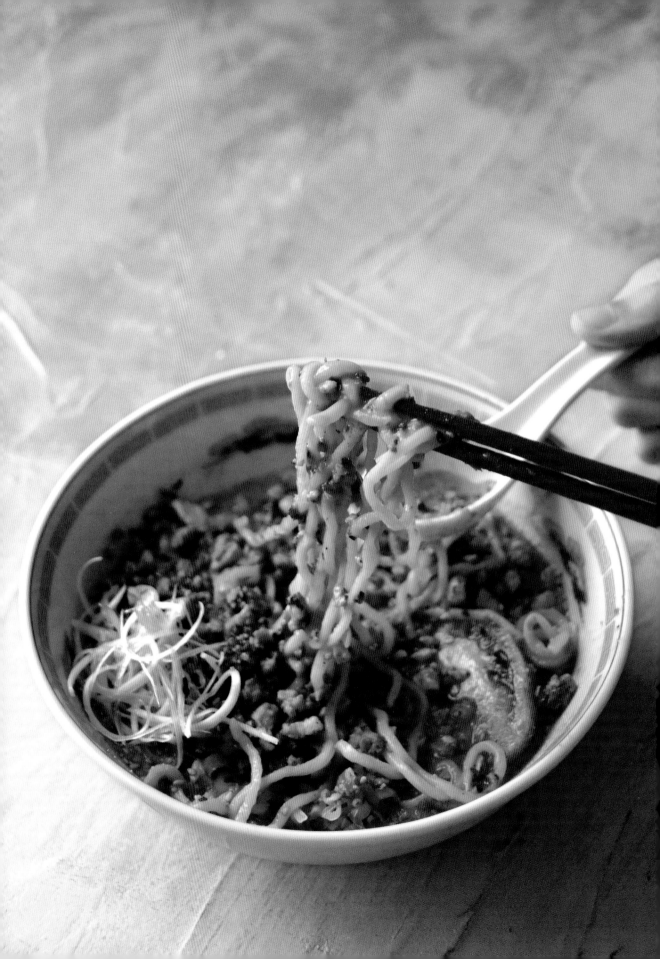

Rice, Noodles and Bread

While rice, noodles and bread aren't exactly superfood staples, eating carbohydrates such as rice porridge or udon noodles at the end of a meal can help weight loss, as it prevents a sudden rise in blood-sugar levels and leaves you feeling satisfied.

Ramen proves to be an ever-versatile template to which layers of superfood goodness can be added. It pairs perfectly with fermented miso and soy sauce or a light and umami-packed dashi stock, all served with a variety of seasonal toppings. This chapter introduces classic noodle soups that use traditional soup stocks (both hot and cold), donburi (a popular rice bowl dish), rice balls, healthy vegan ramen and a sandwich that's a common sight at typical Japanese cafes. Carbohydrates may not be the healthiest elements on the table, but they serve as an ideal partner for highlighting the healthful benefits of superfoods.

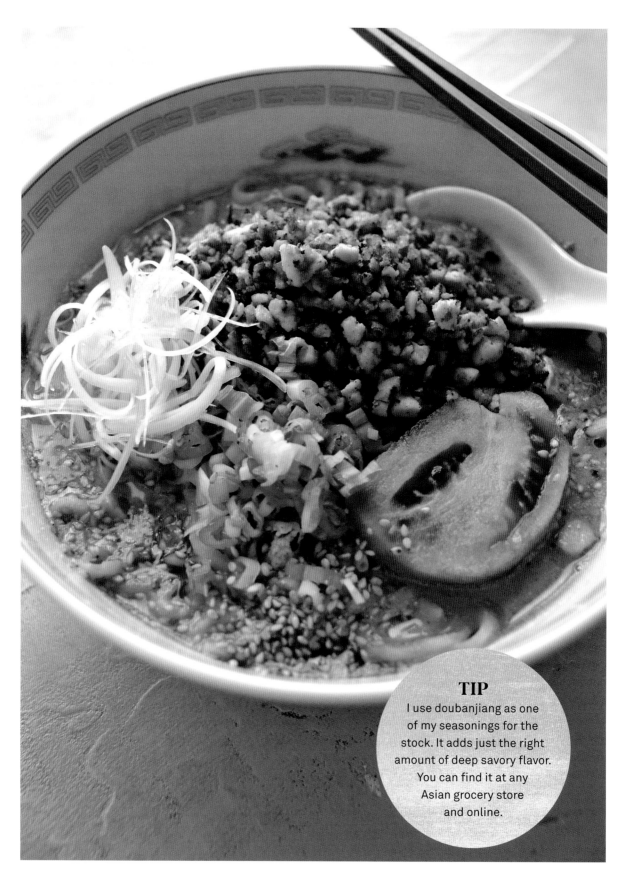

TIP

I use doubanjiang as one of my seasonings for the stock. It adds just the right amount of deep savory flavor. You can find it at any Asian grocery store and online.

Vegan Tantan-Men

Ramen has become the most popular noodle in the world. Each ramen shop has its own signature bowl, and every region throughout Japan has its own variation, a unique ramen style true to the local ingredients. Why has ramen become so popular? For one thing, it's inexpensive, and of course it's a very quick meal. This dish, called tantan-men (men means "noodles"), is the Japanese take on the popular Sichuan dandan noodles. Here I've adapted it into a healthier, vegan version that my family loves. The claims about ramen are true! It's easy to make at home, so give it a try.

PREPARATION TIME: 15 minutes
COOKING TIME: 40 minutes
SERVES 4

4 rehydrated shiitake mushrooms
½ medium tomato
2 scallions, both white and green parts
3 tablespoons sesame oil, divided
One 14-oz (400-g) block firm tofu, cut into
  small cubes
2 tablespoons ginger, minced, divided
2 tablespoons garlic, minced, divided
¾ cup (180 ml) + 2 tablespoons Kaeshi Sauce
  (page 40), divided
¾ cup (180 ml) + 1 tablespoon tahini, divided
1 tablespoon doubanjiang (spicy black bean
  paste), divided
1 tablespoon granulated sugar, divided
7 cups (1750 ml) Kombu Water (page 38)
1 cup (250 ml) Shiitake Dashi Stock (page 39)
1½ tablespoons rice vinegar
Four 5.1-oz (145g) packages dried ramen or
  3.5-oz (100g) fresh ramen noodles (see Tip)
2 teaspoons roasted white sesame seeds
1 teaspoon hot chili oil (optional)

TIP If you're using fresh ramen: Add equal amounts of salt and baking soda to the water and boil for about 2 minutes longer than indicated. When you add the baking soda, be careful as it bubbles up to the top. Drain and rinse the noodles in cool running water.

1. Mince the shiitake mushrooms. Cut the tomato lengthwise into 4 slices. Trim the roots off the green onions and cut the green parts into small pieces. Cut the white parts into thin julienne strips and soak them in a small bowl of water. Set aside.

2. Heat 2 tablespoons of the sesame oil in a skillet over medium-high heat and add the tofu, shiitake and 1 tablespoon each of the ginger and garlic to the pan. Constantly stir and scramble the tofu with a wooden spatula, breaking it up into small pieces until it's cooked through, about 4 to 6 minutes. Add 2 tablespoons of the Kaeshi Sauce, 1 teaspoon each of the doubanjiang and sugar to the pan and continue scrambling over medium heat with the spatula until the liquid is completely absorbed into the meat, about 2 to 3 minutes. This process is very important, as it transforms the tofu into small crumbled pieces similar to ground meat. Set aside.

3. In a large pot, place the stock, the remaining ¾ cups of the Kaeshi Sauce and tahini, 2 teaspoons of the doubanjiang, rice vinegar and sugar and 1 tablespoon each of the sesame oil, garlic and ginger and bring it to a boil. Then reduce the heat to medium-low and simmer for 5 to 7 minutes.

4. Fill four individual ramen bowls with hot water and set them aside. Boil the noodles according to the package instructions. Drain well. Discard the hot water from the bowls and pour the hot stock into each. Add the noodles and top with the tofu crumbles, tomato, green onions and sesame seeds. To serve, drizzle with hot chili oil, if using.

Ground Chicken and Egg Rice Bowl

I loved eating this as a child and still love it today. This style of rice bowl is called *soboro* (or crumbled) in Japanese. It features finely ground chicken that's simmered in flavorful Kaeshi Sauce until the sauce is completely absorbed by the chicken, resulting in a deeply satisfying umami flavor. Served with fluffy scrambled eggs and boiled snow peas over steamed rice, this is a versatile recipe that can be adapted by using any ground meat or tofu or by substituting other steamed vegetables (such as carrots, spinach, broccoli or string beans) for the snow peas. Keep breaking up the meat as it cooks in order to create small, crumbled pieces. I like to garnish the bowl with red pickled ginger strips called beni-shoga, as they lend a nice balance of salty and sour flavor to the dish.

PREPARATION TIME: 15 minutes
COOKING TIME: 25 minutes
SERVES 4

6 oz (175 g) snow peas
Pinch of sea salt
4 eggs, beaten
6 tablespoons Kaeshi Sauce, divided
  (page 40)
2 tablespoons extra-virgin olive oil,
  divided
1 lb (450 g) ground chicken
1 tablespoon granulated or brown
  sugar
4 cups (660 g) cooked, short-grain
  Japanese rice, for serving
2 tablespoons pickled red ginger,
  to garnish (optional)

1. Place the snow peas on a cutting board. Use a knife to trim the ends and remove the thin strings that run the sides with your fingers. In a small pot, bring 2 cups of water to a boil. Add the snow peas and cook about 1 minute until just tender. Drain the snow peas in a colander and run under cold water for 10 seconds to stop the cooking, then drain well. Thinly slice the snow peas lengthwise. Sprinkle with a pinch of salt and set aside.

2. Combine the eggs and 1 tablespoon of the Kaeshi Sauce in a bowl and mix well. Heat 1 tablespoon of the oil in a skillet over medium heat and place the egg mixture in the pan. While cooking the eggs, constantly stir and scramble with a wooden spatula by breaking up the eggs into small pieces until it's cooked through, about 2 to 3 minutes. Set aside.

3. Heat the remaining oil in a skillet over medium-high and add the chicken to the pan. Constantly stir and break up the meat into small, crumbled pieces with a wooden spatula until it's cooked through, about 5 to 7 minutes. Add the sugar and the remaining Kaeshi Sauce and continue breaking up the meat until the liquid is completed absorbed into the meat, about 2 to 3 minutes. Set aside.

4. To serve, place 1 cup of rice in each serving bowl. Divide the remaining ingredients between the four bowls, placing the chicken on one side, the egg on the other side and the peas in the middle. Garnish with pickled ginger, if using.

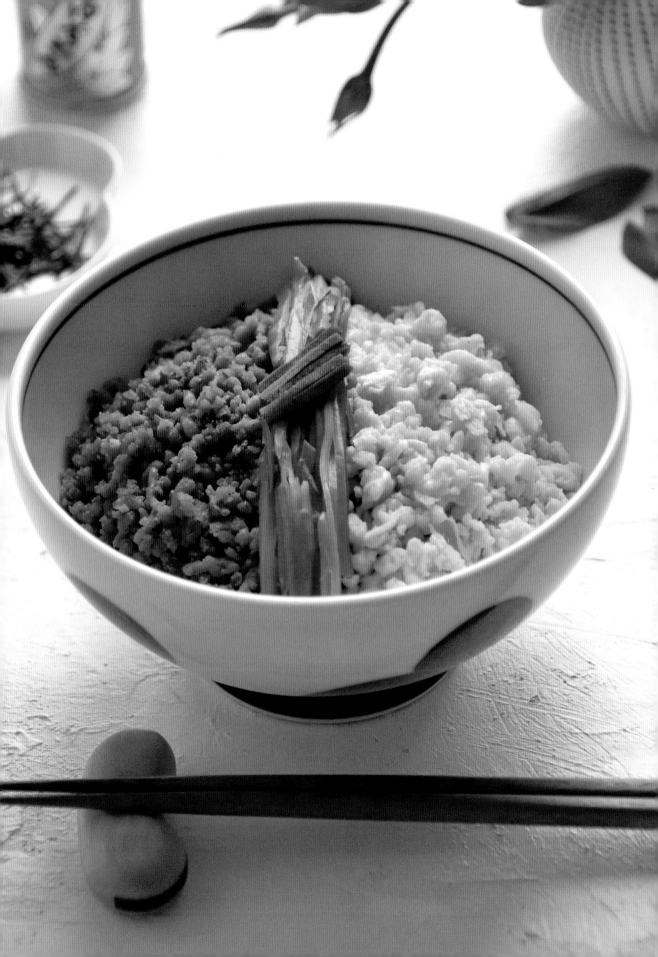

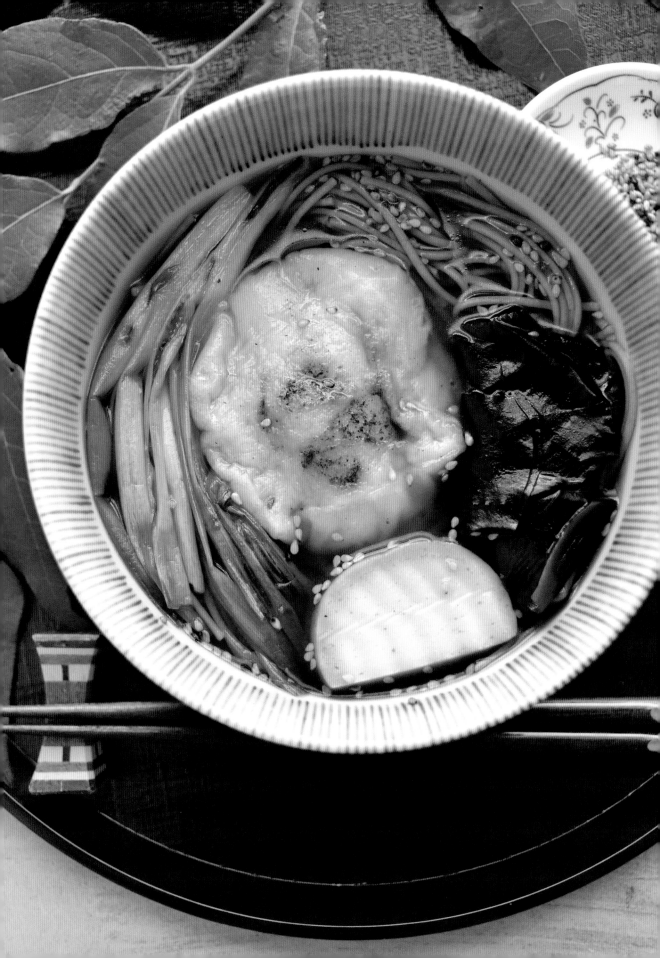

Chikara Soba Noodle Soup
with Wakame, Mochi and Kamaboko Fish Cake

Soba is a traditional Japanese noodle made from buckwheat flour, a bit of whole wheat flour (or yamaimo mountain potato) and water. Soba makers also often add some wheat flour to the dough, to make these fragile noodles a bit more durable. Soba is a good source of vitamin B, potassium and rutin, making it a powerful antioxidant as well as having anti-inflammatory properties. This recipe is one of my favorites—soba served in a savory hot dashi broth topped with chewy mochi rice cakes and leafy wakame seaweed. *Chikara* means power in Japanese, a reference to the combination of soba and mochi—which together pack a punch of stamina and energy. You can also add shrimp or vegetable tempura or fried tofu instead of the mochi: the possibilities are endless!

PREPARATION TIME: 15 minutes
COOKING TIME: 20 minutes
SERVES 4

4 small bundles dried soba noodles
  (12 oz/350 g)
1 teaspoon neutral-flavored oil
4 unsweetened mochi rice cakes
  1.5 x 2.5 in (4 x 7 cm), around 8 oz/
  350 g total
8 scallions, green parts only, cut into
  4-in (10-cm) lengths
3 tablespoons fresh or dried wakame
4 cups (1 liter) Basic Dashi Stock
  (page 36)
½ cup (125 ml) Kaeshi Sauce (page 40)
4 slices kamaboko fish cake (optional)
Pinch shichimi togarashi or cayenne
  pepper (optional)

TIP
The soba noodles are typically packaged in small individual portion bundles. A bundle typically weighs a little over 3 oz (80 g).

1. Fill a large pot two-thirds full with water and bring to a boil. Don't add salt to the water. Cook the soba according to the package instructions or until it's al dente. Drain it and rinse it under cold running water to get rid of the starch. Set aside.

2. Add the oil to a nonstick skillet and heat over medium heat. Add the mochi and cook, covered, for 3 to 4 minutes or until light browned. Flip each slice, lower the heat to medium-low, cover and continue cooking until the other side has cooked through, about 3 to 4 minutes. In the same skillet, add the green onions and cook over medium heat until they're slightly charred on both sides, about 30 seconds to 1 minute.

3. Place a strainer in a bowl, add the fresh wakame and fill the bowl with water, letting it sit for a few seconds. Drain and rinse the wakame under running water until the salt is removed and the wakame doubles or triples in size. Squeeze out the excess water and cut it into bite-sized pieces. If you're using dried wakame, follow the instruction on the package or rehydrate it in a bowl of water for 5 minutes. Drain it, squeeze out the excess water, then set aside.

4. Combine the Basic Dashi Stock and the Kaeshi Sauce in a pot and bring to a simmer over medium-high heat. Add the soba and the mochi to the pot to reheat them in the hot soup for about 1 to 2 minutes. Turn off the heat.

5. To serve, ladle 1 cup of hot soup along with the soba into each bowl and top it with the mochi, wakame and green onions. To make it in an authentic style, add kamaboko fish cakes and shichimi togarashi for spiciness.

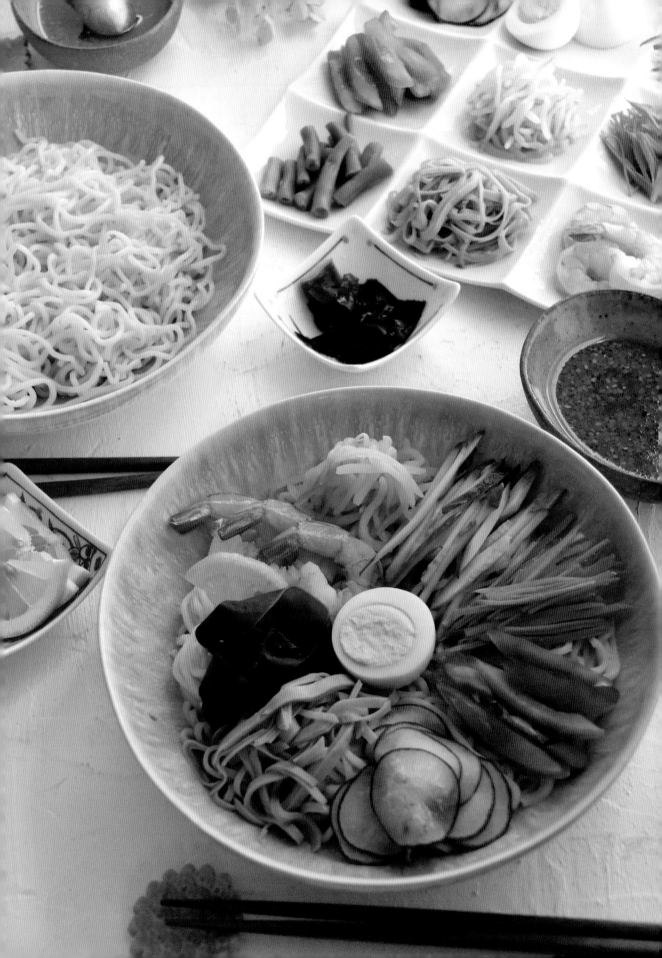

Cold Noodle Salad

Hiyashi chuka cold noodle salad is a Japanese summertime favorite. Chilled, chewy ramen noodles are topped with meat or seafood, fresh vegetables and eggs, then tossed with a vinegary dressing just before serving. In my house, this is a popular weeknight dish when the temperature rises and we're craving something cold and refreshing. Served with lots of crunchy and leafy vegetables, this healthy meal comes together quickly. It's a versatile dish and you can substitute any vegetables and proteins in place of the ones listed here. Whatever is on hand or is easy to find. Other types of noodles also work well, so try making this with konnyaku, vermicelli or your favorite pasta.

PREPARATION TIME: 10 minutes
COOKING TIME: 20 minutes
SERVES 4

12 medium fresh shrimp, about 5 oz (150 g), peeled and deveined
3 tablespoons fresh or dried wakame
1 Japanese or ½ baby cucumber
½ carrot
2 eggs, hardboiled
½ tomato
4 slices cooked ham or turkey
3 radishes
Pinch of sea salt
1 cup (100 g) bean sprouts
8 string beans

DRESSING
4 tablespoons toasted white sesame seeds
4 tablespoons Basic or Kombu Dashi Stock (pages 36, 38)
4 tablespoon Sushi Vinegar (page 52)
2 tablespoons sesame oil
2 tablespoons Kaeshi Sauce (page 40)
½ teaspoon fresh ginger juice
Four 4.25-oz (480-g) bundles fresh ramen noodles (see headnote)
½ lemon, sliced, to garnish (optional)

1. Bring water to a boil in a small saucepan. Add the shrimp and cook for 2 to 3 minutes or until they start to turn pink. Drain and let cool.

2. Place a strainer in a bowl, add the fresh wakame and fill the bowl with water, letting it sit for a few seconds. Drain and rinse the wakame under running water until the salt is removed and the wakame doubles or triples in size. Squeeze out the excess water and cut it into bite-sized pieces. If you're using dried wakame, follow the instruction on the package or rehydrate it in a bowl of water for 5 minutes. Drain it, squeeze out the excess water, then set aside.

3. Slice the cucumber and carrot into fine matchsticks. Peel and cut the eggs in half. Thinly slice the tomato and ham or turkey into strips. Slice the radish and sprinkle the pieces with a pinch of sea salt. Set aside.

4. Boil the bean sprouts for 1 minute, drain and squeeze out the excess water. Boil the string beans for 3 to 4 minutes until soft. Drain and cut into bite0sized pieces, then set aside.

5. In a bowl, combine the sesame seeds, dashi stock, Sushi Vinegar, sesame oil, Kaeshi Sauce and ginger juice. Mix well.

6. In a large pot of boiling water, cook the noodles according to the package directions, using chopsticks or tongs to separate them. Drain and immediately rinse the noodles in cold running water to remove the starch. Drain again well, then divide the noodles among 4 serving bowls.

7. To serve, top the noodles with the shrimp, wakame, cucumber, carrot, egg, tomato, ham/turkey, radish, beans sprouts and string beans. Pour the dressing over and garnish with a slice of lemon, if using.

TIP You can store the dressing for up to 5 days in the refrigerator in an airtight container. It can be used for leafy greens or steamed vegetables such as string beans or corn. It's also great served with chilled tofu, grilled chicken or shrimp.

Traditional Udon Noodle Soup
with Fried Tofu, Eggs, Green Onions and Ginger

Comprising udon noodles with fried tofu, green onions and ginger, kitsune udon is an easy dish that comes together in about 15 minutes. All that's needed to prepare the soup is a Basic Dashi Stock and Kaeshi Sauce. Then add the noodles and toppings. This classic version is topped with a poached egg. It's often called *tsukimi* kitsune udon ("*tsukimi*" means moon viewing) because the poached yolk suggests the harvest moon. As for the toppings, here I'm using light and puffy fried tofu (abraage), available in the refrigerated or freezer section of any Asian grocery store. If you want to make the dish heartier, adding shrimp or vegetable tempura, leafy wakame or even sliced avocado are all great additions as well.

PREPARATION TIME: 10 minutes
COOKING TIME: 15 minutes
SERVES 4

Four 3.5-oz (400 g) packages dried udon or 2.2 lb (1 kg) frozen or refrigerated noodles
4 sheets fried tofu, 2.5 x 5 in (6 x 12 cm) , preferably unseasoned
4 cups (1 liter) Basic Dashi Stock (page 36)
½ cup (125 ml) Kaeshi Sauce (page 40)
Pinch of salt
4 eggs
2 scallions, green part only, cut on the bias
1 tablespoon ginger, peeled and grated
Pinch of shichimi togarashi or cayenne pepper (optional)

1. Fill a large pot half-full with unsalted water and bring it to a boil. Cook the udon noodles according to the package instructions or until they're tender but firm. Drain and rinse them under cold running water to get rid of the starch, then set aside.

2. Place the fried tofu in a colander in the sink and slowly pour boiling water, about 2 cups (500 ml), over it. Then rinse the tofu well with cold water and cut it in half crosswise.

3. Combine the Basic Dashi Stock, Kaeshi Sauce, fried tofu and udon noodles in a pot and bring it to a boil over medium-high heat, about 6 to 8 minutes. Crack the eggs into the pot of hot soup and cook, covered, for 1 to 2 minutes over medium-high heat. Taste the soup and add a pinch of salt, if necessary, then turn off the heat.

4. To serve, ladle 1 cup of the hot soup along with the udon into each soup bowl and top with the fried tofu, green onions, an egg and some ginger. Sprinkle with a pinch of shichimi togarashi (Japanese seven spice), if using.

TIP Udon is available dried, refrigerated or frozen. The texture and thickness of the noodles vary depending on the type, so sample a few to find one you really like. I find that frozen udon is the easiest to cook, but I also enjoy the texture of the dried version.

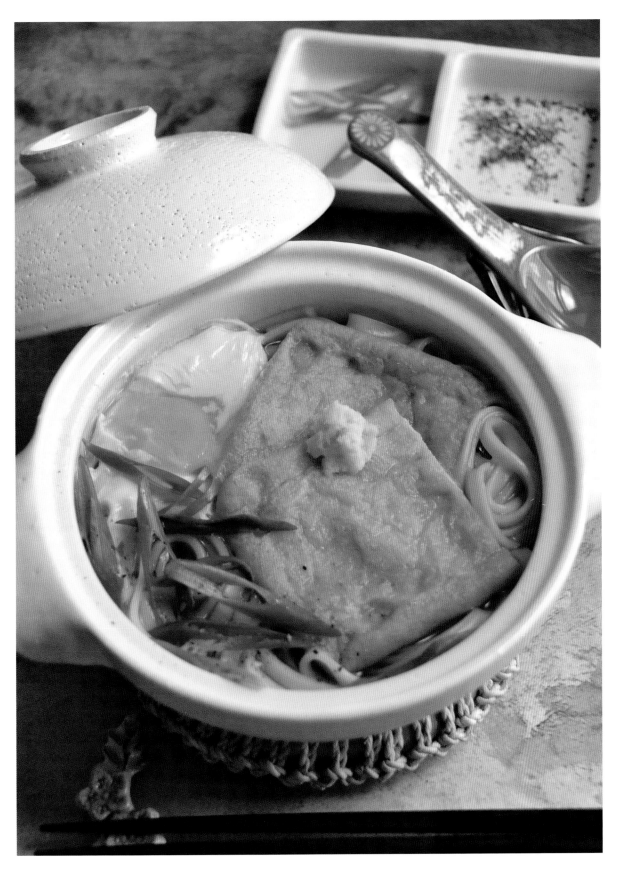

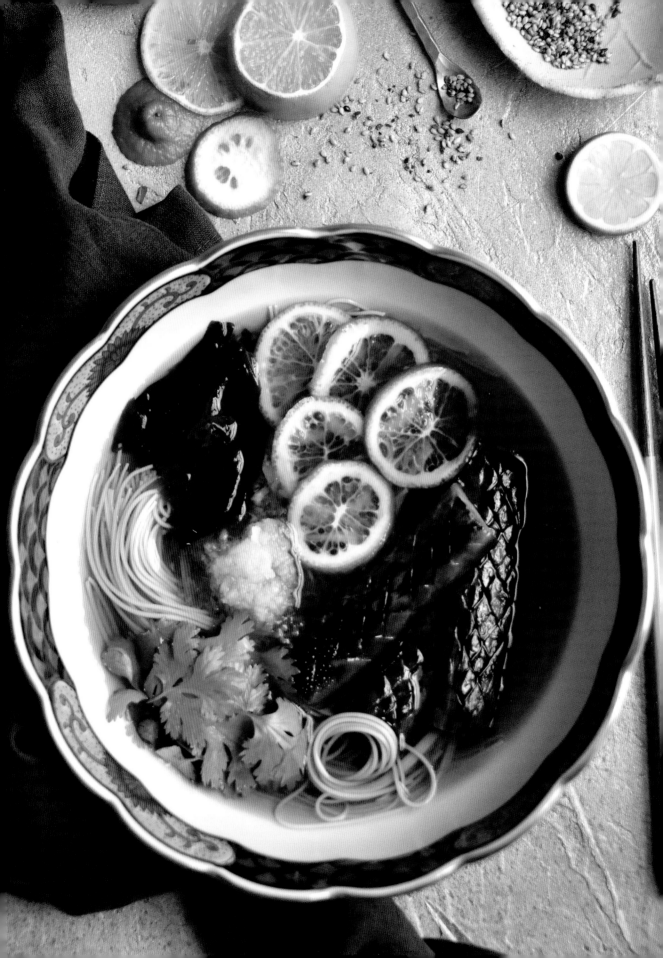

Cold Lime Broth Somen
with Eggplant, Wakame and Grated Daikon

This light, refreshing and aromatic dish is ideal for summer or whenever you're craving simple, cold noodles. While originally served with sudachi limes, regular limes work well and are more widely available, so I often use them instead. This dish combines silky somen noodles, thin wheat noodles and flavorful dashi stock with panfried Japanese eggplant, which are smaller and skinnier with thinner skin than Western eggplant. We grow them in our family garden. Eggplant is high in fiber and vitamins. Japanese cuisine incorporates this Mediterranean favorite into a range of dishes, including miso soups, stir fries, tempura and pickles.

PREPARATION TIME: 15 minutes
COOKING TIME: 20 minutes
SERVES 4

4 cups (1 liter) Basic or Kombu Dashi Stock (pages 36, 38)
½ cup (125 ml) Kaeshi Sauce (page 40)
Three 15-oz (450-g) Japanese eggplants
½ teaspoon sea salt
3 tablespoons fresh or dried wakame
1 small lime
3 tablespoons extra-virgin olive oil
8 bundles somen noodles, 16 oz (500 g)
2 tablespoons grated daikon
2 tablespoons fresh cilantro/coriander leaves

TIP
Two key points for retaining the eggplant's beautiful purple color: sprinkle it with sea salt to draw out the moisture, and cook it quickly over high heat. Use a sharp knife to crosshatch the skin for quick and even cooking, though they'll also cook fine without it.

1. Combine the dashi stock you're using and the Kaeshi Sauce in a large bowl and mix well. Put it in the refrigerator to chill until serving.

2. Cut each eggplant in half lengthwise, then in half crosswise, to make 4 pieces. Using a sharp knife, score the skin of each piece to create shallow, crosshatches (see Tip). Sprinkle the salt over the eggplant, put the pieces on a plate and let them sit for 5 to 10 minutes. Then pat the pieces with a paper towel until they're completely dry and set aside.

3. Place a strainer in a bowl, add the fresh wakame and fill the bowl with water, letting it sit for a few seconds. Drain and rinse the wakame under running water until the salt is removed and the wakame doubles or triples in size. Squeeze out the excess water and cut it into bite-sized pieces. If you're using dried wakame, follow the instruction on the package or rehydrate it in a bowl of water for 5 minutes. Drain it, squeeze out the excess water, then set aside.

4. Thinly slice the lime into ⅛-in (3-mm) slices and set aside.

5. In a skillet, heat the oil over high heat. Add the eggplant, skin side down, and cook for about 1 minute. Use tongs to flip the pieces and cook the other side for 1 minute or until the edges turn golden brown and soften. Transfer the pieces to a dish and let cool.

6. Fill a large pot ⅔ full of unsalted water and bring to a boil. Cook the somen noodles according to the package instructions or until they're tender but firm, to keep them slightly chewy. Drain and rinse them under cold running water to remove the starch, then set aside.

7. To serve, ladle 1 cup of the cold stock along with a portion of the noodles into each soup bowl and top with 3 to 5 slices of lime, 3 pieces of eggplant, the wakame, grated daikon and fresh cilantro/coriander leaves.

Tomato Somen Cold Noodles

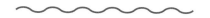

Somen is one of the most popular noodles in Japan. Usually served cold—with dashi soy sauce, grated ginger and finely chopped green onions on the side—it's a dish synonymous with summer. Somen are white wheat noodles made by stretching the dough until it's extremely thin, then cutting it thinly and drying it. While I love the traditional way of eating these noodles, by dipping them into dashi soy sauce, I wanted to change it up a little. I developed this recipe by mixing leftover fresh tomato juice with dashi soy sauce that I had on hand, and tomato somen noodles were born! It's so refreshing that I fell in love with it immediately. I hope you do too.

PREPARATION TIME: 15 minutes
COOKING TIME: 20 minutes
SERVES 4

1 cup (250 ml) unsalted tomato juice
  or tomato puree
⅔ cup (160 ml) Kaeshi Sauce
  (page 40)
3 cups (750 ml) Basic or Kombu
  Dashi Stock (pages 36, 38)
1 tablespoon white sesame oil or
  extra-virgin olive oil
Pinch of salt
½ large tomato
¼ red onion
8 shiso leaves or Italian basil,
  divided
6 oz (175 g) cooked boneless chicken
  breast
3 tablespoons fresh or dried wakame
Eight 1.75-oz (400 g) packages
  somen
1 tablespoon toasted white sesame
  seeds
1 slice of lime, cut into 4 pieces,
  to garnish (optional)

1. Combine the tomato juice, Kaeshi Sauce, the dashi stock you're using and the white sesame oil in a medium bowl and mix well. Taste, adding a pinch of salt if necessary. Cover and put it in the refrigerator to chill for at least 30 minutes or until ready to serve.

2. Cut tomato into bite-sized pieces. Thinly slice the red onion. Cut four leaves of basil into thin strips. Slice the chicken into thin strips or bite-sized pieces, then set aside.

3. Place a strainer in a bowl, add the fresh wakame and fill the bowl with water, letting it sit for a few seconds. Drain and rinse the wakame under running water until the salt is removed and the wakame doubles in size. Squeeze out excess water and cut it into bite-sized pieces. If you're using dried wakame, follow the instructions on the package or rehydrate it in a bowl of water for 5 minutes. Drain it, squeeze out the excess water, then set aside.

4. Fill a large pot ⅔ full with unsalted water and bring to a boil. Cook the somen noodles according to the package instructions or until they are tender but firm. Drain and rinse under cold running water to get rid of the starch, then set aside.

5. To serve, ladle 1 cup of the cold stock along with the somen into each bowl. Top with 1 basil leaf, tomato, onion, chicken and wakame. Garnish with thin strips of basil leaves, a sprinkle of sesame seeds and the lime, if using.

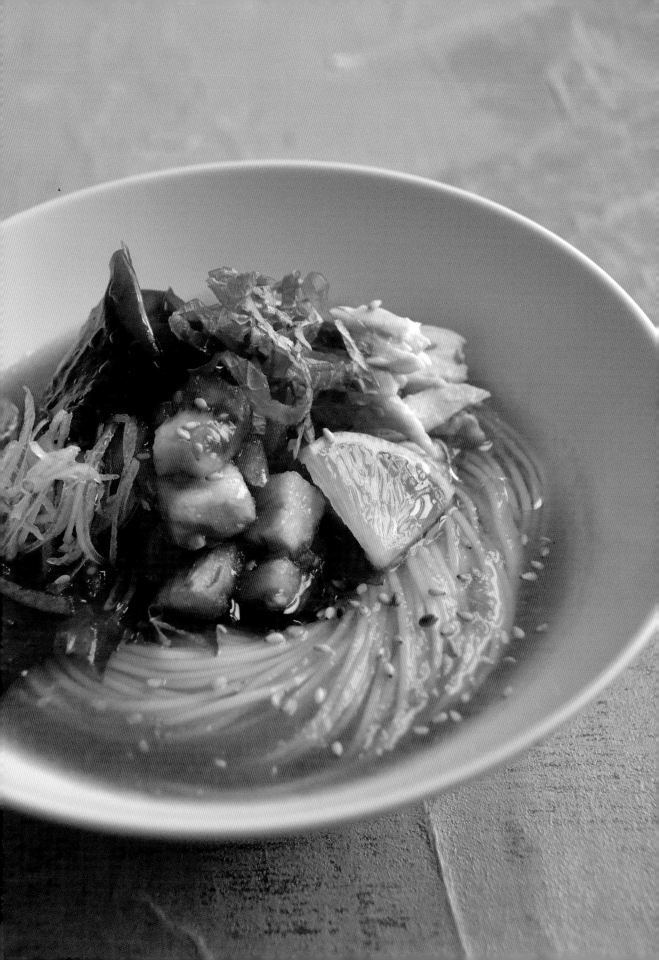

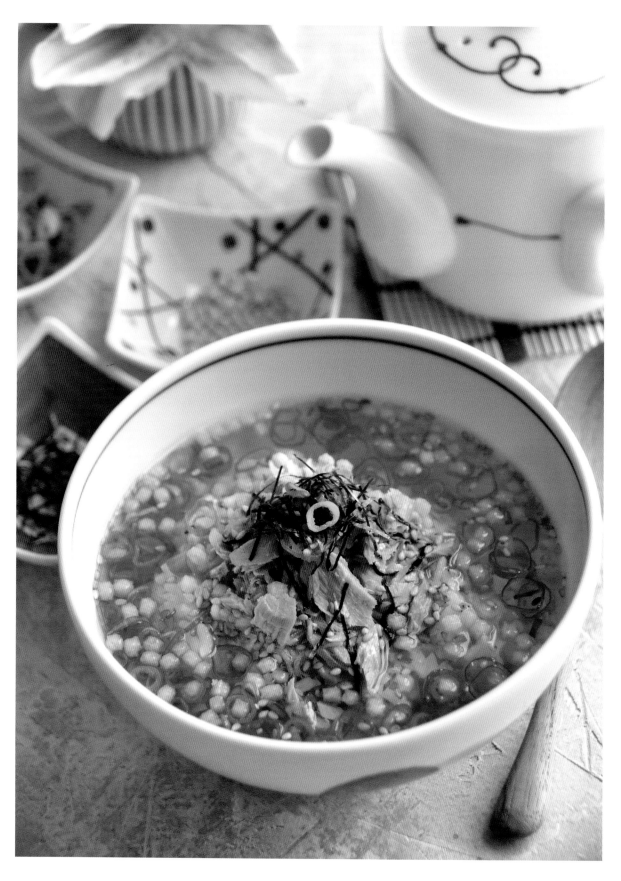

Salted Grilled Salmon Rice Bowl
with Green Tea Dashi

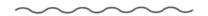

Chazuke is Japanese soul food that became popular duing the Edo period
(1603–1868). It's a soupy rice bowl filled with grilled fish, nori, pickled vegetables
and wasabi and served with hot green tea or hot dashi stock poured over the top.
It was developed as a way to revive day-old rice. You might have doubts about green
tea being served as a broth, but this is a true comfort food enjoyed year-round
in Japan. Chazuke is a versatile dish commonly eaten for the evening meal,
while out with friends and even as a quick breakfast on the go.

PREPARATION TIME: 15 minutes
COOKING TIME: 15 minutes
SERVES 4

2 small salmon filets, ½ lb (250 g),
  salted and grilled
3½ cups (600 g) cooked Japanese
  short-grain rice
2 tablespoons Kaeshi Sauce
  (page 40)
2 cups (500 ml) Basic Dashi Stock
  (page 36)
Pinch of sea salt
2 cups (500 ml) green tea (sencha,
  hojicha or genmaicha)
1 scallion, both the green and
  white part, finely chopped
1 tablespoon shredded nori, to
  garnish (optional)
1 tablespoon rice crackers, to
  garnish (optional)
1 teaspoon toasted white sesame
  seeds, to garnish (optional)

1. To make the salted salmon for this dish, place the skin-on salmon in a container in a single layer. Pat the salmon dry with a paper towel and sprinkle 1 teaspoon of sea salt over each filet, on both sides, then cover tightly. Let it sit in the refrigerator for at least 30 minutes or overnight.

2. Gently wipe the filets to remove any excess salt and moisture, then grill them in a parchment-paper-lined skillet, covered, over medium-low heat for 6 to 8 minutes or until golden brown. When the bottom turns light brown, flip the salmon with a spatula and turn the heat to low. Cook the other side for about 4 to 6 minutes or until it starts to brown. Alternatively, roast the salmon in the oven at 350°F (180°C) for 15 to 20 minutes.

3. Remove the skin and bones from the salted salmon and discard. Use a fork to divide the filets into bite-sized pieces.

4. Warm the rice, if you're using leftovers.

5. Combine the Kaeshi Sauce, Basic Dashi Stock and a pinch of salt in a small pan over medium heat and bring to a boil. Add the tea leaves and hot water, about 160°F (72°C), to a teapot and let the tea steep for 2 minutes or follow the instructions on the package.

6. To serve, put a quarter of the rice in a soup bowl. Place a quarter of the salmon on top of the rice. When all the guests are seated, pour in both the hot stock and the tea to just barely cover the rice. Sprinkle green onion, nori, rice crackers and sesame seeds on top.

Yakisoba with Homemade BBQ Sauce

This yakisoba noodle dish combines beef, vegetables and a thick homemade Japanese barbecue sauce made with traditional dashi stock, seasoned soy sauce and oyster sauce. Traditionally, yakisoba is sold at street festivals all over Japan. There is also a very popular sandwich called yakisoba-pan, which is an American-style hot dog bun filled with yakisoba noodles. It might sound a bit strange, but it's quintessential Japanese soul food and a favorite snack. When you buy yakisoba at stores, it usually comes with a premade sauce or powdered seasoning package, but making your own sauce is just as easy as using premade ones. Plus it tastes better and is healthier. When you first open the package, you'll notice that the noodles are tightly stuck together. I always rinse them first under cold running water in a strainer so they'll be easy to handle and to prevent the noodles from breaking apart while cooking.

PREPARATION TIME: 15 minutes
COOKING TIME: 20 minutes
SERVES 4

2 cups (140 g) shredded cabbage, about 3 to 4 medium leaves
2 cups (200 g) bean sprouts
14 oz (400 g) flank steak or boneless chicken breast
1 tablespoon minced ginger
1 tablespoon minced garlic
4 tablespoons Basic or Second-Brew Dashi Stock (pages 36–7)
⅓ cup (80 ml) Kaeshi Sauce (page 40)
4 tablespoons oyster sauce
4 tablespoons rice vinegar
4 teaspoons Dijon mustard
2 teaspoons brown sugar
Four 5.3-oz packages yakisoba noodles, about 1¼ lbs/600 g, fresh or dried (see Tip)
2 tablespoons sesame oil
4 fried eggs (optional)
1 tablespoon aonori seaweed flakes, to garnish (optional)
4 tablespoons pickled vegetables (optional)

1. Wash the cabbage leaves. Remove the cores and thinly slice the leaves. Wash, drain and dry the bean sprouts with a kitchen towel. Cut the meat into thin strips, about 1 in (2.5 cm) long.

2. In a medium-sized bowl, combine the ginger, garlic, stock, Kaeshi Sauce, oyster sauce, rice vinegar, Dijon mustard and brown sugar. Mix well, then set aside.

3. If you're using fresh yakisoba noodles, put them in a strainer and rinse them under cold running water for about 10 to 15 seconds (see the headnote). Use your fingers to gently separate the noodles, then drain them well. If you're using dried noodles, follow the instructions on the package or cook them in boiling water until tender, then drain and squeeze out excess water. Set aside.

4. In a large skillet, heat the oil, add the meat and cook it over medium-high for 1 to 2 minutes. Then add the noodles to the skillet. Use tongs to separate them, cooking for about 3 to 4 minutes over medium heat. Add the cabbage and bean sprouts to the skillet, and continue cooking for 1 to 2 minutes.

5. Add the sauce to the skillet and continue cooking over medium-high heat for 3 to 5 minutes or until the sauce is almost evaporated.

6. To serve, place the noodles on individual plates and top each with a fried egg, the aonori seaweed flakes and the pickled vegetables, if using.

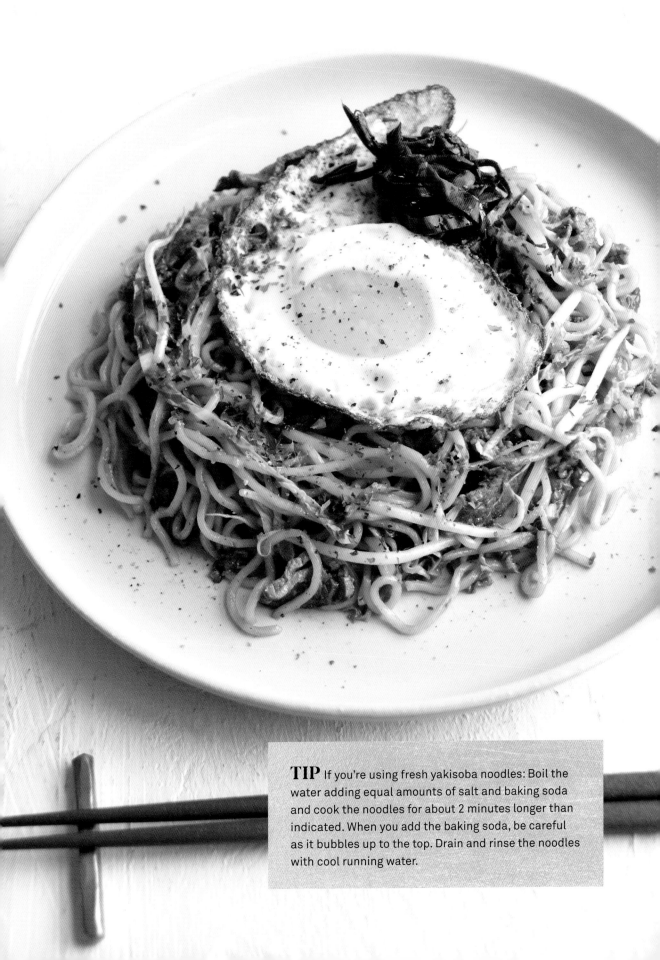

TIP If you're using fresh yakisoba noodles: Boil the water adding equal amounts of salt and baking soda and cook the noodles for about 2 minutes longer than indicated. When you add the baking soda, be careful as it bubbles up to the top. Drain and rinse the noodles with cool running water.

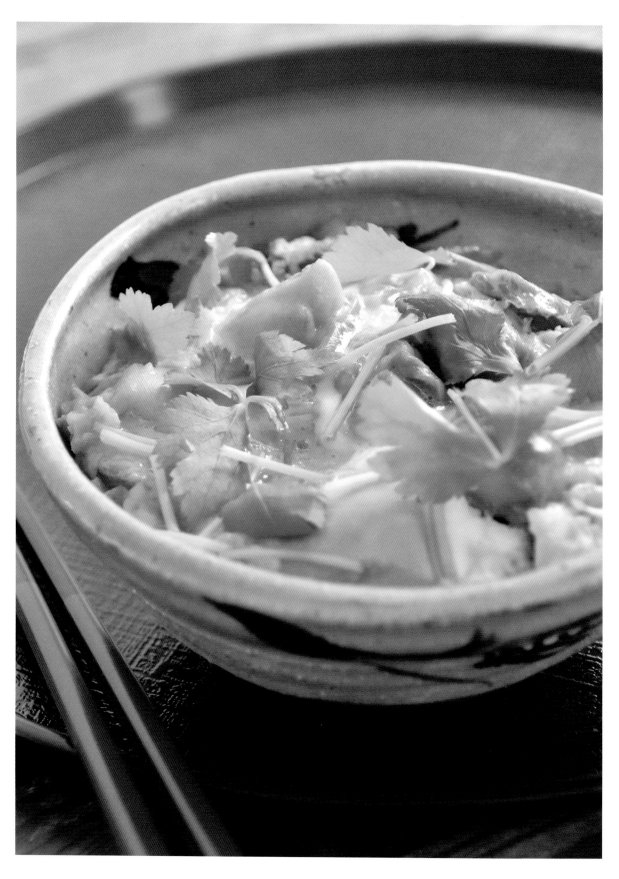

Chicken and Egg Rice Bowl

If you asked me about the best of Japanese soul food, I would definitely mention the ubiquitous chicken and egg rice bowl, *oyako don*. A healthy one-pot wonder, the chicken is simmered in seasoned dashi stock, instead of frying with oil, resulting in a filling though light dish with a great savory flavor. Eggs are poured over the chicken and cooked very gently, then the finished dish is served over steamed rice. When you order this classic at a restaurant, it's usually served in a bowl with a lid, which allows the eggs to continue steaming, giving them a silky, fluffy texture. A key element of making a delicious *oyako don* is not overcooking them. Once you pour the eggs over the chicken, they'll cook in less than a minute. One last note: you can always substitute tofu, beef or shrimp for the chicken, according to your preferences.

PREPARATION TIME: 10 minutes
COOKING TIME: 25 minutes
SERVES 4

2 boneless, skinless chicken thighs, about 1 lb (500 g)
1 onion
1 cup (250 ml) Basic Dashi Stock (page 36)
⅓ cup (80 ml) Kaeshi Sauce (page 40)
8 eggs
4 cups (660 g) cooked Japanese short-grain rice
1 tablespoon cut mitsuba greens or scallions (the green parts), to garnish (optional)

1. Place the chicken thighs on a cutting board and trim away any excess fat. Cut each thigh into bite-sized pieces. Peel the onion then cut it into thin ½-in (1.25-cm) slices.

2. Combine the chicken, onion, Basic Dashi Stock and Kaeshi Sauce in a saucepan over medium-high heat and bring to a simmer. Cook for 7 to 8 minutes, until the chicken is tender and smaller in size. Turn the heat to medium-low once the chicken is cooked.

3. Whisk the eggs in a large bowl. Slowly pour half of the eggs over the chicken and onions. Cook, covered, over medium-low heat while shaking the pan back and forth over the burner. Cook until the eggs are partially set, about 1 minute.

4. Remove the lid and pour in the remaining eggs. Replace the lid and shake the pan back and forth over the burner for another 30 seconds to 1 minute or until the eggs are cooked to your liking (traditionally, they're served slightly runny on top, firm on the bottom).

5. To serve, put some steamed rice in each bowl and pour the chicken and egg over the rice, adding some of the remaining sauce. Garnish with mitsuba or scallion, if using.

Tomato Rice with Kombu and Shio Koji

This rice dish is our family's summertime favorite, especially when tomatoes are in season in our garden. The key is to use fresh, not canned, tomatoes as they're juicier and sweeter. Don't be afraid of putting whole tomatoes in the pot, as they'll break down into a soft, velvety sauce that'll coat the rice with a beautiful red color. In this recipe, I'm introducing Shio Koji (see page 53) as a natural seasoning with intense umami flavor. Koji is the key ingredient in all Japanese fermented products, such as soy sauce, miso and sake. You can purchase Shio Koji at any Japanese grocery store or online. It's available in two forms: either as a white paste that looks similar to rice porridge or as a clear liquid in a bottle. You can easily make it at home too. Shio Koji is a great substitute for salt with both delicious flavor and health benefits that improve digestion and boost the immune system.

PREPARATION TIME: 40 minutes
   (including soaking time)
COOKING TIME: 50 minutes
SERVES 4

1½ cups (340 g) uncooked Japanese
   short-grain white rice
1⅓ cups (330 ml) Basic Dashi Stock
   (page 36)
1 piece of dried kombu, 2 x 6 in
   (5 x 15 cm)
4 tablespoons Shio Koji (page 53), or
   2 teaspoons sea salt
1 tablespoon extra-virgin olive oil
1 medium tomato
2 teaspoons ginger, peeled and
   julienned
2 shiso leaves, cut in a chiffonade
1 teaspoon white sesame seeds
8 shiso leaves to wrap the onigiri,
   optional (see Tip)

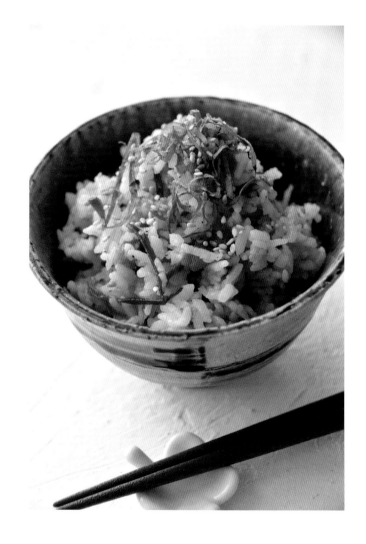

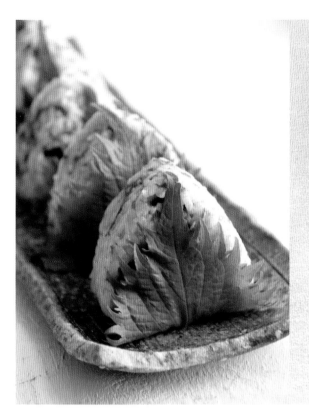

Onigiri

This dish is also great for making onigiri rice balls. To make onigiri, divide the tomato rice into 7 to 8 portions (about ⅜ cup/85 g). Set a small bowl of water on your work surface. To prevent the rice from sticking to your hands, wet them before forming the balls. Place a small portion of rice in one wet hand and, with your other hand, mold the rice into a triangle. Form a triangle shape by rotating and pressing the rice with your fingers a couple of times to create a shape to your liking. Don't squeeze the rice too hard, as you want to keep it soft and fluffy. Or you can simply make them into round balls, gently press them with your fingers a couple of times to be sure they hold together. Wrap each rice ball with 2 shiso leaves (or nori), one on each side, if you like and continue with the remaining rice balls.

1. Rinse the rice in enough water to cover it, lightly stirring the rice with your hands 5 to 6 times, then drain the cloudy water immediately.

2. Refill the bowl with water to cover the rice. Use the palms of your hands to gently press the rice about 10 times, then drain the cloudy water. Repeat this process 3 to 4 times, until the water runs clear. Then, refill the bowl with the washed rice and 1½ cups of water and soak for 30 minutes.

3. While soaking the rice, prepare the seasoning stock by combining 1⅓ cups of Basic Dashi Stock, a strip of kombu, the Shio Koji and extra-virgin olive oil in a small (2.5-qt/2.4-l) heavy saucepan or Dutch oven and soak for 30 minutes.

4. Pierce the tomato with a fork at the stem end and hold it over the open flame on the stove, slowly rotating it for 10 to 15 seconds until the skin bursts. Remove from the flame and let cool on a plate for 1–2 minutes. Peel off the skin with your hand.

5. Drain the rice completely in a colander.

6. Combine the seasoning stock, the kombu strip and the rice in a pot or pan and mix well. Add the tomato and ginger.

7. Cook, covered, over medium high heat for 10 minutes until the water starts to boil. (TIP: If you're not sure if the water is boiling, you can open the lid quickly to check.) If there's any water left on top of the rice, close the lid and continue cooking for a few more minutes.

8. Turn the heat to low and continue cooking the rice, covered, for 15 minutes. (TIP: From this point on, don't open the lid until the rice is fully cooked.)

9. Turn off the heat and with the pot covered, let the rice steam for another 25 to 30 minutes before removing the lid. If you're using a rice cooker, follow the manufacturer's instructions.

10. Remove the cooked kombu from the saucepan and cut it into thin strips. Return the kombu to the pot. Using a rice paddle, gently break it up and mix the tomato with the the kombu and rice. Let it steam for another 7 to 10 minutes with the saucepan covered.

11. Serve in individual bowls. Garnish with shiso and sesame seeds. Enjoy the crunchy texture of the okoge, the thin crust of slightly browned rice at the bottom of the pot created during the cooking process.

Miso-glazed Grilled Rice Balls

~~~~~~~~~~

Crispy and smoky-savory on the outside, soft and fluffy inside, grilled rice balls are a popular and perfect pick-me-up snack. They have a pleasing balance of sweet and salty flavor due to the special sauce that seasons the rice balls during grilling. My family often makes them with a sweet miso glaze that gives them an extra crunchy surface texture with a slightly charred flavor from the glaze.

PREPARATION TIME: 15 minutes
COOKING TIME: 25 minutes
SERVES 4

Neutral-flavored cooking spray
4 cups (660 g) cooked and warm short-grain rice
2 tablespoons sesame oil, divided
4 tablespoons Tama Miso (page 205)
8 large nori sheets, 4 x 7 in (10 x 18 cm) or shiso leaves, to garnish (optional)

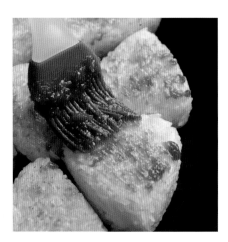

1. **If baking them in the oven:** Line a baking sheet with parchment paper and lightly spray it with the oil. Preheat the oven to 350ºF (175ºC).

2. Divide the rice into 7 or 8 portions, about half a cup of rice per ball.

3. Set a small bowl of water on your work surface. Dip your hands in the water (to prevent the rice from sticking to your hands). Grab one portion of the rice in one hand and mold it into a ball by using your other hand to shape it, rotating the ball a few times until it's round. Then, with the rice in one hand, use the other hand to form three corners, turning it into a triangle. If that proes too difficult, stick to the balls. Gently flatten the rice ball between your hands into a 2-in (5-cm) diameter and about ¾ in (2 cm) thick disc. Gently press it a couple of times to ensure it's firmly formed and not breaking apart. Repeat with the remaining rice balls.

4. Pour 1 tablespoon of sesame oil into a small bown. Using a brush, lightly coat the discs on all sides with the oil.

5. **If you're using a skillet:** Add the remaining 1 tablespoon of sesame oil to the skillet and set it over medium-high heat until the oil is shimmering. Place the rice discs in the skillet, lower the heat to medium and cook for 3 to 5 minutes without touching them until they're a nice light-brown color. Then, turn them over, cover them, lower the heat to medium-low and cook for another 3 to 5 minutes until the second side is light brown.

6. **If you're baking them in the oven:** Place the rice balls on the prepared baking sheet, leaving some space between them and bake them in the preheated oven for about 8 to 11 minutes. Keep an eye on them. Once they become firm to the touch and light brown, turn them over. If not, let them bake for another 1 to 2 minutes. Brush the miso sauce on the exposed side of the rice ball and continue cooking in the skillet for another 30 seconds to 1 minute over medium-low heat or continue baking in the oven until the miso becomes slightly charred. Then flip the pieces and brush the miso on the other side, frying for another 30 seconds to 1 minute until the other becomes slightly charred as well.

7. To serve, place the rice balls on top of nori sheets or shiso leaves on individual plates or simply serve as is without wrappers.

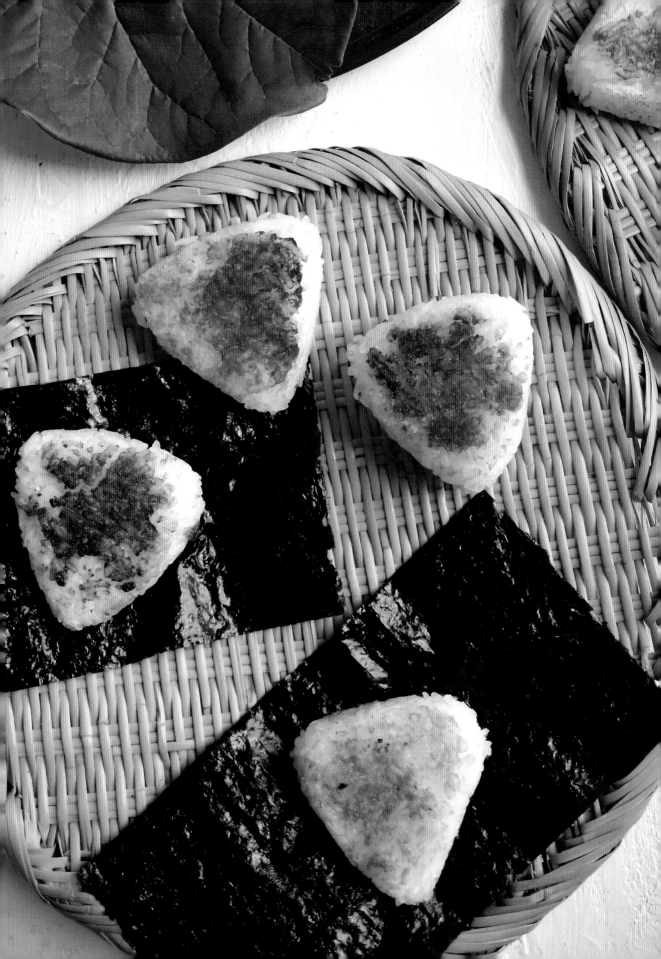

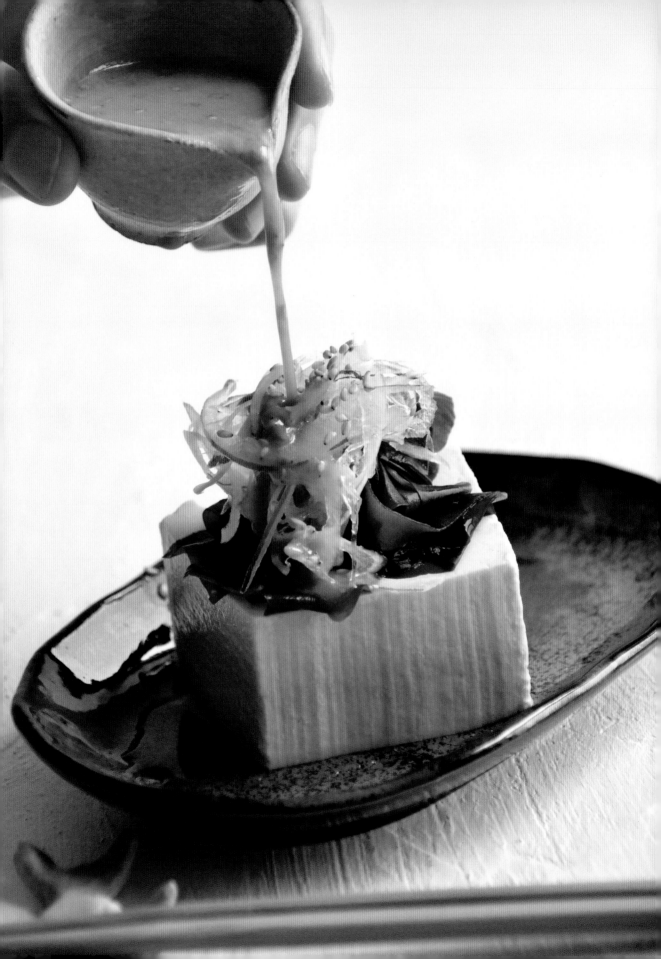

Soy, Sesame and Eggs

Soybeans have been an integral part of the traditional, vegetable-based Japanese diet since ancient times. They're an essential ingredient providing a valuable source of plant-based protein. In their original form, soybeans are not easily digested, so the Japanese have processed them in a variety of ways to incorporate them into their daily diets for centuries. This includes transforming them, through the power of fermentation, into miso paste and natto (a fermented, sticky soybean superfood containing probiotics and vitamin K2 for strong bones, clearer arteries and stronger immune health) slowly boiling them and curdling the liquid to create tofu and yuba (bean curd) and using the squeezed liquid to make soy milk.

Sesame stands in the shadow of soy as an overlooked and underused superfood. High in many beneficial minerals including copper, calcium, manganese, iron, zinc and fiber, it's an essential source of nutrition for vegetarians and vegans. The fiber in sesame is also a specific type of lignan which helps manage cholesterol, prevent high blood pressure and protect the liver from oxidative damage. Eggs, meanwhile, prove the perfect pairing with these two ingredients. So don't forget about their protein power when preparing a superfood supper!

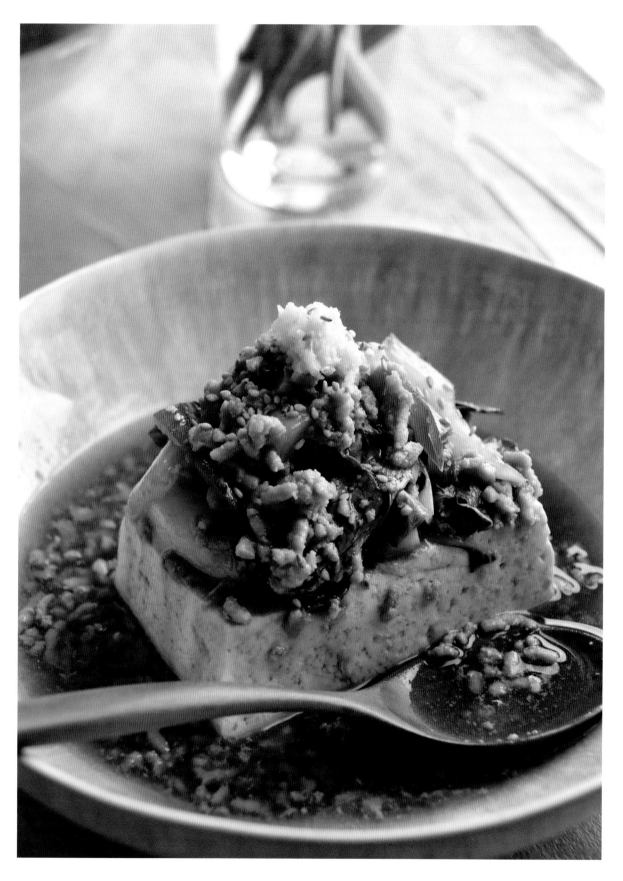

Tofu with Ankake Sauce

My mom often cooked this dish—which is both easy and healthy—on busy weeknights, served over steamed rice. The soft, silky tofu was blanketed in the delicious ankake sauce. This dish is a popular home-cooked meal that pairs a thick, glossy potato-starch-based sauce with seasonal vegetables and often some kind of protein. Hardboiled quail eggs, kamaboko fish cakes and earwood mushrooms are also sometimes added to make a heartier dish. Ankake sauce can be served over steamed rice, noodle soups or panfried noodles. In this recipe, I'm showing you the heathiest way to use everyday ingredients readily available at your grocery store. This is such a versatile recipe, you can adapt it by using any leftover vegetables or meat you have in the fridge. I often make it right before going grocery shopping.

PREPARATION TIME: 15 minutes
COOKING TIME: 25 minutes
SERVES 4

Two 14-oz (400-g) blocks soft tofu
1 large bok choy (7 oz/200 g)
½ red bell pepper
1 cup (250 ml) Basic or Second-Brew
  Dashi Stock (pages 36–7)
6 tablespoons Kaeshi Sauce (page 40)
2 tablespoons sake
Pinch of salt
8 oz (250 g) ground chicken
1 tablespoon potato starch or
  cornstarch
1 teaspoon ginger, peeled and grated
Steamed rice, for serving (optional)

1. Cut the blocks of tofu in half crosswise. Place the pieces in a medium-sized pot with just enough water to cover and simmer, covered, over low heat for 15 to 20 minutes.

2. Cut the bok choy lengthwise first then crosswise into 2-in (5-cm) pieces. Cut the stem end into quarters. Cut the bell pepper into 1½-in (3.75-cm) strips.

3. In a separate medium-sized pot, combine the Dashi Stock, Kaeshi Sauce, sake and salt and bring it to a boil. Add the ground chicken to the pot, lower the heat to medium and, using a wooden spoon, stir constantly for 5 minutes, until the ground chicken is coated and broken into small crumbles. Skim the foam and fat from the surface of the pot using a sieve.

4. Add the bok choy and bell pepper to the chicken mixture and cook, covered, for 2 to 3 minutes over medium-low heat or until the vegetables are tender but firm and have retained their shape.

5. Mix the potato starch with 1 tablespoon of water in a small bowl. Pour it into the pot and whisk until the starch starts to thicken and is well combined with the meat and vegetables. Remove from the heat.

6. To serve, scoop the hot tofu out of the pot with a mesh sieve and drain well. Place the tofu in four individual serving bowls and pour the chicken and the vegetable sauce over it. Serve with steamed rice, if using.

Braised Koyadofu with Flat Peas

Have you ever cooked with freeze-dried tofu before? It may sound a bit strange, but if you try this recipe, I'm sure you'll be hooked. Koyadofu is a traditional preserved food in Japan that originated in the mountaintop Buddhist monasteries on Mt. Koya, near Nara (which today are a very popular tourist destination). It was originally made by leaving fresh tofu outdoors to freeze in wintertime, then hanging it up to dry. Koyadofu comes in rectangular blocks, about the size of a credit card and 1 inch (2.5 cm) thick. Once they are rehydrated, they expand slightly and have a denser, firmer texture than fresh tofu. The sponge-like texture helps soak up all the delicious flavors of a sauce quickly. You can serve this dish hot, cold or at room temperature, and it can be made ahead of time. The flavors will intensify as the tofu draws in the broth. Koyadofu is easier to digest than plain tofu and is an excellent source of protein, iron and calcium. Comforting and loaded with savory flavor, this recipe can be the basis for a delicious vegan supper.

PREPARATION TIME: 10 minutes
COOKNG TIME: 25 minutes
SERVES 4

4 pieces koyadofu, freeze-dried tofu (3 oz/80 g total), see page 15
Neutral-flavored oil, for deep-frying
4 tablespoons potato starch or cornstarch
1 cup (250 ml) Kombu Dashi (page 38)
3 tablespoons Kaeshi Sauce (page 40)
1 tablespoon sake
½ tablespoon maple or agave syrup
2 cups (100 g) flat peas, sugar snap peas or snow peas, ends removed

TIP
This is a great addition to a bento box served at room temperature. To prevent the tofu from getting soggy, squeeze the broth out before packing it.

1. Soak the koyadofu in plenty of water in a medium-sized bowl for 15 to 20 minutes, then wash it, changing the bowl of water 3 to 4 times. Use your hands to gently squeeze the tofu. At first the water will be milky, but it will gradually become clear after washing the pieces for 1 to 2 minutes. Squeeze out the excess water by wringing the pieces gently with your hands. Cut each block of tofu into 4 pieces.

2. Fill a heavy-bottomed medium-sized pot with about 2 in (5 cm) of oil and bring it to 325ºF (160ºC) over medium heat.

3. Put the potato starch in a shallow bowl or on a small plate. Right before the oil has reached 325ºF (160ºC), roll the koyadofu pieces in the potato starch, pressing firmly to be sure the starch sticks to the tofu and that each piece is evenly coated.

4. Gently drop each piece of tofu separately into the oil. Don't overcrowd the pot—if all the pieces don't fit at one time, fry them in batches.

5. Cook over medium heat for about 3 to 4 minutes on each side for a total of 6 to 7 minutes, until the tofu is light golden brown. Drain the tofu on a wire rack.

6. Combine the Kombu Water, Kaeshi Sauce, sake and maple syrup in a saucepan and bring to a boil over medium-high heat. Add the koyadofu and simmer for 8 to 10 minutes over medium-low heat. Add the snow peas and continue simmering for 1 minute more. To serve, place the koyadofu and the snow peas in a bowl with the remaining sauce drizzled over them.

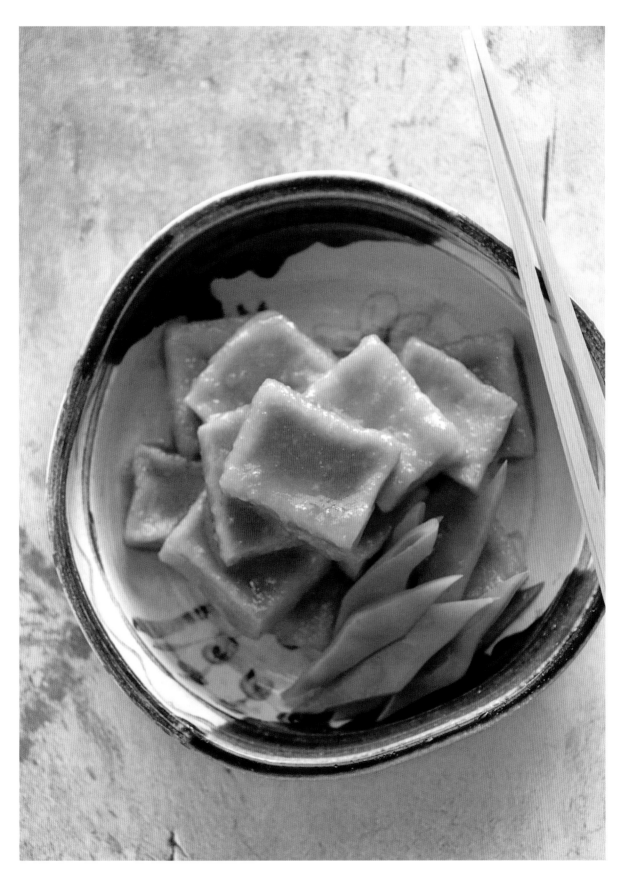

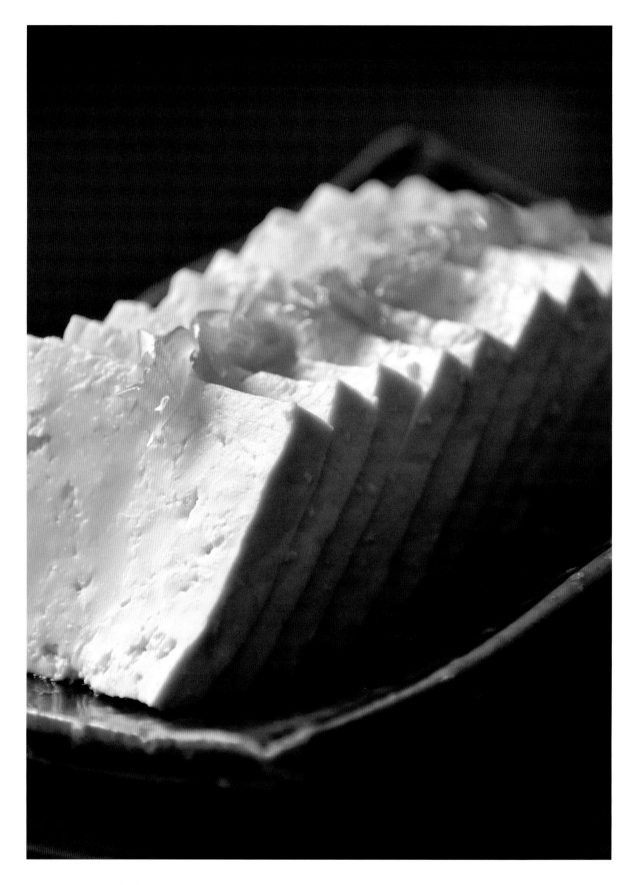

Koji-cured Tofu with Toppings

What makes this tofu so creamy and savory? You guessed it, koji—the all-purpose fungi that brings a strong savory flavor to so many traditional Japanese foods, including miso, soy sauce, rice vinegar, mirin and sake. In this recipe, I'm using Shio Koji, a popular seasoning made with three ingredients: koji, salt and water. It tastes slightly sweet and salty with a mild fermented smell like sweet miso paste. It's easy to make at home (page 53) and is also available in bottled form at Asian markets and health food stores. We often use Shio Koji, with its added bonus of natural umami flavor, as a seasoning instead of salt. The enzymes in Shio Koji also help tenderize proteins. This recipe only requires three simple steps: squeezing the water out of the tofu, rubbing Shio Koji onto the tofu and then letting it sit in the refrigerator for at least three days. As a result, the tofu's texture becomes like a creamy cheese. The first time I cooked this dish for a party, nobody could believe it was tofu! If you're looking for something similar to plant-based cheese, I highly recommend this recipe. It's also a perfect cold appetizer to serve with sliced persimmon as a sake or wine paring, or try tossing it with salads or adding it to a stir fry.

PREPARATION TIME: 5 minutes
COOKING TIME: 10 minutes
MARINADING: 3 to 7 days
SERVES 4

One 14-oz (400-g) block firm tofu
2 tablespoons Shio Koji (page 53)
1 teaspoon wasabi paste, to garnish
 (optional)

1. Place the tofu on a plate with another plate or a wooden cutting board on top of it. The pressure of the weight will draw out excess moisture from the tofu. Put it in refrigerator overnight.

2. Cut the block of tofu in half lengthwise. Sprinkle 1 tablespoon of the Shio Koji on each half of the tofu, rubbing it into the surface with your fingers. Wrap each half in plastic wrap and place them in an airtight container or a reusable food storage bag. Allow them to marinate in the refrigerator for 3 to 7 days.

3. To serve, you can leave the Shio Koji on the tofu or wipe the excess off with a paper towel. Slice the tofu and garnish it with wasabi on top or simply serve sliced tofu with wasabi.

TIP
You can keep koji-cured tofu in the refrigerator for up to 7 days. As you marinate the tofu, it loses its moisture and becomes thicker in texture with a stronger fermented flavor. Eat it within 3 to 5 days for the best flavor. Use firm tofu, not silky or soft, for this recipe. Finally, make sure to drain the water completely for at least 8 hours in the refrigerator for best flavor and texture.

Chilled Tofu Topped with Wakame, Red Onions and Sesame Ginger Vinaigrette

This is the easiest, no-fuss dish you can prepare as a cold appetizer. There's no cooking involved! Served with a variety of toppings and sauces, each cook's selection is unique. If I want to eat this as a main meal of the day, my topping options would be something more filling: sliced avocado with okra, tuna sashimi salad or sliced hardboiled egg. However, if I serve it as an appetizer, I keep it simple, such as this recipe, just plain tofu with sesame vinaigrette. I always keep the rich, creamy and nutty sesame dressing in my refrigerator. I can simply add rice vinegar if I want to sharpen the flavor. Think of the tofu as your blank canvas and be adventurous! Prepare the ingredients ahead of time, keep them chilled in the refrigerator, then add the vinaigrette to the tofu when you're ready to serve.

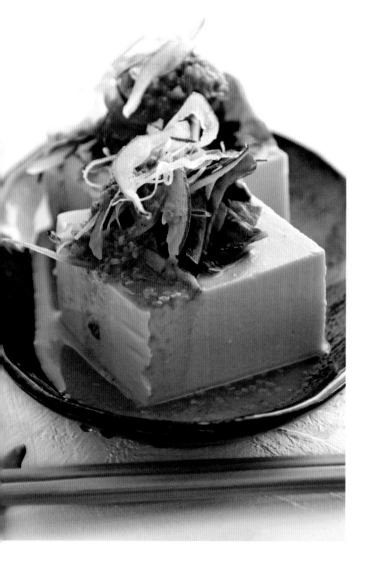

PREPARATION TIME: 10 minutes
COOKING TIME: 10 minutes
SERVES 4 to 5

Two 14-oz (400-g) blocks silken or soft tofu
3 tablespoons fresh or dried wakame
6 tablespoons Goma Sesame Dressing (page 40)
2 tablespoons rice vinegar
2 tablespoons Kombu Dashi Stock (page 38)
½ teaspoon ginger, peeled and minced
4 tablespoons finely sliced red onion

1. Cut each block of tofu crosswise, then lengthwise into 4 pieces.

2. Place a strainer in a bowl, add the fresh wakame and fill the bowl with water, letting it sit for a few seconds. Drain and rinse the wakame under running water until the salt is removed and the wakame doubles or triples in size. Squeeze out the excess water and cut it into bite-sized pieces. If you're using dried wakame, follow the instructions on the package or rehydrate it in a bowl of water for 5 minutes. Drain it, squeeze out the excess water, then set aside.

3. In a small bowl, combine the Goma Sesame Dressing, rice vinegar, dashi and ginger. Mix well.

4. To serve, place the tofu on a serving platter and top with the wakame and the red onion, using a spoon to drizzle the vinaigrette over the top.

Homemade Sesame "Tofu"

Sesame tofu, which is actually not tofu at all as it doesn't contain any soy, has the rich, earthy and nutty flavor of creamy sesame custard. Made from only three ingredients, sesame paste, kuzu starch and Kombu Dashi Stock, it's thickened by kuzu root starch then molded to look like square tofu, which is where the name comes from. It's an ideal healthy appetizer, but who has the time to grind sesame seeds by hand? In this recipe, I include the convenience of using neri goma (Japanese sesame paste) or tahini to achieve the same rich and delicious flavor, and you only spend 15 minutes in the kitchen. For the mold, I used a square lunch box, 2.5 by 4 inches (6 x 10 cm), but you can use any type of small square or rectangular containers or cake molds close to that size.

PREPARATION TIME: 5 minutes
COOKING TIME: 15 minutes
SERVES 4

4 tablespoons kuzu root starch
2 cups (500 ml) Kombu Dashi Stock or Kombu
  Water (page 38)
4 tablespoons neri goma Japanese sesame paste
  or tahini
Pinch of sea salt
1 teaspoon Tama Miso (page 205), to garnish
  (optional)
Wasabi, to garnish (optional)

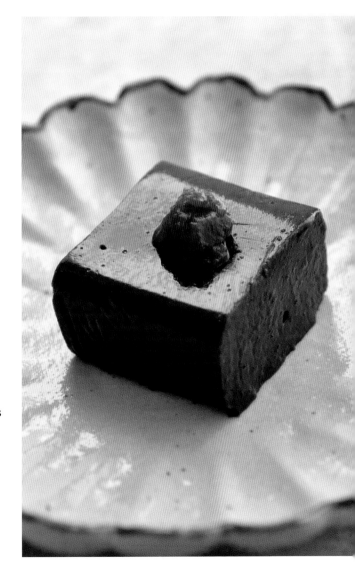

1. Put the kuzu root starch in a blender and blend into a fine powder. Place it in a small saucepan along with the Kashi Dashi Stock and whisk until it's smooth over medium-low heat.

2. Add the neri goma and the salt and cook over medium low. Continue stirring for about 5 minutes. As you continuously stir, reduce the heat to low. The sesame mixture will be watery at first, but as it heats it starts to thicken a lot faster. It will take about 8 to 10 minutes to achieve a creamy, pudding-like consistency, by stirring and smoothing out any lumps over low heat.

3. Wet the inside of the square container that you're using. Pour in the hot sesame mixture and smooth out the top. Bang the container on a countertop a few times to release any air bubbles and let it cool. Transfer the container to the refrigerator to set and cool completely for an hour. Unmold the sesame mixture by flipping the mold on the cutting board and slicing the block into 4 even squares. Serve with the Tama Miso and wasabi, if using.

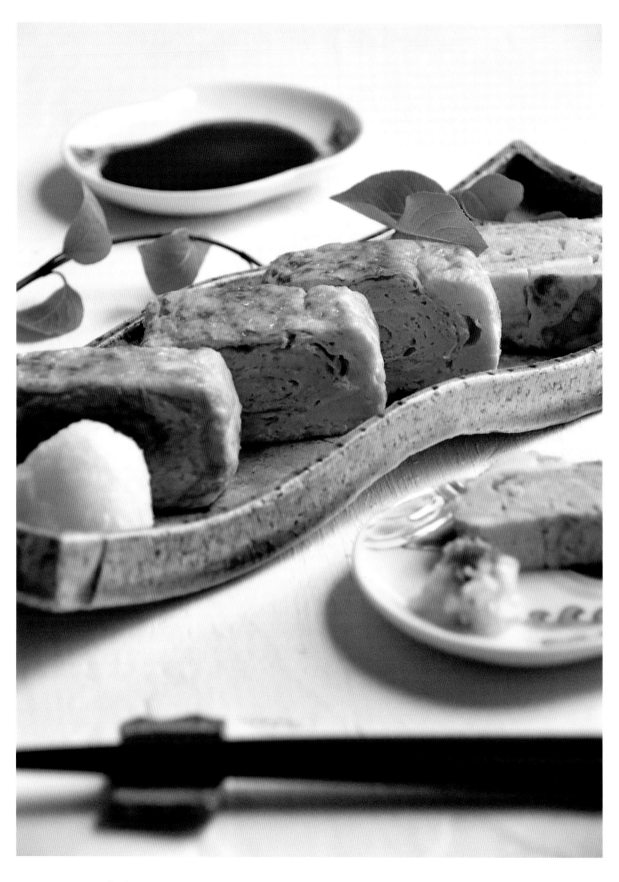

Japanese Rolled Omelet

Eaten for breakfast, school lunches, as part of bento boxes, as a side dish for any meal of the day and even as a filling in sushi and sandwiches, every Japanese family has its own version. Since my family is in the seaweed business, we've always loved the natural flavor of dashi made from kombu. Therefore, our Dashimaki tamago is often flavored with a good amount of dashi stock added to the egg mixture. This results in more flavor, and a slightly custardy texture due to the higher amount of moisture in the egg mixture. When you bite into the eggs, the dashi stock will ooze out and the complex flavors will be a nice surprise. Ideally, use a small nonstick pan, but if you're using a fry pan bigger than 10 inches (25 cm), double the recipe for the best result.

PREPARATION TIME: 5 minutes
COOKING TIME: 10 minutes
SERVES 4

5 eggs
½ cup (125 ml) Basic Dashi Stock (page 36)
2 teaspoons Kaeshi Sauce (page 40)
1 teaspoon granulated sugar
2 tablespoons neutral-flavored oil
2 tablespoons daikon, grated and drained, to garnish
1 tablespoon soy sauce, poured over grated daikon, to garnish

TIP
You can add various proteins, such as shredded ham, tofu or salmon to the egg mixture to turn it into a meal. Adding minced vegetables, such as peppers and mushrooms, or cheddar cheese and nori are other popular fillings to upgrade the flavor and texture for bento boxes.

1. Whisk the eggs just until the yolks and *whites* are slightly blended, don't overmix. Some traces of egg white should be visible for a nice texture when the omelet is cooked.

2. Add Basic Dashi Stock and Kaeshi Sauce to the eggs and mix well. Trying not to create bubbles.

3. Heat the pan over medium heat, adding 1 tablespoon of oil. Wipe off excess oil in the pan with a paper towel.

4. Pour a thin layer of the egg mixture, about ¼ of the total amount, into the hot pan and tilt the pan so it covers the whole surface. When the egg is half-cooked—it will be firm on the bottom but still wet on top—after about 20–30 seconds, pick up the back edge with a chopstick or spatula and roll it up toward the front of the pan. Push the rolled omelet from the back of the pan to the front of the pan three times, finishing with the roll at the back of the pan.

5. Add a little more oil, wiping the excess with a paper towel. Pour ¼ of the egg mixture into the pan and tilt to allow the new layer to spread across the pan, lifting the edge of the rolled omelet with a chopstick or fork at the back of the pan so the egg mixture flows evenly underneath it. When the second layer of egg is half-cooked, roll the omelet toward the front of the pan so it now becomes part of the roll. Roll the omelet back and forth from the front of the pan to the back of the pan three times.

6. Repeat this process twice more, using the remaining egg mixture.

7. Remove the rolled omelet from the pan, cutting it lengthwise into 1-in (2.5-cm) pieces. Add the grated daikon with the soy sauce next to the slices and serve.

Seasoned Tofu with Green Onion Sauce

If you're looking for a tasty tofu dish you can make in less than 10 minutes, you'll enjoy this offering. It might seem almost too simple, but sometimes less is more in bringing out the flavor of ingredients. It can be served as an appetizer or as a main dish. As for the choice of tofu, I generally prefer silken or soft, but depending on availability, I switch it up and sometimes use firm. This dish utilizes an unusual, time-saving technique—the accompanying green onion sauce is cooked at the same time in the same pot as the tofu, but it's kept separate in a small cup placed in the middle of the pot. It's filled to the top with the green onions and katsuobushi, but as it steams in the pot, it releases moisture and cooks down to half its volume, becoming a rich, umami-packed sauce. Of course be sure to use a heat-resistant cup.

PREPARATION TIME: 15 minutes
COOKING TIME: 15 minutes
SERVES 4

Two 14-oz (400-g) blocks tofu (see the headnote)
4 cups (1 liter) water
One piece of dried kombu, 2 x 6 in (5 x 15 cm)
3 scallions, green and white parts, minced
½ cup (10 g) katsuobushi flakes
4 tablespoons Kaeshi Sauce (page 40)

TIP

Place the covered pot on the dining table and serve the hot tofu to each person one piece at a time, so it stays hot. As for the kombu left in the pot, put it in a resealable plastic bag and store it in the freezer until you need it. It can be repurposed by cutting it into thin strips and adding it to your salads and stir fries.

1. Cut each block of tofu into 6 small pieces, about 1½ in (3.75 cm).

2. In a large heavy-bottomed pot, or hot pot nabe pan, add the water, kombu and tofu, leaving an empty spot in the middle of the pot. Set aside.

3. In a heat-resistant tea or coffee cup, combine the green onions, katsuobushi and the Kaeshi Sauce and mix well. Place the cup in the empty spot in the middle of the tofu pot. Make sure that the teacup is above the water level in the pot, to avoid any water seeping in while it's cooking.

4. Put the pot over medium-low heat and bring to a simmer, cooking for about 5 to 7 minutes. Reduce the heat to low and continue cooking for another 1 to 2 minutes. Skim the foam from the surface of the pot using a sieve. Stir the green onion mixture with a spoon. Make sure the sauce is heated through.

5. To serve, place a piece of the tofu on each plate and drizzle with the green onion sauce. Serve each person one to two pieces of tofu at a time, keeping the remaining pieces in the pot so they stay hot.

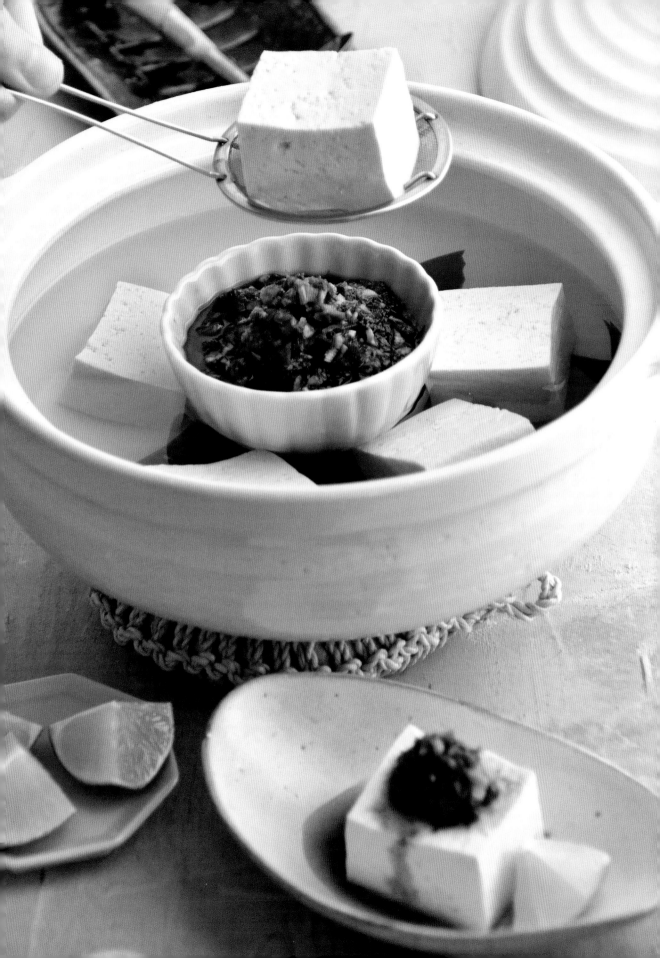

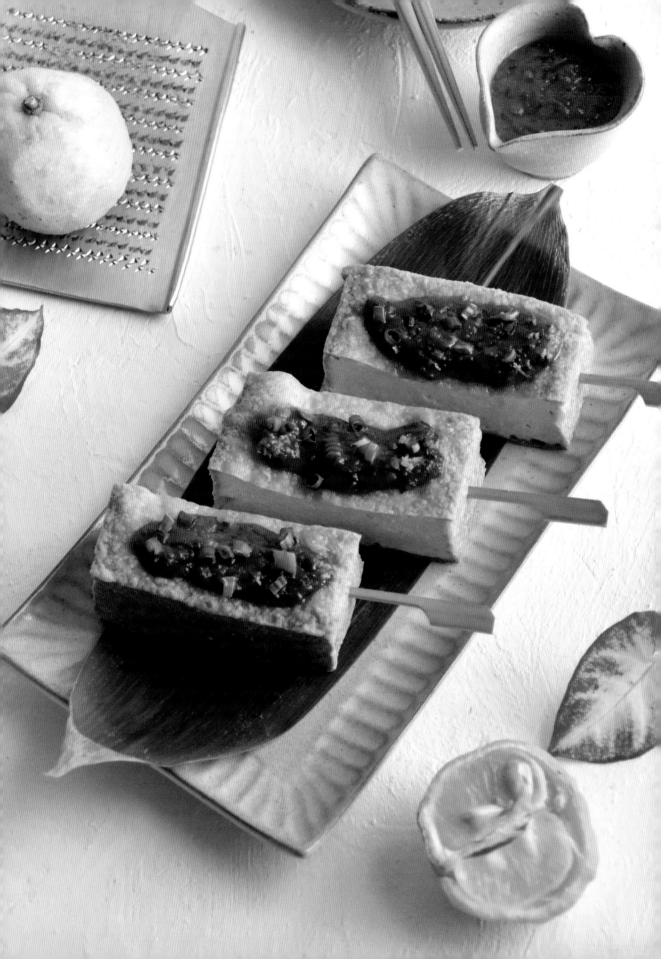

Fried Tofu with Yuzu Miso Glaze

With a crispy exterior and a fluffy-soft interior, fried tofu with a sweet and savory dengaku miso glaze is so addictive you won't be able to stop eating it! Miso contributes an amazing depth of umami flavor to dishes. If this is your first time working with Japanese ingredients such as miso and tofu, this is a great recipe to make. You might be surprised to learn that in Japan tofu is often delivered to homes by bike. Since moving to the United States, I've satisfied my craving for fresh tofu by making my own. Fried tofu is especially easy to make at home. In this recipe, I serve the fried tofu with the sauce on top without grilling it, for an easy preparation. As for the sauce, it's also great with simmered or grilled vegetables such as daikon, eggplant or konnyaku potato cake or to use as a filling for onigiri rice balls.

PREPARATION TIME: 15 minutes
COOKING TIME: 15 minutes
SERVES 4 to 5

2 blocks 14-oz (400-g) medium firm tofu
3½ tablespoons Tama Miso (page 205)
½ cup (125 ml) Basic Dashi Stock (page 36)
2 tablespoons scallions, green parts only, minced
½ teaspoon yuzu or lemon juice
Neutral-flavored oil, for deep frying
6 bamboo skewers
½ teaspoon grated yuzu or lemon zest, to garnish

1. Wrap the tofu in a tea towel. Place the tofu on a plate with another plate or a wooden cutting board on top of it for 15 minutes. The pressure of the weight will draw out the excess moisture from the tofu.

2. Put the miso, Basic Dashi Stock, green onions and yuzu juice in a small saucepan and bring to a boil over medium-high heat, stirring occasionally. Lower the heat and simmer for 30 seconds to reduce the liquid and to thicken it into a sauce. Set aside.

3. Fill a heavy-bottomed pot with about 2 in (5 cm) of oil and heat it to 325ºF (160ºC) over medium.

4. Gently drop each block of tofu into the oil. Don't over-crowd the pot—if both blocks don't fit at one time, fry them one at a time.

5. Cook over medium-low heat for about 4 to 5 minutes on each side, for a total of 8 to 10 minutes or until the tofu is light golden brown.

6. Drain the tofu on a wire rack and then cut each block into 3 pieces crosswise on a cutting board using a sharp knife.

7. To serve, insert a bamboo skewer through the middle of each piece of tofu. Using a spoon, drizzle the sauce on top of the tofu and sprinkle with the yuzu zest.

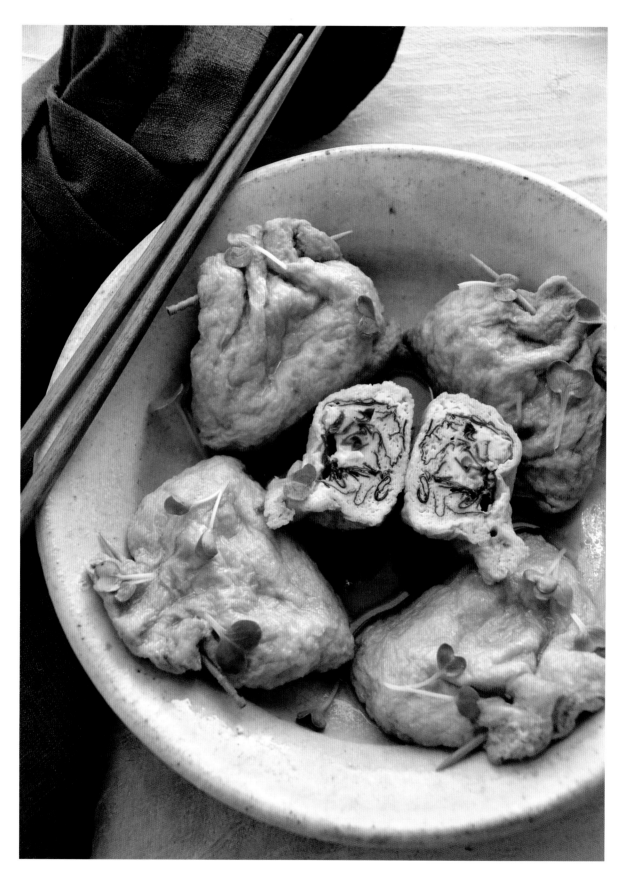

Fried Tofu Pockets with Egg and Wakame

~~~~~~~~~~

Fried tofu pockets, *aburaage*, were so much fun to eat when I was growing up.
I loved the element of surprise because I never knew exactly what it was filled
with until I bit into it. Tofu is sliced lengthwise into thin sheets, then deep-fried
until golden brown. When sliced in half crosswise, there are two small pockets,
which can then be stuffed with whatever you like. If you don't like plain tofu but
would like to eat more soybean dishes, fried tofu is a great alternative. In this
recipe, I introduce light and puffy fried tofu that's stuffed with egg and wakame
then cooked with dashi stock, which absorbs lots of delicious flavor.
You can change up the filling according to your mood and the ingredients you
have on hand. This is also a great addition to a bento box.

PREPARATION TIME: 15 minutes
COOKING TIME: 15 minutes
SERVES 4 (8 pieces)

3 tablespoons fresh or dried wakame
4 sheets of fried tofu, 2.5 x 5 in (6 x 12 cm)
6 medium eggs
¼ cup (65 ml) Kaeshi Sauce (page 40),
  divided
8 toothpicks
1 cup (250 ml) Basic or Kombu Dashi
  Stock (pages 36, 38)
1 teaspoon maple syrup
1 scallion, green and white parts, minced
1 tablespoon kaiware sprouts, to garnish

1. Place a strainer in a bowl, add the fresh wakame and fill
the bowl with water, letting it sit for a few seconds. Drain
and rinse the wakame under running water until the salt is
removed and the wakame doubles or triples in size. Squeeze
out the excess water and cut it into bite-sized pieces. If
you're using dried wakame, follow the instruction on the
package or rehydrate it in a bowl of water for 5 minutes.
Drain it, squeeze out the excess water, then set aside.

2. Place the fried tofu in a colander and slowly pour boiling
water, about 2 cups (500 ml), over both it. Rinse it well with
cold water, squeezing out the excess water. Cut each piece in
half crosswise.

3. Gently open the pocket in each piece of tofu and stand it
up in a small cup with the pocket facing up. Put the wakame
in the bottom of the pocket.

4. Beat the eggs and the Kaeshi Sauce together in a
measuring cup (or in a small bowl with a spout) and mix
well. Gently pour an equal amount of the egg mixture over
the wakame in each tofu pocket.

5. Close the top completely by threading a toothpick
through the tofu in a zigzag pattern. Set the tofu aside and
repeat with the remaining tofu, wakame and eggs.

6. In a medium pot, combine the stock, Kaeshi Sauce and
maple syrup and bring to a boil over medium-high heat. Add
the tofu pockets and reduce the heat to medium-low, cover
with a lid or a piece of fitted parchment paper and cook for
4 to 7 minutes or until the egg mixture is firmly set.

7. To serve, transfer the tofu pockets to a serving plate and
pour the remaining sauce over them. Garnish with the
kaiware sprouts.

Tofu Fritters with Edamame

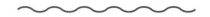

There was a small izakaya pub around the corner from our home growing up. They served delicious homemade fritters—simply made with tofu and shredded seasonal vegetables—and I've enjoyed them ever since. The chef made them to order, so they were piping hot and crispy on the outside, while fluffy inside. To make them, tofu is mashed into a smooth paste, and vegetables are added. They're then formed into patties and deep-fried until golden brown. The classic version always includes hijiki, which lends a nice texture to the soft tofu patty, while also adding healthy nutrients. Here, I use kombu left over from making dashi. Traditionally, we either serve these fritters with a broth or simply eat them as is. Serve these as a side dish or on their own as a snack, but serve them immediately while they're still hot and crispy!

PREPARATION TIME: 30 minutes
COOKING TIME: 25 minutes
YIELDS: 10–12

One 14-oz (400-g) medium-firm tofu
One 5-in (12-cm) square dried kombu,
   rehydrated and shredded
⅓ carrot, peeled and shredded
3 tablespoons shelled frozen
   edamame soybeans
½ teaspoon fresh ginger juice
2 tablespoons Kaeshi Sauce
   (page 40)
1 tablespoon potato starch or
   cornstarch
1 egg, beaten
1 tablespoon Shio Koji (page 53), or
   1 teaspoon sea salt
Neutral-flavored oil, for deep frying
4 tablespoons Tosazu Sauce (see Tip)
   or Ponzu Sauce (page 40)
6 shiso leaves, to garnish (optional)
2 tablespoons grated daikon radish,
   to garnish (optional)

1. Wrap the tofu in a tea towel. Place the tofu on a plate and place another plate or a wooden cutting board on top of it for 30 minutes. The pressure of the weight will draw out excess moisture from the tofu. Pour off the water. If the tofu is still wet, put it in a kitchen towel and gently squeeze the water out.

2. Use a potato masher to mash the tofu into a smooth texture (similar to the consistency of mashed potatoes). Add the kombu, carrots, edamame, ginger juice, Kaeshi Sauce, potato starch, egg and Shio Koji. Mix well. The filling should be creamy yet firm enough to form patties. If it's too wet, add more potato starch.

3. Fill a heavy-bottomed pot with about 2 in (5 cm) of oil and bring it to 325°F (160°C) over medium heat.

4. Form the tofu mixture into small, oval patties about 2 in (5 cm) in size and gently drop them into the oil. Don't over-crowd the pot—if all the pieces don't fit at one time, fry them in batches. Cook over medium-low heat for about 2 to 4 minutes on each side, for a total of 5 to 7 minutes or until the tofu is light golden brown.

5. Drain the fritters on a wire rack and sprinkle with salt while they are hot.

6. Serve immediately, accompanied by Tosazu Sauce or Ponzu Sauce.

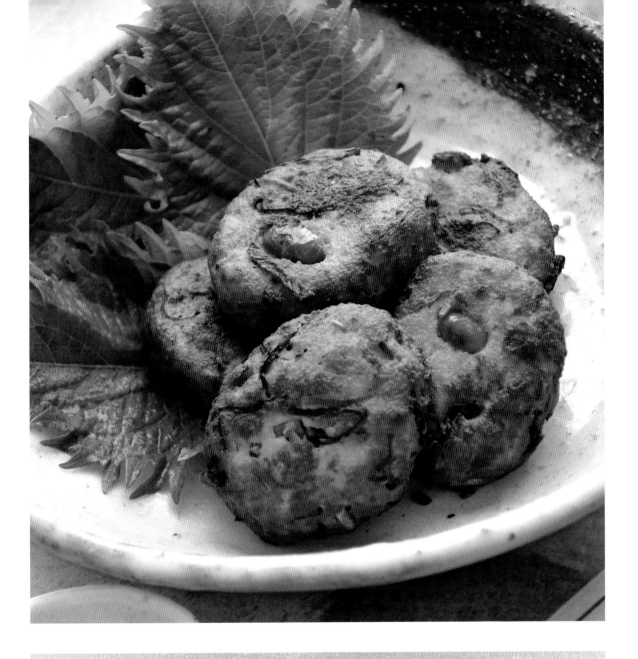

TIP Tosazu is a popular vinegar sauce that is traditionally made with katsuobushi, soy sauce and vinegar. It is often served with sunomono, vinegar-based fish or vegetables dishes that are served as side dishes and small plates in Japanese cuisine. The deep savory flavors from the kombu and katsuobushi add a layer of flavor that is a perfect condiment for dipping white-fish sashimi and fresh oysters, some of my favorite non-cooked dishes. Tosazu is an old-fashioned name for an area in the Shikoku region—where fishermen have long caught katsuo (bonito)—and it is used for cooking their local dishes by infusing the smoky flavor of shaved katsuobushi (bonito flakes) into thevinegar to make it less acidic, and also adding a hint of umami. In this recipe, I am using Basic Dashi Stock for an easy preparation for home cooks. You can make your own Tosazu Sauce by combining ½ cup (125 ml) Basic Dashi Stock (page 36), 2 tablespoons soy sauce, 2 tablespoons rice vinegar, 1 tablespoon katsuobushi into a sterilized glass bottle or jar with a lid. Shake it well to combine all the ingredients and store, tightly covered, in the refrigerator.

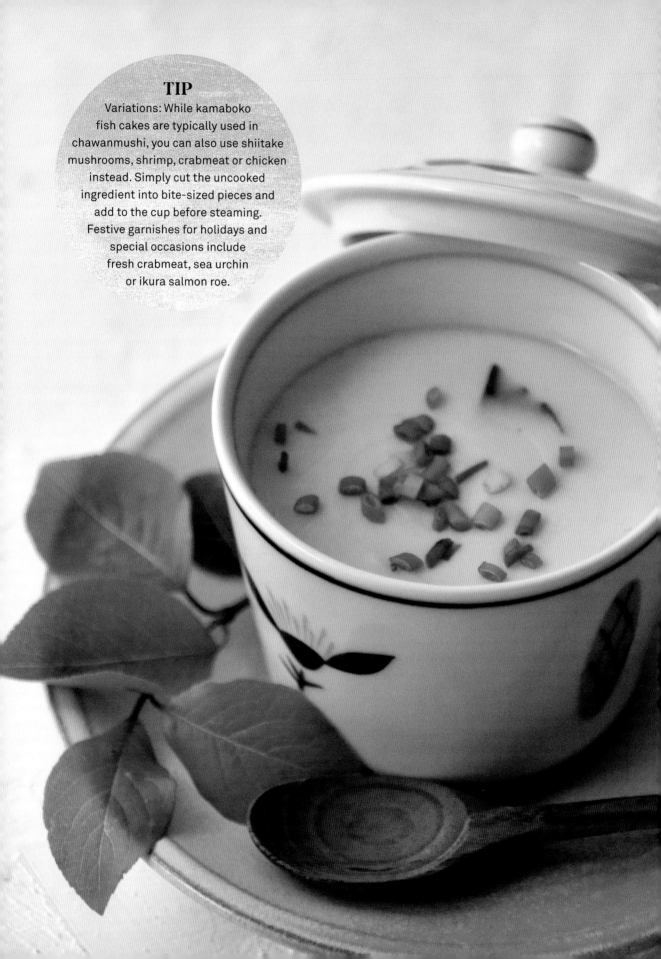

TIP

Variations: While kamaboko fish cakes are typically used in chawanmushi, you can also use shiitake mushrooms, shrimp, crabmeat or chicken instead. Simply cut the uncooked ingredient into bite-sized pieces and add to the cup before steaming. Festive garnishes for holidays and special occasions include fresh crabmeat, sea urchin or ikura salmon roe.

Savory Egg Custard with Mochi and Wakame

Can you imagine serving a steamed egg custard in a small teacup as an appetizer at your next family dinner? Impressive indeed and the meal has barely started! Traditionally served in a small ceramic cup covered with a lid, you open it releasing a rush of dashi-scented steam, then eat a spoonful of the creamy custard and discover the numerous bite-sized surprises hidden within: shrimp, shiitake mushrooms, chicken and bamboo shoots. You never know what you'll discover inside the custard, which is what I love about this dish. You can use your favorite teacups for making this dish, and I'll show you how to finish the custards, so they're perfectly set, if you don't have a food steamer.

PREPARATION TIME: 20 minutes
COOKING TIME: 30 minutes
SERVES 4

3 eggs
1½ cups (375 ml) Basic Dashi Stock (page 36)
2 tablespoons Kaeshi Sauce (page 40)
3 tablespoons fresh or dried wakame
1 unsweetened mochi rice cake, 1.5 x 2.5 in (4 x 6 cm)
1-in (2.5-cm) piece kamaboko fish cake
3 tablespoons frozen edamame soybeans
1 tablespoon chives, chopped, to garnish

1. Add the water to your steamer and heat the pan over medium heat. If you don't have a steamer, use a large pot with a lid to create a water bath. Place four empty teacups into a pan and add water to the pan to reach about ⅓ of the way up each cup. Remove the cups from the pan and place it over medium heat.

2. In a medium bowl, whisk the eggs and add the Basic Dashi Stock and Kaeshi Sauce, mixing well. Strain the mixture through a sieve into a clean bowl and set aside.

3. Place a strainer in a bowl, add the fresh wakame and fill the bowl with water and let it sit for a few seconds. Drain and rinse the wakame under running water until the salt is removed and the wakame doubles or triples in size. Squeeze out the excess water and cut it into bite-sized pieces. If you're using dried wakame, follow the instruction on the package or rehydrate it in a bowl of water for 5 minutes. Drain it, squeeze out the excess water, then set aside.

4. Cut the mochi and kamaboko into 4 pieces each.

5. Place the wakame, mochi, kamaboko and edamame in chawanmushi cups or teacups. Gently pour the egg mixture into each, dividing it evenly. Place the lids on the chawanmushi cups or cover each teacup with aluminum foil or plastic wrap. Carefully place the cups into the steamer or pan over medium heat for 9 to 10 minutes.

6. Check to see if the custard is set by inserting a toothpick into the center of the cup. If it comes out clean, the custard's done, and if it has egg mixture stuck to it, continue steaming until the center is set, another 1 to 2 minutes. Don't overcook the custard, as that will result in air pockets and a too firm texture instead of the desirable smooth, silky texture.

7. Carefully remove the cups from the steamer or the pan by lifting them with tongs or using a potholder or kitchen towel. They'll be extremely hot so use caution when handling them. Sprinkle some chives on top.

8. Serve the chawanmushi cups with their lids in place or remove the foil from the teacups, with each cup placed on an individual plate with a spoon.

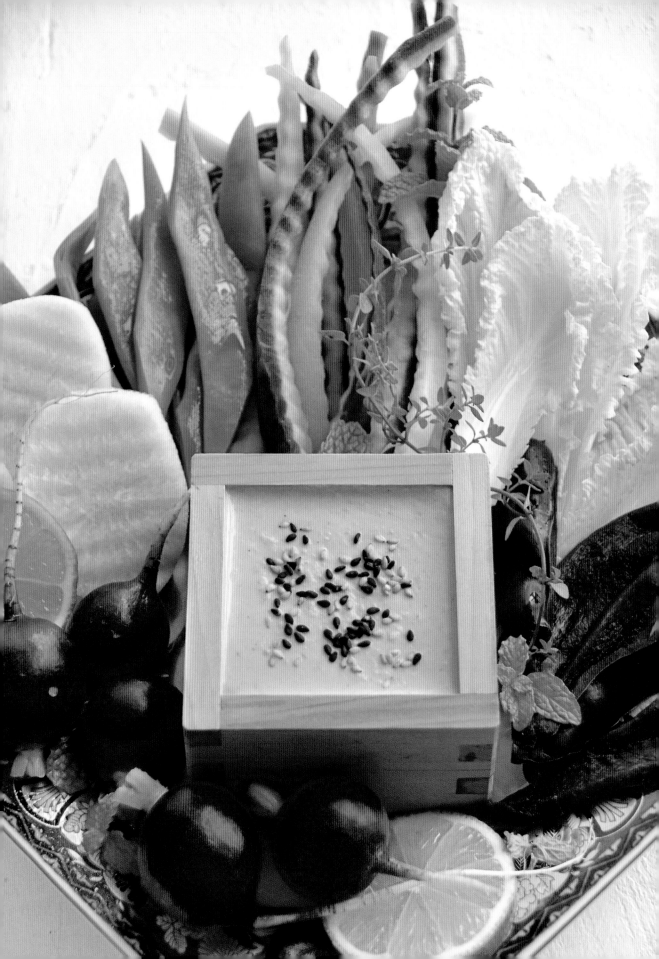

Don't Forget the Veggies!

Highlighting the healthful benefits of vegetables is a defining feature of Japanese cuisine. Emphasizing the natural flavors of plant-based ingredients and products, especially those that are in season is one of the joys of mastering adaptable four-season preparations. Regional specialties and preparations add to the healthsome, wholesome goodness.

Spring vegetables (crunchy bamboo shoots are among my favorite) are known for their strong, slightly bitter taste, which is said to improve metabolism and enliven the taste buds. Summer vegetables like cucumbers and eggplants contain a lot of water, so they help cool the body down from the heat. Fall brings various kinds of mushrooms and sweet persimmons. Finally, winter vegetables, such as daikon, lotus root and burdock root, store sugar to protect themselves from the cold weather. Here, I introduce a variety of traditional vegetable dishes that are easy and quick to prepare at home using popular Japanese vegetables you can easily find at your local farmers' market or grocery store.

Mixed Mushroom and Watercress Salad
with Walnut Miso Dressing

My grandmother had a walnut tree across the street from her house, and I often picked them fresh from the tree. She had a big grinding bowl to crush them into a paste, adding soy sauce, miso and sugar to make a sweet and savory sauce to drizzle over the vegetables she harvested on her farm. The crunchy texture pairs perfectly with fresh vegetables. This vegan recipe is cooked in the *nibitashi* style—braising the mushrooms in a Kombu Dashi Stock, letting it absorb all the flavors—a simple preparation that allows the vegetables to shine.

PREPARATION TIME: 10 minutes
COOKING TIME: 20 minutes
SERVES 4

8 oz (250 g) mixed mushrooms (buna shimeji and enoki)
1 bunch (4 oz/100 g) watercress
1½ cups (375 ml) Kombu Dashi Stock (page 38)
Pinch of salt
⅓ cup (35 g) walnuts, plus 2 table-spoons to garnish
1½ tablespoons soy sauce
1 tablespoon maple syrup
1 tablespoon Tama Miso (page 205)

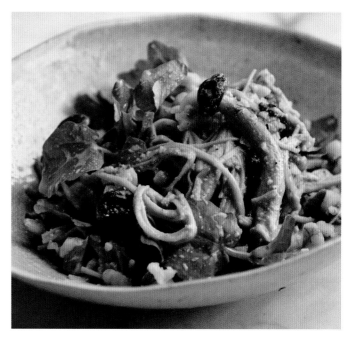

TIP For more intense umami flavor, let the mushrooms marinate in the stock in the refrigerator overnight. Save the stock from cooking the mushrooms for making soups later. You can add tofu, beaten egg and vegetables to make quick, healthy soups. Store the stock in the refrigerator for up to 3 days or in the freezer for a month.

1. Cut off the base of the cluster of mushrooms and separate them into individual stalks. If you're using an alterante type of mushroom, slice them thinly. Cut the watercress into 2-in (5-cm) pieces.

2. In a saucepan, combine the mushrooms, stock and salt and bring to a boil over medium-high heat. Cook for 5 to 7 minutes, until the mushrooms are soft. Transfer the mushrooms and the stock to a bowl and allow it to cool for 15 minutes or until it reaches room temperature.

3. Finely chop the walnuts into tiny pieces on a cutting board and transfer to a medium-sized bowl. Combine the soy sauce, maple syrup and miso in a bowl and mix well.

4. Strain the mushrooms, reserving the stock. Add the mushrooms to the bowl of sauce, then the watercress. Toss, then serve in individual bowls or a salad bowl. Crush the remaining walnuts and sprinkle them over the salad as a garnish, if you wish.

Shredded Daikon Salad
with Flying Fish Roe and Seaweed Flakes

I had this tasty salad for the first time in the mid-1990s at a tiny izakaya pub in New York. The orange-colored fish roe were popping in my mouth, and the crisp, thinly shredded daikon added a great crunchy texture. It was dressed in a creamy mayonnaise sauce that was so delicious I couldn't put my chopsticks down. The next day I re-created the recipe at home and I've been making it ever since. For garnish, I use black sesame seeds, aonori seaweed flakes and shichimi chili peppers. Hope you love it as much as I do!

PREPARATION TIME: 10 minutes
COOKING TIME: 10 minutes
SERVES 4

1 lb (450 g) daikon
⅓ cup (80 g) tobiko flying fish roe
¼ cup (65 ml) Japanese mayonnaise
1 teaspoon rice vinegar
½ teaspoon soy sauce
½ teaspoon toasted black sesame seeds, to garnish
½ teaspoon aonori seaweed flakes, to garnish
Shichimi Japanese chili pepper or cayenne pepper, to taste (optional)

1. Peel and shred the daikon using a mandolin or grater to get about 3 cups. Soak them in a bowl of water.

2. Combine the roe, mayonnaise, rice vinegar and soy sauce in a large bowl and mix well.

3. Drain the daikon then transfer it to a dish towel and squeeze out the excess water.

4. Add the daikon to the dressing bowl and mix well.

5. To serve, sprinkle the sesame seeds, aonori flakes and a touch of shichimi chili pepper for heat over the salad.

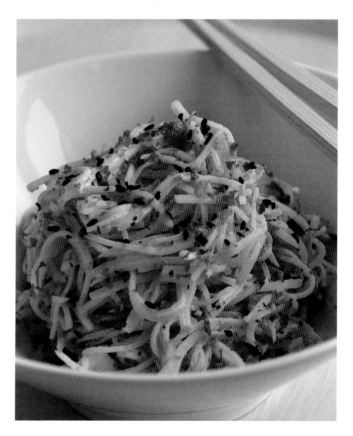

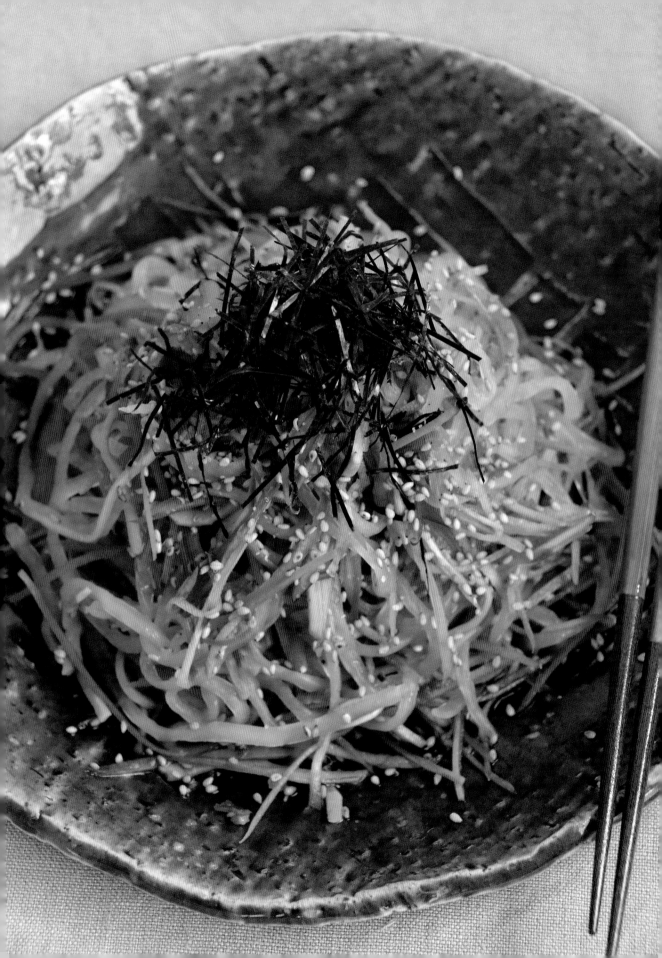

Konnyaku Noodle Salad
with Umeboshi Dressing

~~~~~~~

Also known as shirataki noodles (see page 31), thin, translucent, jelly-like konnyaku noodles are made from konjac yam and are a low-calorie, low-carb form of pasta. Two important things to remember when cooking them: if you're using fresh noodles, you'll need to drain, rinse and boil them for 2 to 3 minutes over high heat to get rid of the pungent smell. The smell may seem a bit strange to a first-timer but after rinsing and boiling, it'll disappear. For the dried version, simply rehydrate them in hot water for 5 minutes before cooking them or follow the instructions on the package. The second thing to remember? The noodles have no flavor of their own, so they need to be seasoned with flavorful dressings or sauces. Here I use an umeboshi preserved plum dressing. Umeboshi are overlooked when it comes to Japanese superfoods. They have medicinal properties, as their powerful acidity has an alkalinizing effect on the body and helps in neutralizing fatigue. They also stimulate digestion and promote the elimination of toxins. All in one salad!

PREPARATION TIME: 10 minutes
COOKING TIME: 20 minutes
SERVES 4

One 12-oz (350-g) package fresh
 or 6.2-oz (176 g) dried konnyaku
 noodles
2 carrots
2 Japanese or baby cucumbers
6 slices (6 oz/175 g) cooked ham
6 umeboshi preserved plums
 with their pits or 3 tablespoons
 umeboshi paste
⅔ cup (80 ml) Ponzu Sauce (page 40)
2 tablespoons maple syrup
¼ cup (65 ml) extra-virgin olive oil
2 tablespoons toasted white sesame
 seeds
2 teaspoons nori, finely shredded

1. If you're using fresh konnyaku noodles, discard all the water from the package and wash them under running water for a minute or so. Then in a small pot of boiling water, cook them for 2 to 3 minutes. Drain them well and squeeze out the excess water. If you're using dried konnyaku, follow the instruction on the package or rehydrate them in a bowl of hot water for 5 minutes. Drain well, squeeze out excess water, then set aside.

2. Slice the carrots, cucumber and ham into fine matchsticks.

3. If using umeboshi, remove the seeds and mash them into a fine paste with the side of your knife blade on a cutting board. Use a wide knife blade, if possible.

4. In a medium-sized bowl, combine the umeboshi paste, Ponzu Sauce, maple syrup, extra-virgin olive oil and sesame seeds and mix well. Add the noodles, carrots, cucumbers and ham and mix well again.

5. To serve, sprinkle shredded nori on top.

Crispy Vegetarian Spring Rolls

This is one of the most popular appetizers I make when I host home parties and pop-up dinner events. Everybody loves these crispy, spring rolls filled with lots of vegetables and a savory sauce inside. They combine the crunch of bamboo shoots with the soft texture of mixed vegetables, and the glossy potato starch gravy is a nice finishing touch binding everything together. The key to creating crispy spring rolls is to fry them twice, at two different temperatures. The first time, they're fried over medium heat, 325ºF (160ºC), for 6 to 7 minutes, until light brown. The second time they're fried at a hotter temperature, 375ºF (190ºC), for about 1 minute, until they're golden brown. Use a thermometer that clips onto the side of the pot to gauge the temperature. The two different stages of frying first cook the filling through then crisp up the wrappers perfectly. If you are not familiar with bamboo shoots, they are truly a great ingredient to try in these spring rolls. They bring a very nice crunchy texture, and an authentic Japanese flair to the dish. You can find boiled bamboo shoots in the refrigerated section of Japanese grocery stores, or sold thinly sliced in cans available at any Asian market and at health food stores. If you can't find boiled bamboo shoots, you can substitute with a medium-sized zucchini.

PREPARATION TIME: 30 minutes
COOKING TIME: 15 minutes
SERVES 4

½ cup (25 g) vermicelli noodles
2 leaves napa cabbage
2 shiitake mushrooms, stems removed
6 oz (175 g) boiled bamboo shoots, or 1 medium zucchini
¼ green bell pepper
½ carrot
2 tablespoons sesame oil
1 teaspoon ginger, peeled and minced
1 teaspoon garlic, minced
⅔ cup (160 ml) Basic or Second-Brew Dashi Stock (pages 36–7)
3 tablespoons Kaeshi Sauce (page 40)
2 tablespoons potato starch or cornstarch
Neutral-flavored oil, for deep-frying
8 spring roll wrappers
3 tablespoons water
Chives, chopped, to garnish (optional)
2 tablespoons mayonnaise (optional)
1 tablespoon yellow mustard (optional)
2 tablespoons rice vinegar (optional)

1. Soak the vermicelli noodles in hot water for 5 minutes until they're soft. Drain them and cut them into 2-in (5-cm) pieces. Cut the cabbage, shiitake, bamboo shoots, bell pepper and carrot into thin, long strips.

2. Heat the oil in a skillet on high and fry the vegetables, ginger and garlic for 3 to 4 minutes.

3. In a small bowl, combine the stock, Kaeshi Sauce and potato starch and mix well. Then, add the mixture to the skillet and cook for another 1 to 2 minutes over medium-high heat.

4. Add the vermicelli noodles (and zucchini, if you're using it) to the skillet and cook over medium heat for 1 minute, until the liquid is reduced by half. Transfer the filling to a container and let it cool in the refrigerator for 15 to 20 minutes. Divide the filling into 8 portions.

5. Fill a heavy-bottomed pot with about 2 inches of oil and bring it to 325ºF (160ºC) over medium heat.

6. Fill a cup with water and set it by your work surface. Gently peel off one wrapper, keeping the rest under a damp paper towel.

7. Lay the wrapper on a large plate and place one portion of filling just below the center of the wrapper.

8. Fold the left and right sides of the wrapper in toward the filling.

9. Fold the bottom over the filling toward the top and roll the wrapper to cover the filling tightly.

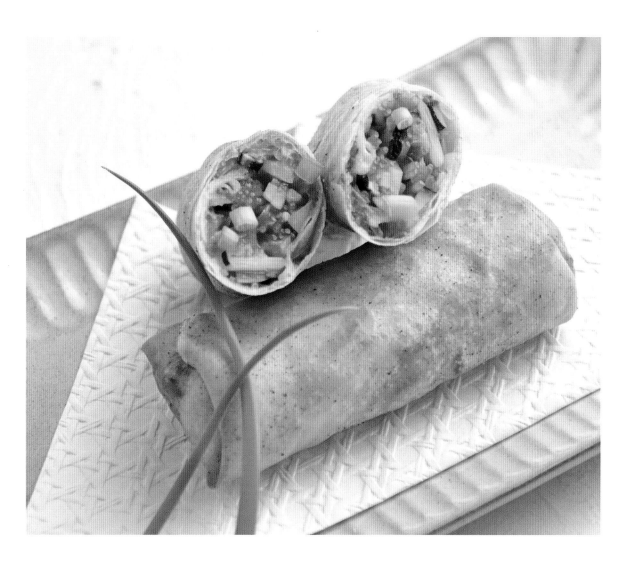

10. Dip your index finger in the water and run it along the edge of the wrapper, then firmly press to seal. Repeat with the remaining wrappers and filling.

11. Heat the oil to 325°F (160°C). Gently drop the spring rolls one at a time into the oil and cook for 2 to 3 minutes, until light brown. Flip them, using chopsticks or tongs, and fry the other side for 2 to 3 minutes, also until light brown. Don't overcrowd the pot—if all the pieces don't fit at one time, fry them in batches.

12. Remove them from the pot, put them on a plate and increase the heat to bring the oil temperature up to 375°F (190°C). Gently drop the rolls back into the oil and cook for 1 minute, until golden brown and crispy. Drain the spring rolls on a wire rack. To make the dipping sauce, combine the mayonnaise, mustard and vinegar in a small bowl and mix well.

13. Place the spring rolls on a large plate and garnish with the chives on top. Serve with the dipping sauce on the side.

TIP Store leftover bamboo shoots in the refrigerator for up to a week in a covered container filled with water, changing the water every day. Or slice them thinly and store them in a resealable plastic bag in the freezer for up to a month. They're a nice addition to stir fries.

To prepare the zucchini as a substitute for bamboo shoots, trim off the ends, scoop out the seeds, then cut it into 2-inch (5-cm) matchsticks.

Lotus Root Chips
with Aonori Seaweed Sprinkles

Lotus root, the edible root of the pink lotus flower, is widely used in Asian cuisine. These irresistibly delicious roots are crunchy and crispy like water chestnuts, even after cooking. They also boast a wide range of health benefits such as boosting the immune system and improving digestion, and they're high in fiber as well. The flavor is naturally sweet, so if you get tired of potato chips, lotus root chips are a fun new alternative to try out. You can find lotus root at any Asian market either whole or presliced and packaged in the refrigerated section. These lotus root chips are not only great for snacking, they also add an extra crunchy texture and unique presentation to salads. For the garnish, I use aonori seaweed flakes. Aonori is dried green laver or seaweed crushed into tiny flakes. It's a great finishing touch, lending a beautiful aroma to the food.

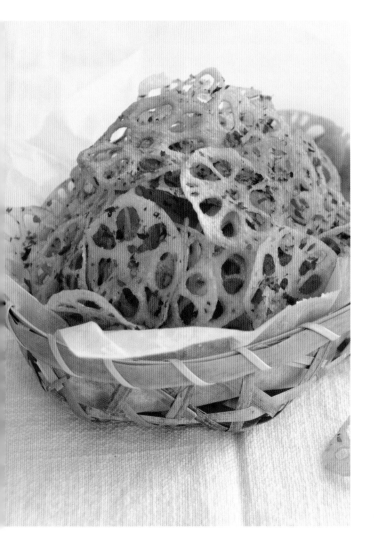

PREPARATION TIME: 10 minutes
COOKING TIME: 20 minutes
SERVES 4

2 fresh lotus roots, about 1 lb (500 g)
Neutral-flavored oil, for deep-frying
¼ teaspoon sea salt
½ tablespoon aonori seaweed flakes,
  to garnish

1. Peel the lotus root. The skin is thin and easy to peel. Cut into thin slices, using either a mandoline or a sharp knife. Soak the slices in a bowl of water for 10 minutes.

2. Fill a heavy-bottomed pot with about 2 in (5 cm) of oil and bring it to 360°F (180°C) over medium heat.

3. Drain the lotus root slices and pat them dry with a paper towel.

4. Fry in batches over medium-low heat until they're crispy and light brown, about 1 to 2 minutes. Use tongs to remove them immediately, otherwise they'll continue to cook and will quickly burn. Transfer to a rack set over a rimmed sheet pan, sprinkling immediately with the salt and aonori seaweed flakes. Let them cool, then serve them in a basket or bowl.

Braised Burdock Root
with Carrot and Kombu

This braised burdock root and carrot dish is crunchy, earthy and savory. Since I regularly have leftover kombu from making dashi, I add some to my kinpira gobo to boost the flavor and texture. So what is kinpira? It's a Japanese cooking technique in which thinly sliced ingredients are first stir-fried in oil then simmered with sweet and savory soy sauce. This popular dish takes just a few steps and proves a perfect pairing with steamed rice. Because kinpira gobo is one of the most common side dishes in Japan, home chefs add their own spin to individualize this classic. My grandmother always added lots of chili flakes and more sugar, but my kid-friendly version isn't particularly spicy. It's a forgiving recipe you can make in your own style as long as you know the basic steps.

PREPARATION TIME: 15 minutes
COOKING TIME: 15 minutes
SERVES 4

Half burdock root (6 oz/175 g)
1 carrot
1 piece kombu, 4 x 6in (10 x 15 cm) leftover
  from making dashi stock
1 tablespoon extra-virgin olive oil
3 tablespoons Kaeshi Sauce (page 40)
1 teaspoon sesame oil
1 tablespoon white sesame seeds
Steamed rice and miso soup (optional)

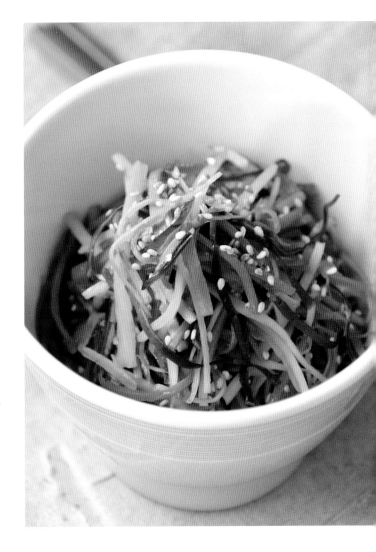

1. Peel and slice the burdock root, carrot and kombu into thin 2-in (5-cm) strips. Soak the burdock in water for 10 minutes, changing the water a couple of times to get rid of the bitterness, then drain well.

2. Heat the oil in a frying pan and fry the burdock for a couple of minutes over medium-high heat. Add the carrots and kombu to the pan and fry for 3 to 5 minutes more.

3. Add the Kaeshi Sauce and cook over medium-low heat until the liquid is almost evaporated, 1 to 2 minutes.

4. Add the sesame oil and sesame seeds and fry for 30 seconds over medium-low heat. Turn off the heat. Serve with steamed rice and miso soup, if you like.

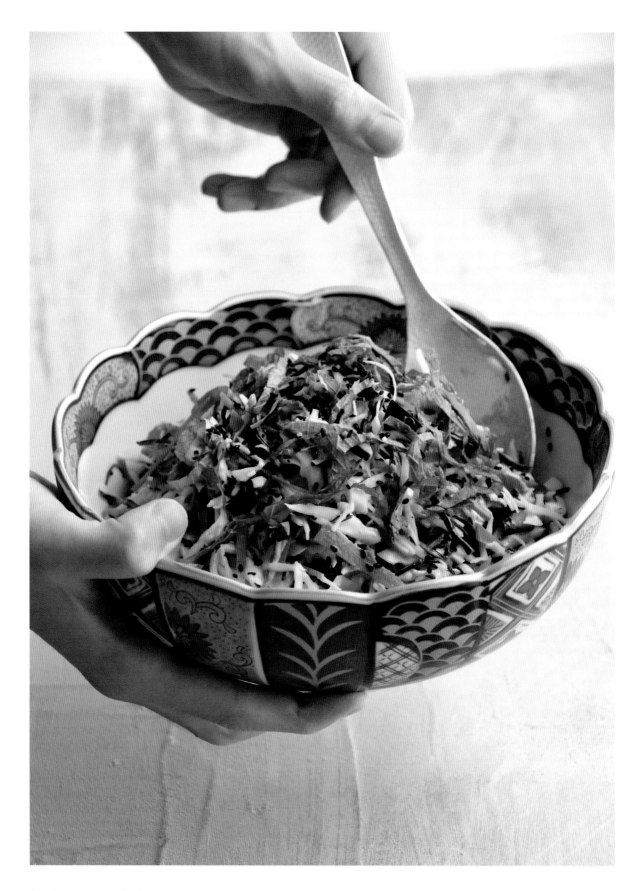

Japanese-style Coleslaw

No barbecue is complete without a big bowl of fresh, crisp coleslaw. If you're in the mood to try something different from the ordinary coleslaw, I've got you covered! This Japanese-style coleslaw is bright and crunchy with a tangy flavor that's well balanced with its sweet and sour dressing made from Japanese mayonnaise and an umeboshi pickled plum. I know it sounds a bit exotic, but the pickled plum works just like vinegar, cutting the richness of mayonnaise while adding a boost of flavor that brightens up the slaw in the most unexpected way. While you can buy preshredded cabbage, I prefer mine superfresh, so I shred it myself using a Japanese mandoline (or a box grater). Then, the shredded ingredients are soaked in cold water for 10 minutes to make them extra crunchy. They are then drained and stored, undressed, in a large container in the refrigerator (for up to 2 days) until you are ready to serve, if you have a plan to make this for your next party. The quick dressing can also be stored in the refrigerator (in a glass jar) until you are ready to put the salad together, making this a perfect make-ahead dish for your next party. I use Japanese mayonnaise for the dressing, as it is bit more eggy and richer in flavor than Western mayonnaise.

PREPARATION TIME: 15 minutes
COOKING TIME: 20 minutes
SERVES 4

¼ green cabbege (7 oz/200 g)
⅛ purple cabbage (4 oz/100 g)
⅔ carrot
½ Fuji apple
2 tablespoons extra-virgin olive oil
2 tablespoons Sushi Vinegar (page 52)
3 tablespoons Japanese mayonnaise
  or Western mayonnaise
1 umeboshi preserved plum with pit
  or ½ tablespoon umeboshi paste
1 teaspoon maple syrup
2 tablespoons black sesame seeds,
  toasted
4 shiso leaves, cut in a chiffonade,
  to garnish (optional)

1. Core then shred the cabbages. Peel and shred the carrot. Soak everything in a large bowl filled with cold water for 10 minutes. Shred the apple (with the skin on) and soak it in a small bowl of water, with a pinch of salt added, for 10 minutes. Drain both bowls well and store the cabbage, carrots and apple in a large, covered container in the refrigerator until you're ready to serve the slaw.

2. Remove the pit from the umeboshi, then mash it into a fine paste with the side of your knife blade on a cutting board. Use a wide knife blade, if possible.

3. In a small glass jar or a container with a lid, combine the umeboshi, oil, vinegar, mayonnaise, maple syrup and sesame seeds. Mix well.

4. Remove the slaw from the refrigerator and toss it with the dressing, making sure the dressing coats all the ingredients evenly. Taste for seasoning and add additional salt or vinegar, if needed.

5. To serve, garnish the slaw with the shiso, if you like.

Edamame Hummus

In Japan, fresh edamame soybeans are readily available in summer. I'm a big fan of classic hummus made with chickpeas and was quite surprised to discover how light and refreshing it is when made with edamame instead. My version includes miso instead of herbs and spices, to add authentic Japanese flavors. Adding Kombu Water and miso lends a naturally sweet and savory flavor that's a nice riff on classic hummus. This is my popular go-to appetizer when I host events. I normally make the dip a day in advance and keep it in the refrigerator until I'm ready to serve it. Then I go to a local farmers market to find gorgeous-looking seasonal vegetables to serve with the dip.
To top it all off, I use white sesame oil.

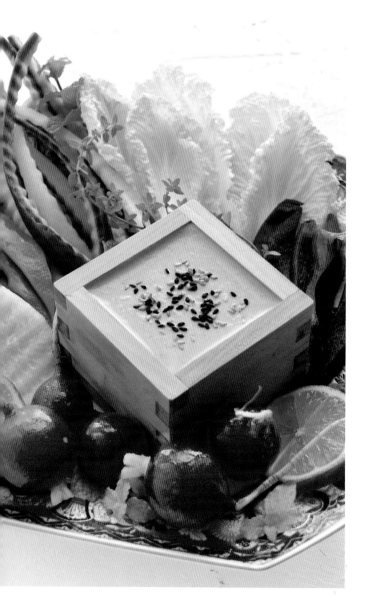

PREPARATION TIME: 5 minutes
COOKING TIME: 15 minutes
SERVES 4

1 cup (150 g) frozen, shelled edamame
    soybeans
2 tablespoons nerigoma sesame paste or
    tahini
⅔ cup (160 ml) Kombu Water or Basic Dashi
    Stock (pages 36, 38)
1 tablespoon fresh lemon juice
1 clove garlic
1 tablespoon Tama Miso (page 205)
2 tablespoons white sesame oil or extra-
    virgin olive oil
¼ teaspoon sea salt
Pepper, to taste
½ teaspoon toasted black and white sesame
    seeds, to garnish
Mixed vegetables sticks, crackers or tortilla
    chips, to serve (optional)

1. Fill a medium-sized pot ⅔ full with unsalted water and bring to a boil. Boil the edamame for 4 to 5 minutes, rinse them under cold running water, then set aside.

2. Puree the edamame, nerigoma, Kombu Water, lemon juice, garlic, miso and oil in a food processor until it reaches a smooth, creamy consistency. Taste it and add salt and pepper, if needed.

3. To serve, pour the dip into a bowl and sprinkle the sesame seeds on top. Serve it with assorted vegetables sticks, crackers or tortilla chips on the side, if using.

Cherry Tomato and Avocado Salad
with Shredded Nori, Shiso and Sesame Dressing

We grow so many cherry tomatoes in our garden in Japan, we consume them in salads, sauces and as juices almost every day when they're in season. This creamy, simple little salad—with its various flavor profiles—adds variety to the sudden bumper crop. This preparation is called *gomaae*, in which vegetables are simply tossed with Japanese-style creamy sesame dressing. You can use any type of seasonal vegetables for this appetizer. If you can't find shiso, you can use fresh coriander leaves, arugula or kale. This is an easy and quick five-ingredient recipe. Just be sure to have the sesame dressing ready in the refrigerator!

PREPARATION TIME: 5 minutes
COOKING TIME: 10 minutes
SERVES 3 to 4

20 cherry tomatoes (about 1 lb/450 g)
1 ripe avocado
3 tablespoons Goma Sesame Dressing
   (page 40)
5 shiso leaves
1 tablespoon shredded nori

1. Cut the cherry tomatoes in half. Cut the avocado in half, remove the skin and the pit, and cut into bite-sized pieces. Tear the shiso leaves with your hands.

2. In a medium-sized bowl, combine the tomatoes, avocado, shiso leaves, and Goma Sesame Dressing and mix well. To serve, sprinkle shredded nori on top.

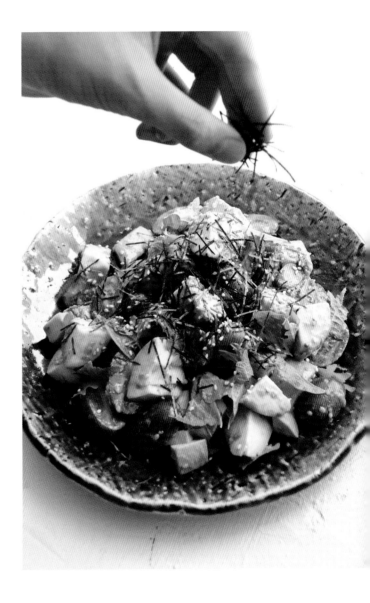

TIP
This dish is generally an appetizer, but it can easily be served as a main dish. Make an open-face sandwich by spreading a thin layer of mayonnaise on toasted sourdough bread, then pile a few spoonfuls of the salad on top.

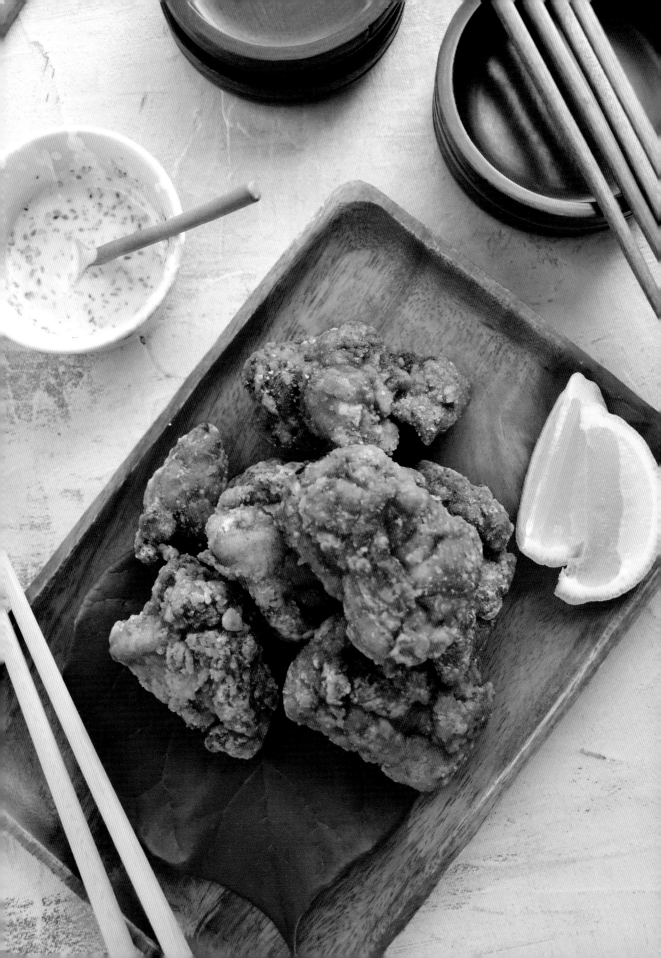

Healthy Meat Dishes

Eating high-quality protein is essential for health and longevity. Japanese cuisine has shifted from a primarily plant-based diet to one that includes animal proteins. Meat is essential in keeping bones strong and blood vessels healthy and flavorfully fits into the newer and wider conception of a well-balanced Japanese diet.

There are a number of beloved classic Japanese meat-based dishes, usually inspired by foreign cuisine but developed with unique Japanese cooking methods and flavors. Japanese-style beef curry, hamburgers and pork cutlets, for example, are very common in Japan and are now spreading worldwide. Here I introduce some of the most popular meat dishes (such as karaage fried chicken, gyoza and yakitori) that often appear in Japanese lunch boxes. Since they're also delicious eaten cold, I always make extra. Or I'll freeze the leftovers for a tasty, healthy and quick weeknight meal down the road.

Miso Marinated Chicken with Bok Choy

If you have only cooked with miso as an ingredient for soup, try this miso grilled chicken. You will realize that miso has so much more to offer as a way to make any food tastier. By marinating chicken in miso, an extra layer of deep umami flavor is added, as well as giving it a nice caramelized finish when grilled. Miso is also linked to a variety of health benefits, including better digestion and a stronger immune system. Please note that since miso marinades tend to burn while cooking, it is important to remove it before cooking—the flavor will remain, as it has already penetrated the chicken during the marinating step. I always make a double batch of this dish and save some for my son's school lunch for the next day. It is just as delicious to eat at room temperature as it is warm, making it a perfect dish for your bento box. I often serve this chicken on a bed of crunchy bok choy along with steamed rice for a quick weeknight supper. You can store uncooked, marinated miso chicken in the refrigerator for up to two days or in the freezer for 1 month.

PREPARATION TIME: 10 minutes
MARINADING TIME: 8 hours to two days
COOKING TIME: 20 minutes
SERVES 4

4 chicken thighs, 2 lbs (1 kg), boneless and skinless
8 tablespoons Tama Miso (page 205)
2 large bok choy
Pinch of sea salt
2 tablespoons extra-virgin olive oil
Steamed rice (optional)

1. Using a small, sharp knife, remove any excess fat from the chicken and pierce the skin with a fork. Using your fingers, rub the chicken well with the Tama Miso, then put it in a medium-sized freezer-safe resealable bag. Press the air out of the bag and seal it tightly. Place it in the refrigerator to marinate for at least 8 hours or up to 2 days.

2. Cut the bok choy stems into quarters. Cut the leaves into 2-in (5-cm) pieces.

3. Remove and discard the miso from the chicken with a paper towel or with your hands, then set aside.

4. Add the oil to a skillet and heat it over medium until the oil shimmers. Place the chicken in the pan and grill it over medium heat for 4 to 6 minutes or until golden brown over. Turn the chicken over, pressing it down with a pot lid, if you wish. Grill for another 4 to 6 minutes over medium-low heat until the second side is golden brown.

5. Add more oil if it's needed, then add the bok choy to the pan. Cover and cook over medium-low heat until it's tender, about 1 to 2 minutes. Add a pinch of salt to the bok choy and chicken. Check the chicken by piercing it with a fork. When its juices run clear, it's done. Remove the chicken and the bok choy from the pan. Cut the chicken into ½-inch (1.25-cm) slices and serve it with bok choy over steamed rice, if you wish.

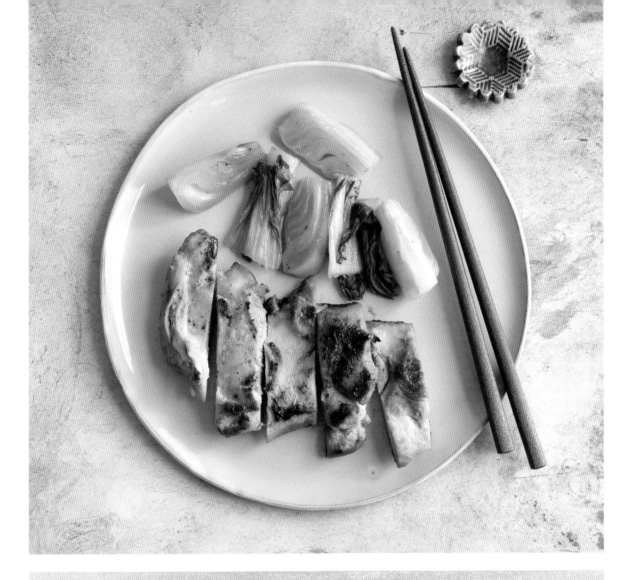

Tama Miso

Tama Miso is a family recipe that has been handed down and is my go-to miso seasoning. It adds a wonderful velvety texture, and a sweet-savory flavor works well with any dish. It also is a good marinade for meat and fish as it acts as a tenderizer.

MAKE : approx. ¾ cup (185 ml)
SHELF LIFE: Store in an airtight container in the refrigerator for up to 2 weeks.

½ cup (125 ml) awase miso (page 15)
4 tablespoons granulated sugar
3 tablespoons mirin
3 tablespoons sake
1 egg yolk

1. Combine the miso, sugar, mirin and sake in a small saucepan and bring to a boil over medium-high heat.

2. Reduce the heat to medium-low, add the yolk to the pan and cook for 5 to 7 minutes. Using a spatula, continually stir until all the ingredients are well mixed, the sugar is dissolved, and you start to see small bubbles around the edge of the pan. When the yolk is fully cooked and the sauce takes on a thick, velvety texture, turn off the heat.

3. Transfer to a sterilized bottle or glass jar with a lid. Let cool to room temperature, then store, tightly covered, in the refrigerator.

Glazed Chicken Meatballs

This recipe has been in my family for over four decades. My mom first came across it at a local cooking school she attended in the 1970s. Every time she returned from class, she'd re-create the same dishes at home, so we got to try something new and delicious for the first time. With a few tweaks over the years, we still enjoy these juicy and flavorful chicken meatballs cooked in a rich dashi soy sauce with fresh ginger. These meatballs are the ultimate comfort food, and I hope you like them as much as I do.

PREPARATION TIME:15 minutes
COOKING TIME: 25 minutes
SERVES 4 (20 meatballs)

12 scallions, green and white
  parts divided
1¼ lbs (600 g) ground chicken
1 egg, beaten
½ teaspoon salt
4 tablespoons potato starch or
  cornstarch
¼ cup (65 ml) Basic Dashi Stock
  (page 36)
¼ cup (65 ml) Kaeshi Sauce
  (page 40)
3 tablespoons granulated sugar
2 tablespoons sake
1 tablespoon fresh ginger juice
1 tablespoon extra-virgin
  olive oil
1 teaspoon toasted white
  sesame seeds, to garnish

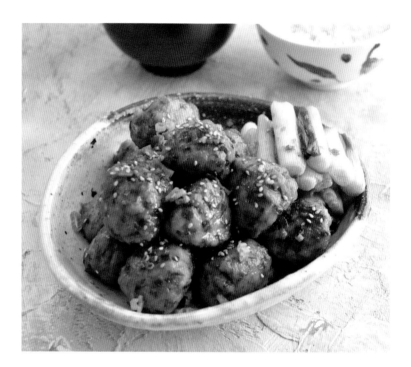

1. Trim the scallions and finely mince 7 of them, both the white and green parts, reserving 1 tablespoon for garnish. Cut the remaining 5 scallions, both the white and green parts, into 2-in (5-cm) lengths.

2. Combine the ground chicken and the minced green onions in a medium-sized bowl, adding the egg, salt and potato starch and mixing well with your hands until it turns paler in color and sticky. Chill the meat mixture in the refrigerator for 15 to 20 minutes before shaping it into balls.

3. In a small bowl, combine the Basic Dashi Stock, Kaeshi Sauce, sugar, sake and ginger juice, then mix well and set aside.

4. For each meatball, scoop out 2 tablespoons of mixture and roll it between your hands to form a smooth ball.

5. Heat the oil in a large skillet over medium-high heat. Place the meatballs in the pan and fry them for about 4 to 6 minutes. Turn them over, frying for another 3 to 5 minutes. Add the Kaeshi Sauce to the skillet and simmer covered for 4 to 5 minutes. Coat the meatballs with the sauce by gently shaking the pan over medium-low heat. Add the green onions to the skillet, cover and simmer for 1 minute more.

6. Arrange the meatballs on a serving dish and drizzle them with some of the sauce. Sprinkle with the chopped green onions and sesame seeds. For a complete meal, serve with rice and miso soup.

Pan-seared Chicken
with Garlic Soy Sauce and Butter Glaze

Juicy, tender, flavorful chicken without needing to marinate it? The secret is to lightly dredge the chicken in flour. This extra step helps seal in the moisture while it's cooking. I use extra-virgin olive oil first and then finish it off with Kaeshi Sauce and Basic Dashi Stock and a touch of butter and garlic to create a deliciously velvety glaze.

PREPARATION TIME: 10 minutes
COOKING TIME: 20 minutes
SERVES 4

4 chicken thighs, 2 lbs (1 kg), boneless and skinless
3 tablespoons all-purpose flour
4 tablespoons Kaeshi Sauce (page 40)
1 tablespoon Basic Dashi Stock (page 36) or water
1 tablespoon minced garlic
1 tablespoon extra-virgin olive oil
1 tablespoon unsalted butter
Freshly ground black pepper, to taste
4 cups (20 g) mixed salad greens
1 medium or 8 cherry tomatoes, cut into bite-sized pieces (optional)

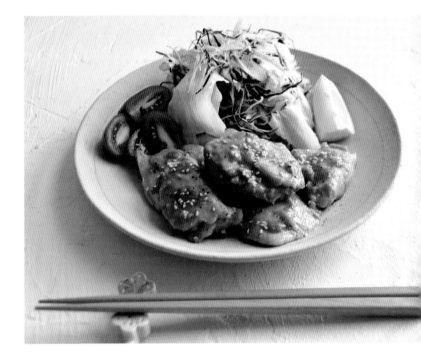

1. Place the chicken thighs on a cutting board and trim away any excess fat with a knife. Cut each thigh into four pieces, about 2 in (5 cm) each.

2. In a medium-sized bowl, dredge the chicken in the flour, then shake off any excess and set aside

3. Combine the Kaeshi Sauce, stock and garlic in a small bowl and mix well.

4. Add the oil to a skillet over medium-high heat until it shimmers. Place the chicken in the pan and cook for 4 to 5 minutes, without moving it, until it's golden brown. Turn the chicken over and cover the pan. Cook for another 5 to 6 minutes over medium-low heat, until the second side is golden brown.

5. Add the Kaeshi Sauce mixture and butter to the pan. Cover and cook over medium heat 1 to 2 minutes, adding freshly ground pepper. Check the chicken by piercing it with a fork. When its juices run clear, it's done. Remove the chicken from the pan. Serve it with salad and tomatoes and pour the remaining sauce from the pan over the chicken. For a complete meal, serve it with pasta, noodles or steamed rice.

Japanese-style Beef Stew with Potatoes, Carrots and Onions

Beef stew with potatoes, onions and carrots, nikujaga, is as popular as sushi and ramen in Japanese cuisine. Traditionally, thinly sliced beef (short ribs) is used for this recipe, but I started using ground beef one day when I did not have short ribs on hand. Since it came out as good as the version made with sliced beef, and ground beef is widely available, I have started making this version more often these days. You can also use ground chicken. I also add konnyaku noodles (or shirataki noodles), thin, translucent, jelly-like noodles made from konjac yam. You can find konnyaku noodles in Japanese markets and online and they are either sold as fresh noodles (soft, packed in water and kept in the refrigerated section), or as dried noodles. I have tried making this without konnyaku noodles, but my son insists that it is more delicious with the noodles added. I guess I have to agree with him—if you can get your hands on the konnyaku noodles, I highly recommend adding them. Serve with a bowl of steamed rice or cooked noodles and you're sure to have leftovers for lunch the next day.

PREPARATION TIME: 10 minutes
COOKING TIME: 25 minutes
SERVES 4

½ onion
14 assorted baby potatoes (7 oz/200 g)
½ carrot
½ cup (100 g) fresh konnyaku noodles (page 31, see Tip)
1 teaspoon extra-virgin olive oil
7 oz (200 g) ground beef
¼ teaspoon ginger, peeled and minced
½ cup (125 ml) Basic or Second-Brew Dashi Stock (pages 36–7)
½ tablespoon granulated sugar
5 tablespoons Kaeshi Sauce (page 40)
1 tablespoon sake
1 tablespoon minced scallions, green part
Steamed rice, for serving (optional)

1. Peel the onion and cut half of it into ½-inch (1.25-cm) pieces. Rinse the potatoes and cut them in half. Cut the carrot on the bias into oval planks.

2. If you're using fresh konnyaku noodles, discard all the water from the package and wash them under running water for 1 minute. In a small pot of boiling water, cook the noodles for 2 minutes, then drain well. If you're using dried konnyaku, rehydrate it in a bowl of hot water for 5 minutes, then drain well.

3. In a medium pot, add the oil and turn the heat to medium. Add the beef and ginger and stir until the beef changes color. Leaving the beef in the pot, wipe the excess oil with a paper towel.

4. Add the onion, potatoes, carrot and noodles to the pot and combine it with the beef. Add the stock, sugar, Kaeshi Sauce and sake and bring to a boil over medium-high heat. Skim the surface with a sieve. Reduce the heat to low, cover the pot and simmer about 10 to 12 minutes or until the potatoes and carrots are soft and the liquid is reduced by half.

5. Serve the stew with steamed rice, if you wish, sprinkling the green onions on top.

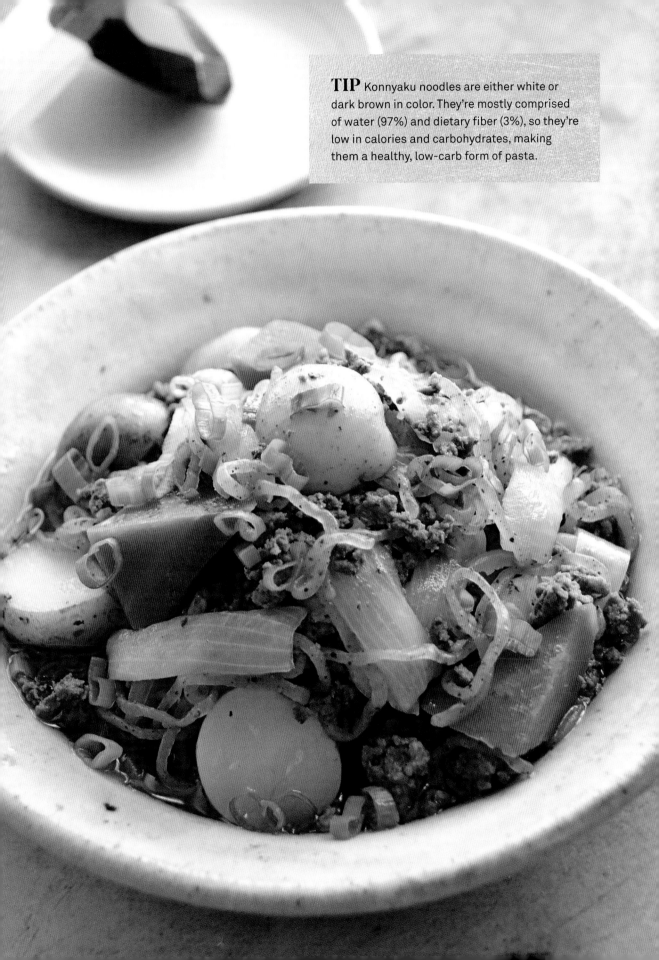

TIP Konnyaku noodles are either white or dark brown in color. They're mostly comprised of water (97%) and dietary fiber (3%), so they're low in calories and carbohydrates, making them a healthy, low-carb form of pasta.

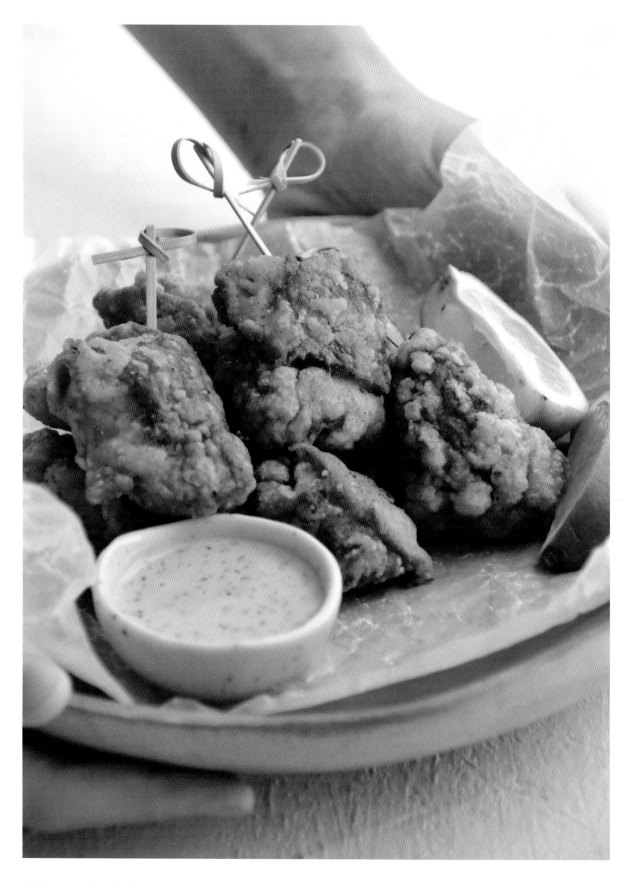

Japanese Fried Chicken Nuggets

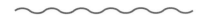

Japanese-style fried chicken, *Karaage*, is one of the most popular soul foods in Japan. You can find Karaage everywhere, at local convenience stores, Izakaya Japanese pubs, ramen shops, and even Karaage specialty restaurants. We cannot get enough of this mouthwateringly crispy, golden brown Japanese fried chicken. But guess what? It is very easy to make at home and it is the perfect dish for you to try if you have never made Japanese food! Not only is my recipe very simple to make, but all the ingredients are easy to find even if you don't have access to Japanese ingredients! Note that potato (or corn) starch plays an important role in this recipe. First, it acts as a thickener; then, very importantly, it creates the crispy texture on the chicken, so be sure that the pieces of chicken are well-coated! Finally, fried chicken must be eaten as soon as it's done—it will quickly lose its crispiness.

PREPARATION TIME: 20 minutes
COOKING TIME: 20 minutes
SERVES 4

4 chicken thighs, 2 lbs (1 kg), boneless and skinless
¼ cup (65 ml) soy sauce
1 tablespoon garlic, grated
1 tablespoon ginger, peeled and grated
1½ cups (375 g) potato starch or cornstarch, divided
Neutral-flavored oil, for deep-frying
¼ lemon, in wedges, to garnish

MAYO DIPPING SAUCE (OPTIONAL)
2 tablespoons mayonnaise
1 tablespoon rice vinegar
½ tablespoon soy sauce
1 teaspoon roasted white sesame seeds
Pinch of chili pepper, to taste

1. Place the chicken thighs on a cutting board and trim away any excess fat with a knife. Cut each thigh into four pieces, about 2 in (5 cm) each.

2. Combine the chicken, soy sauce, garlic and ginger in a large bowl, using your hands to moisten the meat, then let it sit for 15 to 20 minutes.

3. Add ½ cup of the potato starch to the bowl and mix it together with your hands until the chicken pieces are coated with the starch.

4. Fill a heavy-bottomed medium-sized pot with about 2 in (5 cm) of oil and bring it to 325°F (160°C) over medium heat.

5. Roll the chicken pieces in the remaining 1 cup of potato starch, pressing firmly to be sure the starch sticks and that each piece is evenly coated. Shake off the excess starch after coating it and lay the chicken on a plate.

6. Use a spider, sieve or slotted spoon to lower the chicken into the oil. Don't overcrowd the pot. If all the pieces don't fit at one time, fry them in batches.

7. Fry over medium-low heat for about 4 to 6 minutes on each side, for a total of 8 to 12 minutes, until the chicken is light golden brown. Check the chicken by piercing with a fork. When its juices run clear, it's done. For safety, chicken should be cooked to 165°F (75°C).

8. Drain the chicken on a wire rack with a paper-towel-lined tray beneath it to absorb the oil.

9. Serve immediately with lemon wedges. If you want to serve it with a dipping sauce, combine the mayonnaise, rice vinegar, soy sauce, sesame seeds and chili pepper in a small bowl and mix well.

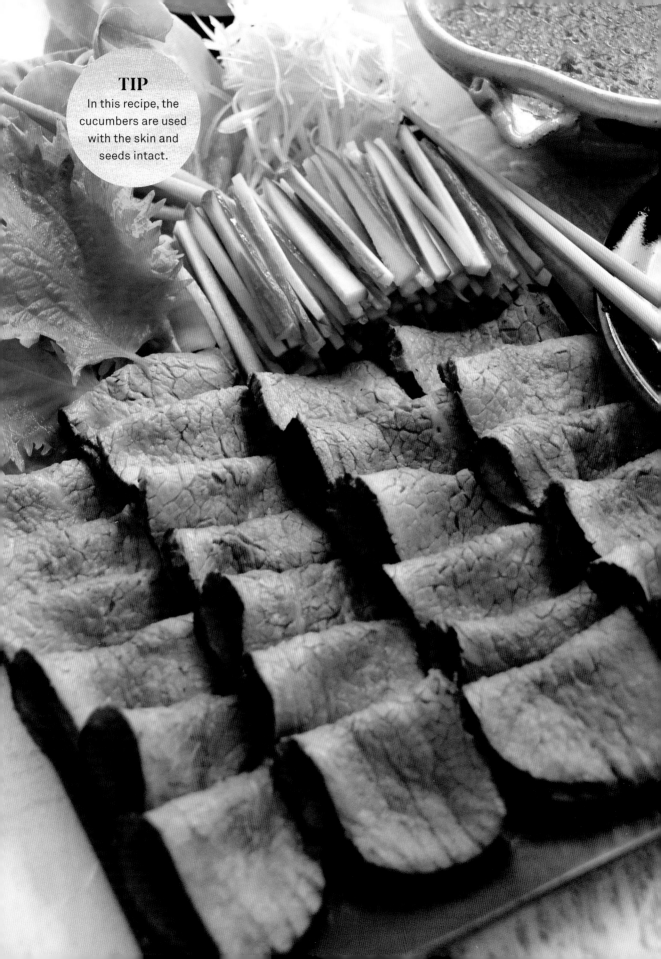

TIP

In this recipe, the cucumbers are used with the skin and seeds intact.

Japanese-style Roast Beef

〜〜〜

The fermented food I most regularly use, besides miso and soy sauce, is koji. Because koji is known for its health benefits—it's naturally packed with probiotic properties and helps strengthen the immune system—I've become obsessed with incorporating it into a variety of dishes. Here I use Shio Koji to marinate the beef. It not only lends a salty flavor, it tenderizes the meat with its natural enzymes. Be sure to remove the excess Shio Koji from the beef before cooking it to prevent it from burning. I often serve this as a weekend dinner, with a thick and flavorful onion sauce and crunchy cucumber and green onion toppings, which are a perfect garnish. Serve this with steamed rice or mashed potatoes, if you prefer.

PREPARATION TIME: 1 hour
(including marinating)
COOKING TIME: 45 minutes
SERVES 4

1½ lbs (750 g) beef eye round or boneless rump roast
4 tablespoons Shio Koji (page 53)
4 scallions, white parts only
2 Japanese or baby cucumbers
3 tablespoons extra-virgin olive oil, divided
12 butter lettuce leaves (optional)
12 shiso leaves (optional)
4 chives (optional)
Steamed rice (optional)

ONION SAUCE
1 cup (250 ml) Basic Dashi Stock (page 36)
2 tablespoons Kaeshi Sauce (page 40)
2 tablespoons Tama Miso (page 205)
2 tablespoons garlic, minced
1 medium onion, grated
2 tablespoons unsalted butter

1. Remove the beef from the refrigerator about 1 hour before cooking. Using a small, sharp knife, remove any excess fat from the beef and pierce the skin with a fork. Using your fingers, rub the beef well with the Shio Koji. Wrap the beef in plastic wrap to marinate for at least 30 minutes and up to 1 hour at room temperature.

2. Preheat the oven to 350ºF (175ºC). Cut the green onions into thin julienne strips and soak them in a small bowl of cold water for 10 minutes. Drain the water, then set aside. Cut the cucumbers into 2-in (5-cm) matchsticks, then set aside.

3. Wipe the Shio Koji off the beef with a paper towel and brush the meat with 1 tablespoon of the oil.

4. In a skillet, heat the remaining oil over medium-high heat and add the beef. Cook each side of the meat for about 1 to 2 minutes, until it's golden brown. Turn it and repeat on every side until all of the meat is golden brown. Place the beef in a roasting pan in the preheated oven. Cook until it's reached your desired degree of doneness: 130ºF/54ºC (rare), 135ºF/57ºC (medium-rare), 140ºF/60ºC (medium), and 155ºF/70ºC (well-done). Place the thermometer all the way into the center of the beef when getting a reading.

5. Remove the beef from the oven. Put it on a plate, cover it with aluminum foil and let it rest for 20 minutes before cutting.

6. Meanwhile, make the Onion Sauce by combining the stock, Kaeshi Sauce, miso, garlic and onion in a pot and bringing it to a boil over medium-high heat. Continue cooking and stirring the sauce, reducing the liquid by half, about 6 to 8 minutes. Add the butter and cook for an additional 1 to 2 minutes over medium-low heat, then turn off the heat.

7. To serve, slice the beef thinly on a cutting board (if juice runs from the beef, add it to the sauce for extra flavor). Serve the slices with the green onions and cucumbers on the side, along with steamed rice, butter lettuce, shiso leaves and the chives, if you like.

Braised Pork Belly with Daikon and Egg

Braised pork belly is a popular regional dish that originated in the Nagasaki area on the northwestern coast of Kyushu. My first visit to Nagasaki was on a high school field trip. I still remember my first bite of the pork belly—it was sensational! The soft texture and deep savory, sweet flavor was so rich, I'd never tasted anything like it before. This is a slow-cooked meal, and while it might take a bit longer to prepare, the cooking process is mostly hands-off simmering on the stovetop. Some people boil the pork before adding the seasonings, but I fry it first so it won't fall apart in the stock. Adding sake to the stock tenderizes the pork and ginger and adds great flavor to the sauce. You can serve a slice of pork as a ramen topping or donburi-style—an oversized rice bowl topped with slices of pork belly and egg. For an extra savory flavor, refrigerate the pork overnight.

PREPARATION TIME: 20 minutes
COOKING TIME: 2.5 hours
SERVES 4

1 lb (500 g) pork belly
1 tablespoon uncooked rice, any type
½ lb (225 g) daikon radish, peeled
  and cut into ½-in (1.25-cm) pieces
2½ cups (625 ml) Basic Dashi Stock
  (page 36)
One 1-in (2.5-cm) piece ginger,
  peeled and sliced into ⅛-in (3-mm)
  pieces
1 cup (250 ml) sake
⅓ cup (80 ml) Kaeshi Sauce (page 40)
2 tablespoons rice vinegar
1 piece Japanese dried chili pepper,
  seeds removed (optional)
1 bunch cilantro/coriander leaves
  and stems (about 50 g), divided
4 eggs
Steamed rice, for serving (optional)

1. Combine 4 cups of water, the pork belly and uncooked rice in a medium-sized pot. Cover and bring to a boil over medium-high heat, then reduce the heat to low and simmer for 1 hour. Skim the foam and fat from the pork with a sieve.

2. Wash the meat with water and drain it in the sink. Cut it into 1-in (2.5-cm) cubes.

3. Drain the pot and return the pork to it, adding the daikon, stock, ginger, sake, Kaeshi Sauce, rice vinegar, chili pepper and coriander, reserving 2 tablespoons of coriander leaves for garnish.

4. Cook the meat, covered, over medium heat for 1.5 hours. Skim the foam and fat from the pork with a sieve. If the stock boils down below the level of the pork, add more stock or water to cover.

5. In the meantime, add water to a small saucepan, cover, and bring to a boil. Gently add the eggs and cook for 7 minutes over medium-high heat. Use a spoon to roll and move the eggs a couple of times in the pot. Drain the eggs, let them cool, then gently peel them and set aside.

6. Add the eggs to the pot and cook over low heat for another 2 minutes. Gently spoon the sauce over everything.

7. To serve, cut the eggs in half lengthwise. Divide the pork, daikon and eggs between four plates and pour the remaining sauce from the pot over everything. Garnish with the cilantro/coriander leaves and serve it with steamed rice, if you like.

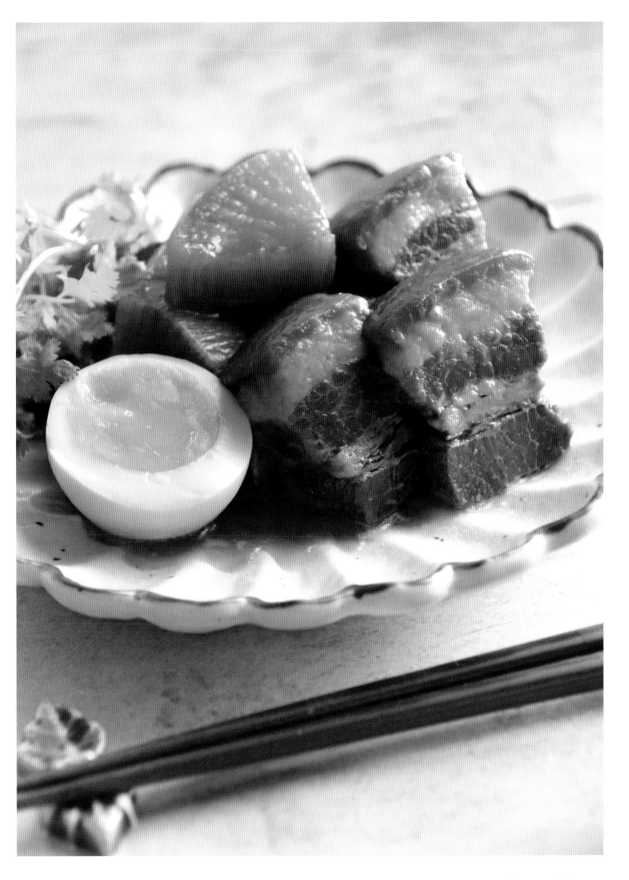

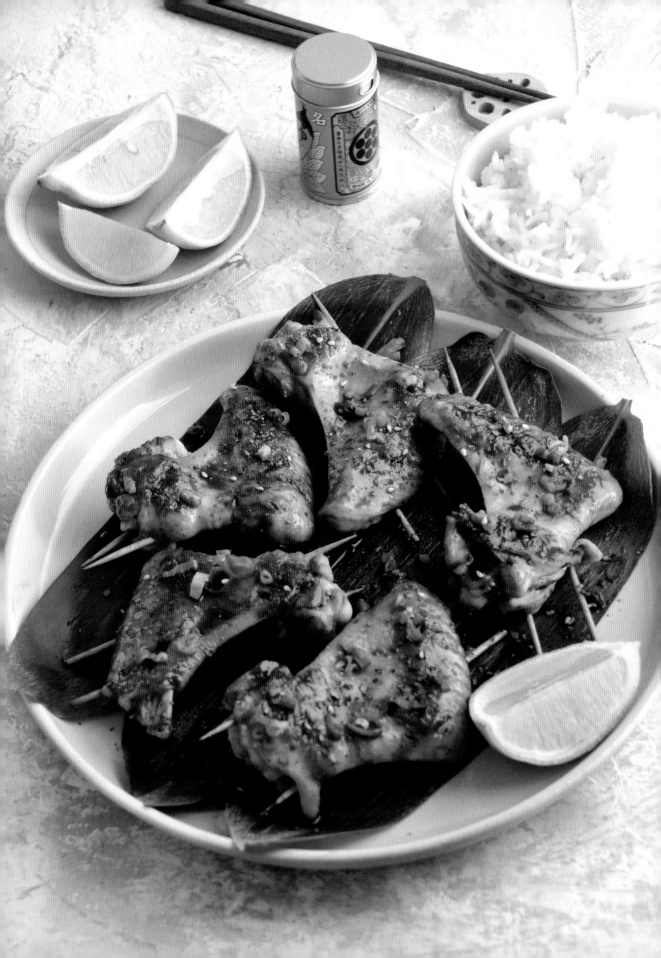

Yakitori Grilled Chicken Wings

⌇⌇⌇⌇⌇⌇

Yakitori is chicken cut into bite-sized pieces, skewered with bamboo sticks, seasoned with a sweet and savory sauce, then grilled over charcoal. It started to appear in the Edo era (1603–1868) and was originally designed as a portable food eaten at festivals. Today it's a popular street food often sold from small food carts on the grounds of Buddhist temples and in izakaya pubs and specialty restaurants. This recipe makes *yakitori* with chicken wings using an easy homemade sauce. It might take some practice to cut the wings open, but it'll help them grill faster and more evenly. But if you'd rather skip the skewering, go ahead and grill the chicken wings as is. I remove the wingtips, as they're not very meaty. But they're wonderful for making chicken stock, so I often store them in an airtight container in the freezer until I'm ready to use them.

PREPARATION TIME: 20 minutes
COOKING TIME: 30 minutes
SERVES 4

24 bamboo skewers
12 whole chicken wings (2½ lbs/1100 kg)
⅓ cup (80 ml) Kaeshi Sauce (page 40)
2 tablespoons granulated sugar
½ teaspoon sea salt
2 tablespoons extra-virgin olive oil
1 tablespoon scallions, minced, to garnish
1 lemon, quartered, to garnish
Shichimi togarashi chili pepper or cayenne pepper, to sprinkle (optional)

1. Soak the bamboo skewers in water for 20 minutes. This prevents them from burning.

2. Place the chicken on a cutting board with the skin side down. Using a sharp knife, score a line along the top of the larger bone. Using your fingers, pry the midwing open and flatten it. Repeat the same process with the other bone. (If this proves too hard, you can skip these steps and grill the unskewered chicken wings as is.)

3. Bring the Kaeshi Sauce and sugar to a boil in a small saucepan over medium-high heat, stirring often, then lower the heat to a simmer until the liquid is reduced and the sauce is thickened, about 1 minute. Set aside.

4. Thread each chicken wing onto two parallel skewers so that the bone's perpendicular to the skewers. The skewer should be inserted between the bone and the skin. Sprinkle salt over the entire piece.

5. Preheat a large-sized oiled grill pan. Place the chicken, skin side down, on the grill pan and cook the chicken on medium until it's browned, about 7 to 10 minutes. Turn the skewers over and cook until the other side is browned too. Or grill the non-skewered chicken wings, turning them until they're browned on both sides, about 12 to 15 minutes total.

6. Using a brush, glaze the chicken with the sauce 3 to 4 times on each side while the heat is on medium-low. When the chicken is completely coated with the sauce and a crust starts to form, turn off the heat.

7. To serve, drizzle some of the sauce over the chicken and sprinkle it with shichimi togarashi chili pepper and chopped scallions, along with lemon wedges on the side. For a complete meal, serve with rice and miso soup.

Steamed Shumai Chicken Dumplings

Shumai are traditionally made with ground pork and minced yellow onions, then steamed and served in a small bamboo basket with a vinegary, soy sauce dipping sauce that includes a touch of spicy yellow mustard. In this recipe, I'm showing you a slightly different style of shumai which uses mochigome, a short-grain japonica glutinous rice, instead of traditional shumai wrappers. These are a great beginner's dumpling because they're so much easier to make than gyoza. Mochigome has a high starch content with a sweet flavor and a sticky and soft texture. This recipe is the white version, using plain mochigome. Over the years, I've tweaked the recipe and added my own spin by switching from pork to chicken for a healthier option, as well as adding some oyster sauce for extra savory flavor.

PREPARATION TIME: 25
COOKING TIME: 25
SERVES: approx. 30 to 32 pcs.

1 cup (200 g) mochigome (see headnote)
1 medium onion, finely minced
2 tablespoons potato starch or cornstarch
1 lb (500 g) ground chicken or pork
1 tablespoon fresh ginger juice
1 tablespoon soy sauce
1 tablespoon oyster sauce
½ teaspoon sea salt
2 tablespoons sesame oil
2 tablespoons Basic Dashi Stock (page 36), for dipping
⅓ cup (80 ml) Ponzu Sauce (page 40), for dipping
1 tablespoon hot Japanese or Chinese mustard (optional)

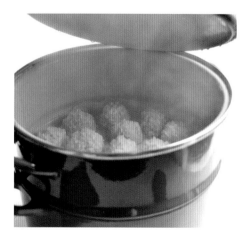

1. Rinse the mochigome in a strainer under cold water for 1 minute. Soak it in 4 cups of water for 1 hour before cooking, then drain and set aside.

2. Combine the onion and potato starch, then mix well.

3. Add the chicken, ginger juice, soy sauce, oyster sauce, salt and sesame oil to the bowl with the onion. Mix well with your hands until it turns paler in color and is sticky. Scoop out 1 tablespoon of the filling mixture and roll it between your hands to form a ball. Place it on a plate, then repeat the process with the remaining mixture. Let the meatballs chill in the refrigerator for 10 minutes.

4. Place the mochigome in a small bowl. Using your hands, gently wrap the meatballs in rice, patting them all around to form a golf-ball-sized portion.

5. Add a few inches of water to a medium-sized pot with a steamer basket set inside.

6. Place cabbage leaves or a round of parchment paper in the steamer basket and place the shumai on top ½ inch (1.25 cm) apart. Don't overcrowd the pot. The rice will slightly expand while it's steaming, so be sure there's enough space between the dumplings. If all the pieces don't fit at one time, steam them in batches. Cover the pot and steam the shumai over medium heat for 20 to 22 minutes, adding water if necessary to maintain the same level. Test one by piercing it with a fork. When the juices run clear, it's done.

7. For the dipping sauce, combine the dashi stock and the Ponzu Sauce in a small bowl and mix well.

8. To serve, transfer the shumai to a serving plate and serve them with steamed rice, Ponzu Sauce and a dollop of yellow mustard, if you like.

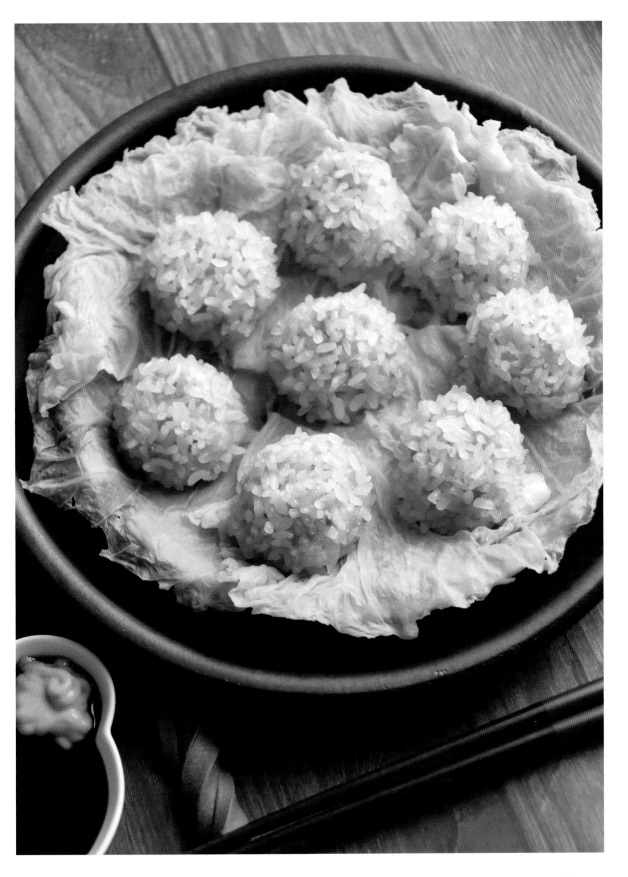

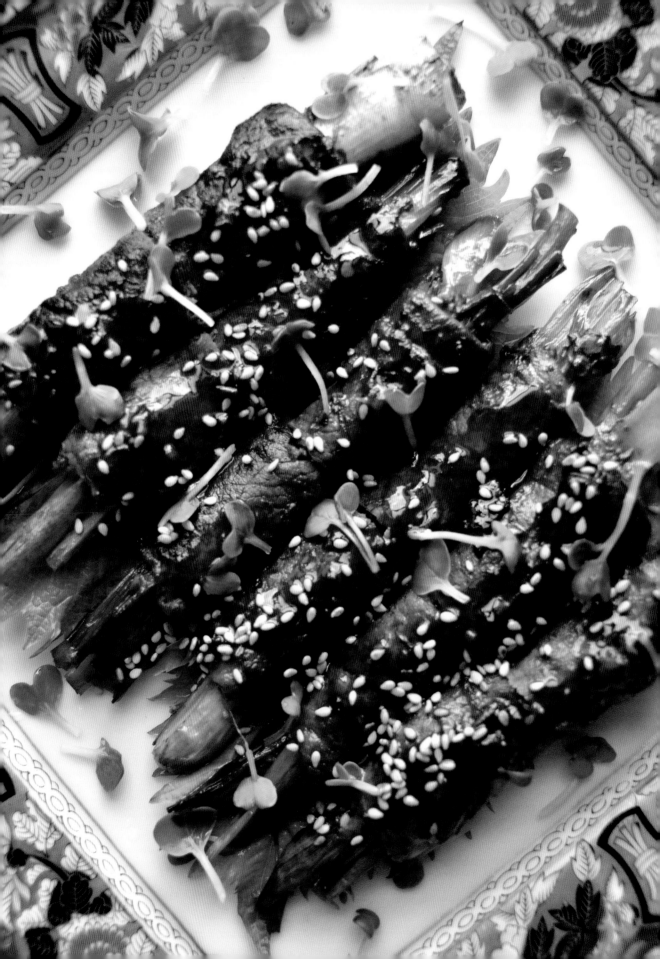

Green Onion Beef Rolls

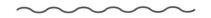

Beef rolls are a classic Japanese homestyle main dish. Cut vegetables are wrapped with thinly sliced beef and cooked in a savory seasoned soy sauce. There's no single winning formula: my mom's version is always made with carrots and green bell peppers, but I like my beef rolls made with green onions instead. The reason is that the green onions take no time to cook and there's less cutting required, so the dish comes together a little more quickly on a weeknight. Leftovers are perfect for packing in a bento box the next day. You'll just need to get or prepare thinly sliced shabu-shabu-style beef (boneless ribeye). You can find this at most Japanese or Asian markets. Those thinly sliced meats are used for Asian-style hot pots and if you're unable to find them, ask your local butcher to slice the meat very thinly for you or partially freeze the meat and then carefully slice it thinly with a sharp knife.

PREPARATION TIME: 10 minutes
COOKING TIME: 25 minutes
SERVES 4

10 scallions, the white and green
  parts, roots trimmed
1 lb (500 g) shabu-shabu-style beef
  (see the headnote)
Pinch of sea salt
1 tablespoon oyster sauce
2 tablespoons Kaeshi Sauce
  (page 40)
1 tablespoon brown sugar
1 tablespoon sake
1 teaspoon mince garlic
2 tablespoons sesame oil
½ teaspoon white sesame seed,
  toasted, to garnish
1 tablespoon kaiware radish sprouts
  or microgreens
Steamed rice (optional)

1. Cut the green onions in half-length crosswise.

2. Lay out a slice of beef on a cutting board with the long side facing you. Place 3 to 4 pieces of the green onions, alternating with white and green parts, across the lower edge, then tightly roll the beef over the green onions. Repeat with the remaining ingredients. Sprinkle the beef rolls with a pinch of salt.

3. In a small bowl, whisk together the oyster sauce, Kaeshi Sauce, brown sugar, sake and garlic.

4. Preheat a lightly oiled skillet over medium-high heat. Place the beef rolls with the seam facing down. Cook over medium-high heat about 2 to 3 minutes per side, rotating until the entire roll has cooked through, about 5 to 6 minutes total.

5. Add the sauce and rotate the beef rolls to coat them evenly. Heat on medium-low for about 1 to 2 minutes, then transfer the beef rolls to a cutting board.

6. Turn the heat to medium-low and thicken the remining sauce. When the sauce is reduced by half, turn off the heat. Cut the rolls into a half on a cutting board.

7. To serve, place the beef rolls on a plate and drizzle with the remaining sauce from the skillet. Sprinkle with the kaiware sprouts/microgreens and sesame seeds and serve with steamed rice.

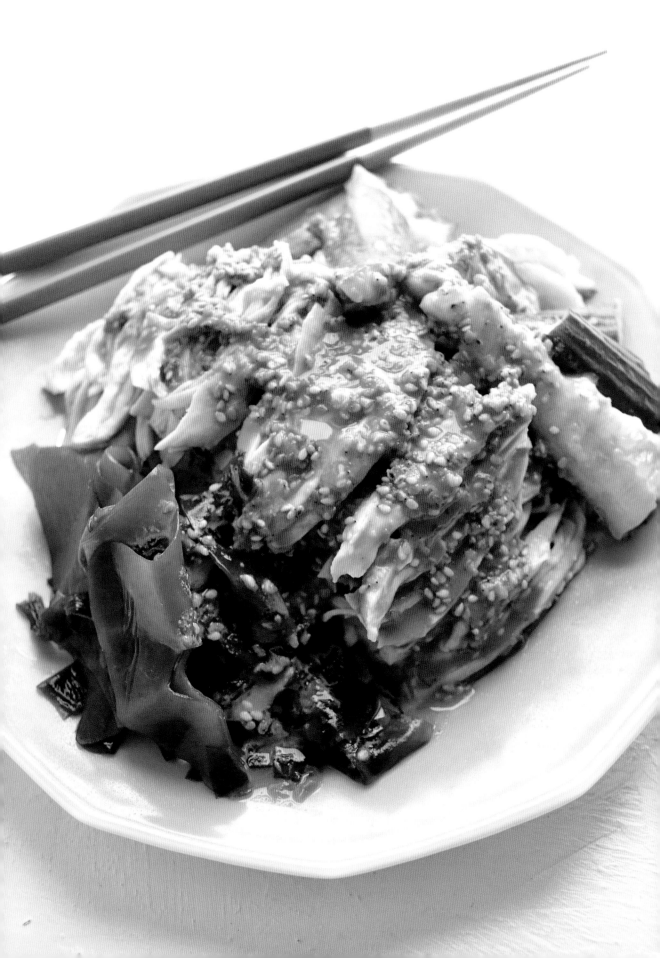

Sake-steamed Chicken
with Wakame and Goma Sesame Dressing

~~~~~

When it comes to chicken, I generally prefer thighs over breasts for their flavor, versatility and affordability. But without a doubt, this Japanese-style sake-steamed chicken is just made for highlighting the plump and meaty pleasures of chicken breast. Sake not only tenderizes the chicken, it also adds a hint of sweetness. Steaming these chicken breasts with the sake- and kombu-infused ginger and scallions results in a very moist and aromatic dish. By combining the kombu's umami glutamate with the chicken's inosinic acid, the flavor is given a superfood upgrade. If you've never steamed chicken before, this is the recipe to try: simple, healthy and delicious.

PREPARATION TIME: 10 minutes
COOKING TIME: 40 minutes
SERVES 4

2 scallions, white and green parts
1 cup (250 ml) water
1 cup (250 ml) sake
1 piece of dried kombu, 2 x 6 in
  (5 x 15 cm)
2 lbs (800 g) chicken breasts,
  boneless and skinless
½ teaspoon salt
2 tablespoons ginger, peeled and cut
  into matchsticks
2 Japanese or baby cucumbers
⅓ cup (60 g) fresh or dried wakame
½ cup (125 ml) Goma Sesame
  Dressing (page 40)
¼ teaspoon hot chili oil
2 tablespoons unsweetened peanut
  or almond butter
2 tablespoons rice vinegar
1 tablespoon reserved chicken
  steaming liquid

1. Trim the scallions and cut them in half. Combine the water, sake and kombu in a medium-sized pot with a steamer basket.

2. Rinse and pierce the chickens with a fork. Pat it dry with a paper towel. Season the chicken with salt on both sides and place it in a steamer basket, adding the green onions and ginger on top. Cover the pot and steam the chicken over medium heat about 18 to 20 minutes, adding ½ cup of water, if necessary, to maintain the same level. Steam the chicken until the juices run clear when pierced with a knife. then turn off the heat.

3. Remove the steamer basket from the pot and allow the chicken to cool for 10 minutes. Reserve the steaming liquid for the dressing.

4. Put the cucumber on the counter. Smash the cucumbers by using a rolling pin or a meat mallet until they're broken into rough, irregular pieces.

5. Place a strainer in a bowl, add the fresh wakame and fill the bowl with water, letting it sit for a few seconds. Drain and rinse the wakame under running water until the salt is removed and the wakame doubles or triples in size. Squeeze out the excess water and cut it into bite-sized pieces. If you're using dried wakame, follow the instruction on the package or rehydrate it in a bowl of water for 5 minutes. Drain it, squeeze out the excess water, then set aside.

6. To prepare the sesame dressing, combine Goma Sesame Dressing, chili oil, peanut butter, rice vinegar and reserved chicken steaming liquid in a small bowl until well combined.

7. To serve, shred the chicken and arrange it on plates with the cucumbers and wakame. Drizzle the dressing over everything or serve it on the side.

Crispy Gyoza Dumplings
Filled with Pork, Shrimp and Cabbage

Crispy outside and juicy inside, gyoza have always been one of my favorite foods both to make and eat. Gyoza was regularly in our dinner rotation when I was a kid. My mom always asked my sisters and me to help, and it was a major production, as we made at least 100 dumplings. When I make gyoza at home today, I of course can't make just a few but instead produce multiple batches so I can stock the freezer—a quick lunch or dinner is only minutes away! You can store uncooked gyoza in the refrigerator for up to 2 days or in the freezer for up to a month. This is a classic gyoza recipe, a combination of pork, shrimp and cabbage, that my family has been making for years. Chicken or tofu can be substituted for the pork. You can find round dumpling wrappers in Asian markets or increasingly in mainstream markets as well.

PREPARATION TIME: 20 minutes
COOKING TIME: 40 minutes
MAKES: 32 to 36 pieces

12 medium fresh shrimp, about
  5 oz (150 g), peeled and deveined
3 green cabbage leaves
4 scallions, the white and green
  parts
5 oz (150 g) ground pork, chicken,
  or firm tofu
2 shiitake mushrooms
1 tablespoon garlic, minced
1 tablespoon ginger, peeled and
  minced
1½ tablespoons sesame oil,
  divided
3 tablespoons Kaeshi Sauce
  (page 40), divided
¼ teaspoon sea salt
2 tablespoons rice vinegar
2 tablespoons Basic Dashi Stock
  (page 36)
36 round dumpling wrappers,
  approx. 4 in (10 cm) in diameter
¾ cup (185 ml) water
1 teaspoon all-purpose flour
Chili oil (optional)

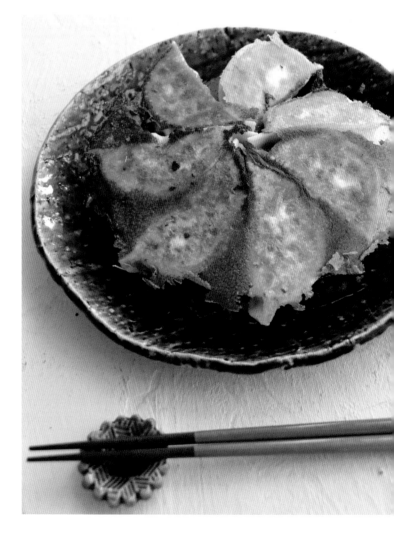

1. Finely mince the shrimp. Core the cabbage and chop the leaves then the green onions and shiitake mushrooms.

2. In a medium-sized bowl, add the shrimp, cabbage, pork, green onions, shiitake mushrooms, garlic, ginger, 1 tablespoon of the Kaeshi Sauce and the salt. Mix well with your hands. Divide the mixture into 32 to 36 equal portions, about 1 tablespoon of the filling for each dumpling.

3. In a small bowl, whisk together the rice vinegar, Basic Dashi Stock and the remaining Kaeshi Sauce to make the dipping sauce, then set aside.

4. Set a small bowl of water on the counter. Put one portion of the filling, about 1 tablespoon, on a dumpling wrapper in the middle. Dip a finger in the water bowl and wet the entire edge of the wrapper. Fold it in half and wrap the filling by making 3 pleats on one side to form the dumpling. If it's too difficult to make the pleats, then just fold the dumpling in half and press the edges to seal them.

5. Place a nonstick skillet over medium heat and coat it with a tablespoon of sesame oil. Arrange the gyoza dumplings in a circle and fry them for 2 minutes, until the bottoms become slightly brown.

6. In a small bowl, whisk together the water and flour until it's smooth. Pour this mixture into the pan until it covers the gyoza a little more than halfway. Cover the skillet and cook over medium heat for about 8 to 10 minutes, or until the filling is fully cooked. Check for doneness by piercing one with a fork. When the juices run clear, it's done. At this point, all the water should be evaporated and the wrappers will have become transparently light brown and have crispy edges. If any water remains in the pan, remove the lid and set it over medium-low heat until it evaporates.

7. Drizzle the remaining sesame oil around the edges of the skillet and cook the dumplings over medium-low heat for another 2 to 3 minutes, until the bottoms are golden brown and crispy.

8. Use a spatula to loosen the gyoza from the skillet. Place a dinner plate upside-down over the skillet and holding both sides tightly together, quickly flip the plate and skillet over to transfer the gyoza to the plate. The crispy, golden brown sides are now facing up. Alternately, simply transfer the gyoza to a serving plate one by one using a spatula or tongs. Serve with the vinegar dipping sauce on the side and add chili oil if you prefer it on the spicy side.

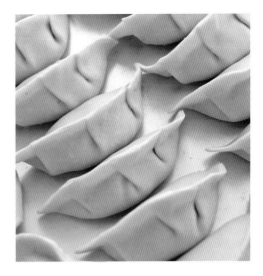

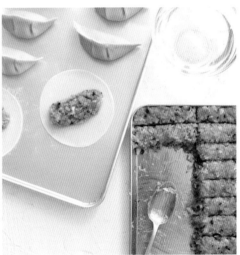

TIP Cover the dumpling wrappers with a damp paper towel to keep them moist. Leftover wrappers can be stored in the freezer, well-wrapped in plastic, for up to a month.

Drizzling oil around the edge of the skillet (see Step 7) is a Japanese technique that results in crispy gyoza and helps to release them easily from the skillet.

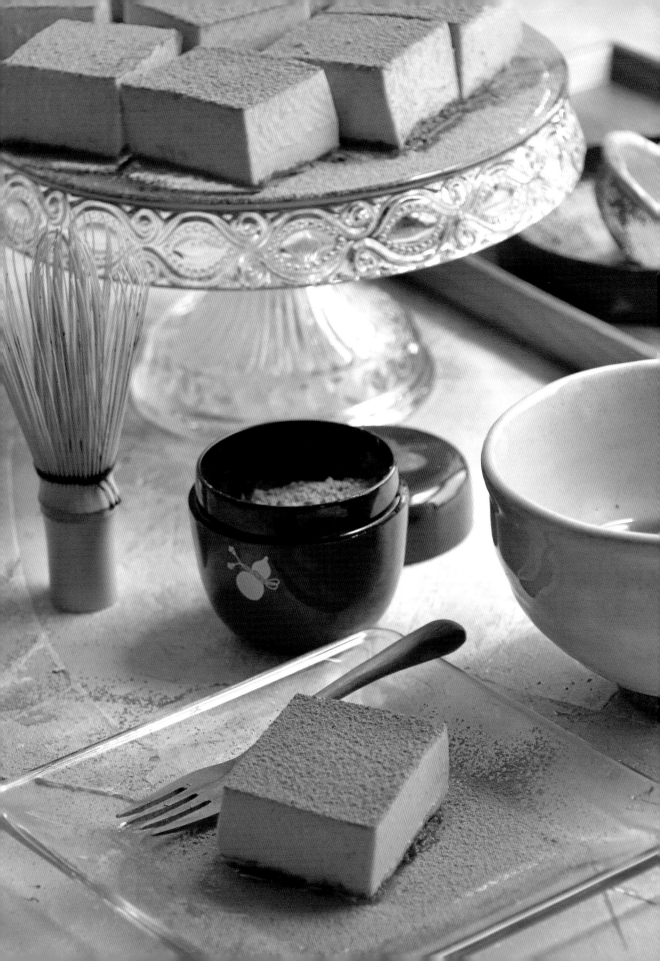

Healthy Desserts

Matcha, amazake and sesame have become the new superfood stars for dessert or whenever you're craving a sweet treat. Matcha is a brightly-colored, powdered green tea that's fragrant and bittersweet. Considered one of the world's healthiest beverages, it contains natural antioxidants that may help protect against cancer, lower the risk of heart disease, support healthy brain function as well as boost the immune system and reduce stress. Matcha recipes include basic desserts such as cookies, gluten-free muffins and cheesecake.

Another popular superfood is amazake, an energy drink served either hot or cold. It contains high levels of natural glucose, is a good source of probiotics, vitamins, and amino acids and is known to improve digestion. Nonalcoholic amazake made from rice koji is naturally sweet so you can enjoy delicious and healthy desserts without feeling guilty.

Finally, nutty sesame paste (neri goma) is a popular ingredient in both sweet and savory Japanese dishes. It's highly nutritious and includes protein, vitamins, minerals, fiber and antioxidants. Here I show you how to make easy and delicious sesame pie with a twist, using an unexpected ingredient found in the Japanese pantry. Try not to eat the whole thing!

Mochi with Black Sesame Sauce

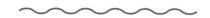

This mochi is made with shiratamako flour—a type of glutinous, or sweet, rice flour—mixed with liquid, then boiled in water for a few minutes until it softens. I learned how to make the bite-sized dessert balls in my home economics class when I was in elementary school. It's a simple and fun recipe, one that you can get your kids involved in making at home. You can use either glutinous rice flour or sweet rice flour, but if you can get shiratamako flour instead, try that first because it'll result in a chewier, more refined texture. In this recipe, I serve the mochi with nutty, sweet and savory black sesame sauce topped with crunchy walnuts. Both ingredients are excellent sources of heathy fats, fiber and protein that may enhance heart and bone health. Enjoy these classic treats served with a cup of green tea at the end of a meal.

PREPARATION TIME: 10 minutes
COOKING TIME: 25 minutes
SERVES: approx. 32 mochi balls

3 tablespoons black nerigoma sesame paste or tahini
4 tablespoons Kombu Water (page 38)
¾ cup (185 ml) soy milk or almond milk or water, divided
1 tablespoon maple syrup
1¼ cups (150 g) shiratamako flour (see the headnote)
½ teaspoon toasted white sesame seeds, to garnish (optional)
1 tablespoon walnuts, chopped, to garnish (optional)

TIP Serve these immediately as the texture will become hard within an hour. Store in a container, with water to cover, in the refrigerator for up to 3 days or in a resealable plastic bag (without water) in the freezer for up to a month. Reheat the refrigerated mochi in boiling water for 15 seconds or frozen ones for a minute before serving.

1. In a small bowl, combine the nerigoma, Kombu Water, 4 tablespoons soy milk and maple syrup and mix well. Set aside.

2. In a medium-sized bowl, combine the shiratamako flour and half the soy milk. Use a spatula to mix it until the dough is partially combined. At this stage, the dough will still be dry and there will be crumbs or powdery lumps visible.

3. Slowly add the remining soy milk to the bowl, continually mixing until the dough is well-combined and smooth, about 3 to 4 minutes. At this stage, the dough should no longer be dry. If it is or still has visible crumbs, add a splash of soy milk to the dough.

4. Use your hands to firmly knead the dough in the bowl until the mixture resembles clay and doesn't stick to the bowl or your hands. The dough should be free of lumps and have a soft and smooth texture, similar to that of an earlobe.

5. To form the mochi balls, scoop out half a tablespoon of dough. Roll the dough between your hands to form a smooth ball. Then use a fingertip to create an indentation in the center of the ball. This will allow it to cook evenly.

6. Fill a pot halfway with water and bring to a boil. Lower the heat to medium and gently place the mochi in the boiling water. Don't overcrowd the pot. If all the balls don't fit, cook them in batches. Use a wooden spoon to stir the pot once so that the mochi don't stick to one another, cooking for about 2 to 3 minutes. When they start to float to the surface, cook for another 30 seconds, then scoop them out with a mesh sieve. Rinse them in cold running water for 30 seconds in a strainer.

7. To serve, place the mochi (8 per serving) in individual bowls and drizzle the sesame sauce over the top. Sprinkle with sesame seeds and walnuts, if using.

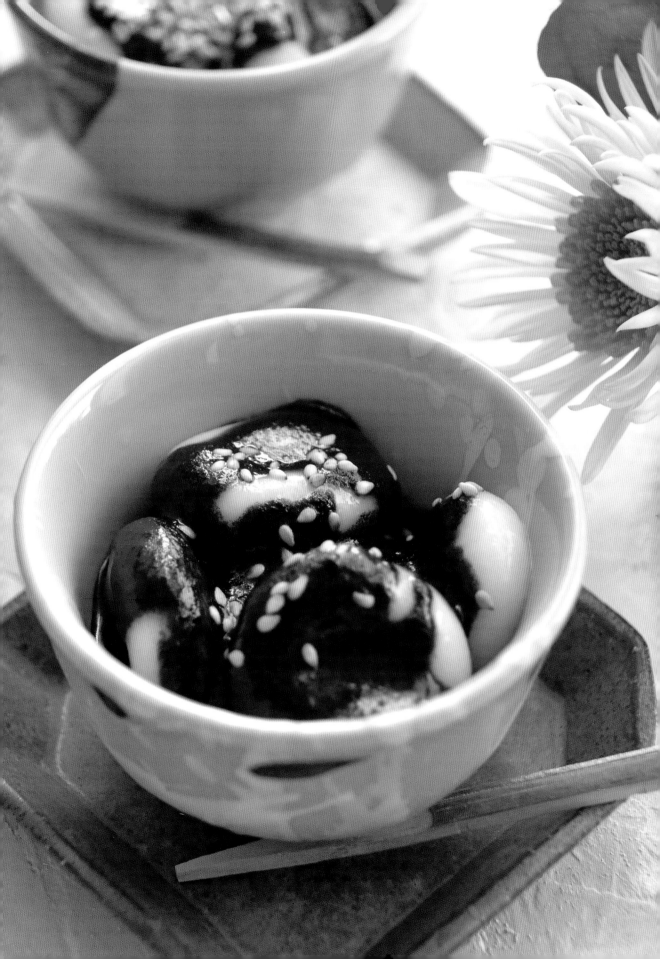

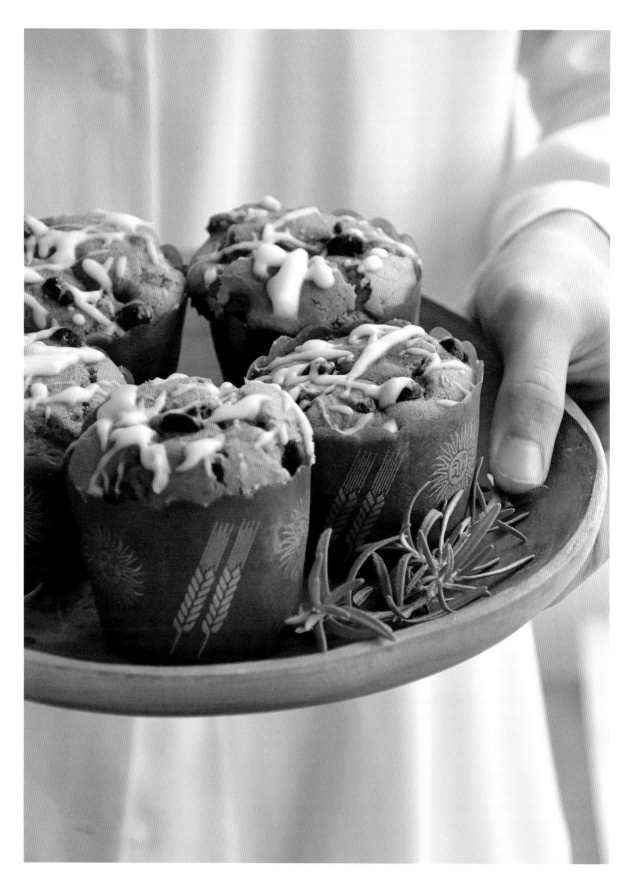

Matcha Mochi Muffins
with Adzuki Sweet Red Beans

~~~~~~~~~

Slightly crunchy like the exterior of a madeleine and chewy like a mochi rice cake, this unique muffin will become addictive as soon as you take your first bite. I developed this recipe because I wanted to create gluten-free cupcakes for my friend's birthday. After several tests, I came up with the perfect ratio of sweet glutinous rice flour to substitute for the original wheat flour. Since it lends chewiness and a great texture to dishes, I'm always fond of using it instead of all-purpose flour. If you eat these muffins the same day they're baked, the top stays rather hard and crunchy, but if you let them sit overnight, somehow the texture changes and becomes a bit moister. I add sweet adzuki red beans, tsubuan, inside the muffins for an extra layer of flavor.

PREPARATION TIME: 15 minutes
COOKING TIME: 40 minutes
SERVES: 8 muffins

8 paper cupcake liners
2 tablespoons matcha green tea powder
1 cup (150 g) mochiko sweet glutinous rice flour (see the headnote)
3 tablespoons almond flour
1 teaspoon baking powder
½ cup (100 g) granulated sugar
2 eggs
⅔ cup (160 ml) heavy cream
8 tablespoons adzuki sweet red beans (about 5 oz/150 g)

SUGAR GLAZE (OPTIONAL)
3 tablespoons powdered sugar
2 tablespoons cream cheese,
1 tablespoon whole milk

1. Line a muffin tin with 8 paper cupcake liners.

2. Preheat the oven to 375°F (190°C).

3. In a medium bowl, sift or whisk the matcha powder, mochiko sweet rice flour and baking powder together. Set aside.

4. In another medium bowl, using a stand mixer fitted with a paddle attachment, beat the sugar and eggs on high speed for 1 minute or until smooth and creamy.

5. In another medium bowl using a stand mixer fitted with a paddle attachment, beat the very cold heavy cream on high speed for 1 to 2 minutes or until it forms stiff peaks.

6. Pour the dry ingredients into the egg mixture and beat on low speed until just about combined. Add the whipped cream to the bowl, using a spatula and gently fold the whipped cream into the muffin mixture until well combined.

7. Spoon the batter into the lined muffin cups, filling each only halfway. Spoon about 1 tablespoon of adzuki beans into the middle of each, then fill with additional batter to cover the adzuki beans, filling to just below the top.

8. Sprinkle a few adzuki beans over the muffin tops.

9. Bake the muffins for 25 to 30 minutes or until a toothpick inserted in the center comes out clean. Let the muffins cool for 15 minutes in the muffin tin, then transfer them to a wire rack.

10. Make the Sugar Glaze (if using) by stirring together the cream cheese and the powdered sugar in a small bowl until well-combined. Add the milk slowly, stirring it until mixed well. Drizzle the cream cheese icing over the muffins using a spoon.

Matcha Green Tea Almond Cookies

~~~~~~~~~~

I'm very excited to share one of my favorite cookie recipes with you.
For those who do not have much of a sweet tooth, like me, these cookies are everything
you're looking for: light, buttery and flaky, but with a hint of bitterness from
the matcha green tea powder that sets them apart. This recipe will yield about
2 dozen cookies, but I always end up making a bigger batch as people always ask if
I have more cookies. I am showing you two different shapes, smooth balls and crisscross
marks (same baking time). You can easily bake a double batch with minimal extra effort,
just make sure to increase the baking time accordingly and bake until the edges are just
starting to brown. After they have cooled completely, I like to lightly dust with sweet
matcha green tea powder (combining matcha and powdered sugar 1:1) for an added
layer of intense matcha flavor. But if additional bitter flavors strike you as too intense,
you can certainly skip this process. You can store baked matcha cookies for up to 10 days
at room temperature in an airtight container, or in the freezer for up to 10 weeks.

PREPARATION TIME: 20 minutes
COOKING TIME: 40 minutes
MAKES: About two dozen cookies

½ cup (115g) unsalted butter,
  softened to room temperature
⅓ cup (70 g) granulated sugar
1 beaten egg
1½ tablespoons matcha green tea
  powder
½ cup (50 g) almond flour
¼ cup (30 g) cornstarch
¾ cup (100 g) all-purpose flour
½ teaspoon matcha green tea
  powder, for dusting (optional)
½ teaspoon powdered sugar, for
  dusting (optional)

1. Line the baking sheet with a silicone baking liner or with parchment paper.

2. Preheat the oven to 325ºF (160ºC).

3. Put the butter and the sugar in a large mixing bowl and beat it with a hand mixer until it's creamy and lightened in color (or in a stand mixer with the paddle attached).

4. Add the egg, matcha green tea powder, almond flour and cornstarch to the butter mixture and beat until combined. Then add the all-purpose flour and mix well.

5. For each cookie, scoop out 1 tablespoon of dough. Roll the cookie dough between your hands to form a smooth ball. If you want to make a crisscross pattern, press down on each cookie with the back of a fork. Space the balls of dough 1 in (2.5 cm) apart on the baking sheet.

6. Bake for 20 to 22 minutes or until golden brown. Let the cookies cool on the sheet for 10 minutes before transferring them to a wire rack. For strong matcha flavor, combine matcha powder and powdered sugar in a small bowl and mix well, dusting the cookies with the sweet matcha powder, if desired. Make sure they're completely cooled, after about 30 minutes, before dusting.

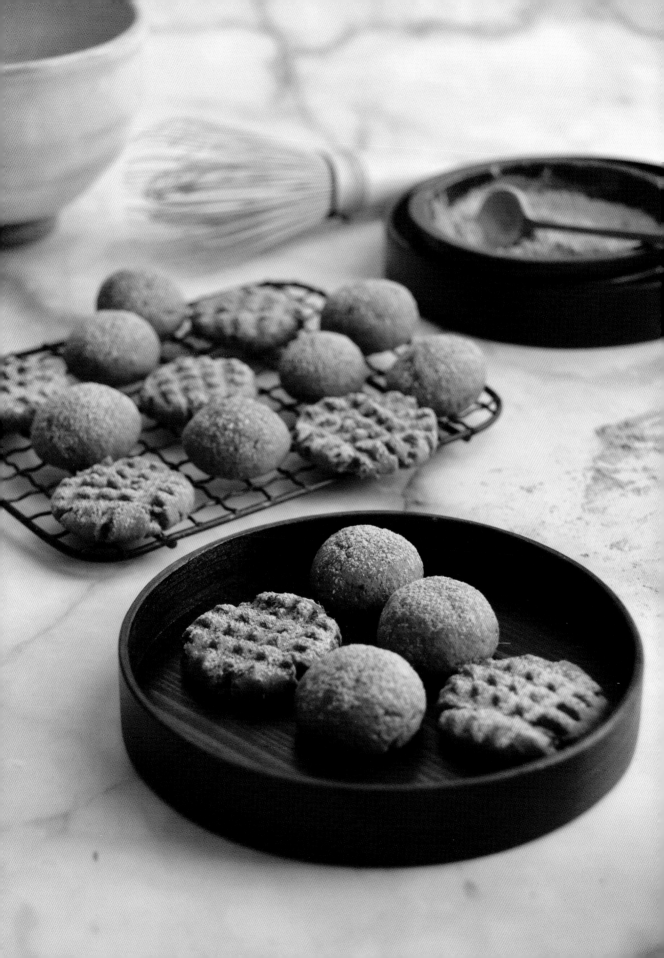

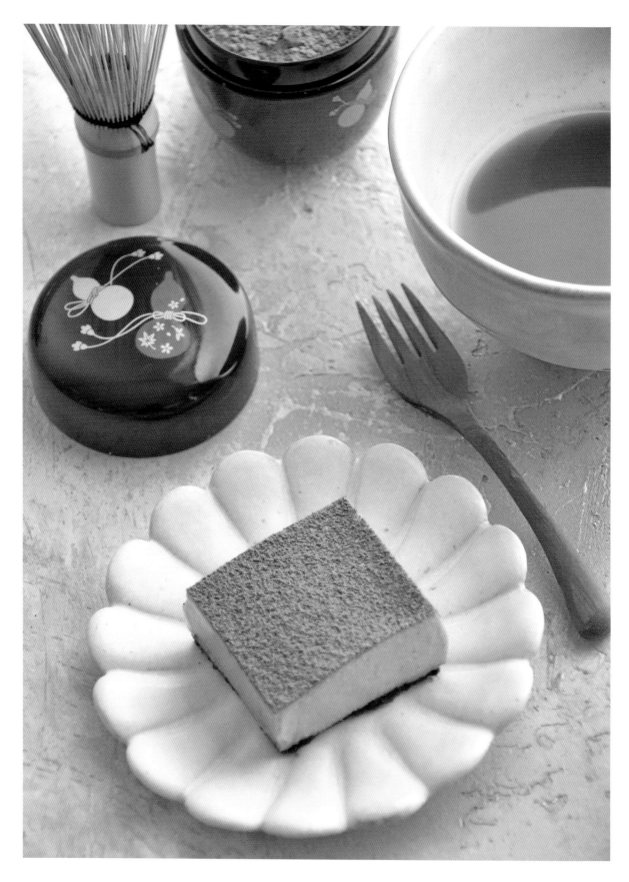

Matcha Green Tea Cheesecake

Are you looking for a last-minute, no-fuss homemade dessert recipe? If so, this matcha cheesecake is for you. I've made this many times through the years, and it comes out perfectly every time. This smooth and creamy cheesecake is packed with matcha green tea powder, known to be rich in antioxidants and other health benefits. It has been used in tea ceremony rituals since the 12th century in Japan. This recipe requires just three easy steps: first is to make a crust in a food processor, press into a pan and bake. By baking the crust, it will firm up and be easy to serve. Then, make the cheese filling in a blender and pour it on top of the crust. The last step's easy: let it set. I use kombu dashi stock as a secret ingredient to add a lightness to the cheese filling with a hint of umami flavor; last is to dust matcha powder on top. Enjoy the hint of bitter notes combined with the earthy flavor of matcha in this creamy cheesecake with a relaxing cup of green tea to calm your mind and body.

PREPARATION TIME: 10 minutes
COOKING TIME: 25 minutes
SERVES 8

1¼ cups (145 g) graham cracker crumbs
½ cup (110 g) unsalted butter, melted
4 tablespoons water
2 teaspoons unflavored powdered gelatin
1 cup (230 g) cream cheese, at room temperature
1 cup (230 g) mascarpone cheese, at room temperature
⅓ cup (75 g) granulated sugar
¼ cup (65 ml) Kombu Water (page 38)
1 cup (250 ml) heavy cream
3 tablespoons matcha green tea powder, divided

1. Preheat the oven to 325°F (160°C). Combine the graham cracker crumbs and the melted butter in a food processor. Blend on low speed until well combined, then press the mixture into the bottom of an 8-in (20-cm) springform pan.

2. To bake the crust, place it in the preheated oven for 10 minutes.

3. Place the water in a small bowl and sprinkle the gelatin on top. Let it stand for 5 minutes, until it's dissolved.

4. In a saucepan over medium-low heat, combine the cream cheese, mascarpone cheese, sugar, Kombu Water, heavy cream and gelatin, stirring until the sugar is completely dissolved, about 4 to 6 minutes. Transfer the cheese filling to a food processor and blend on medium speed until it's smooth and creamy, about 2 minutes.

5. Add 2 tablespoons of the matcha powder to the blender and blend it again for 1 minute. Strain the matcha cheese filling through a fine mesh strainer 2 to 3 times, then pour it into the crust, using a spatula to smooth the top.

6. Cover it tightly with plastic wrap and refrigerate it for at least 3 hours. Use a knife to loosen the cheesecake from the rim of the pan then release the springform pan and place the cake on a serving plate. Carefully sift the remaining 1 tablespoon of matcha green tea powder through a strainer to dust the top of the cheesecake. Use a knife to cut into slices for serving.

Sesame Cream Pie

This rich and nutty sesame pie is great to serve after an authentic Japanese meal. It's made with three of the most popular traditional ingredients: neri goma (Japanese sesame paste), tofu and kombu dashi. You can substitute with tahini if you don't have neri goma. I love to use a secret ingredient in my desserts—a splash of Kombu Dashi Stock, which adds a savory note as well as a lightness to sweet dishes.

PREPARATION TIME: 15 minutes
COOKING TIME: 50 minutes
SERVES 8

One 9-in (23-cm) prepared pie crust, unbaked
1 tablespoon water
1½ teaspoons unflavored powdered gelatin
⅓ cup (80 ml) white neri goma sesame paste or tahini
4 oz (100 g) soft tofu
¼ cup (55 g) maple syrup
1½ cups (375 ml) heavy cream, divided
⅓ cup (80 ml) Kombu Water (page 38)
2 tablespoons granulated sugar
1 teaspoon toasted white sesame seeds,
  to garnish

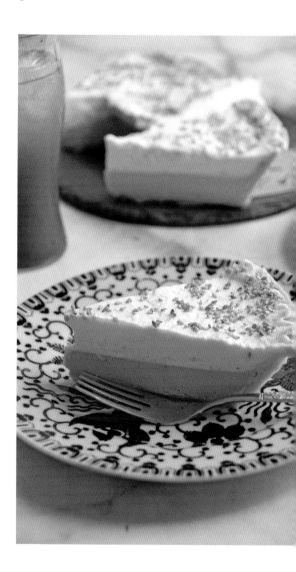

1. Bake the pie crust according to the package instructions, preferably until it's golden brown.

2. Place the water in a small bowl and sprinkle the gelatin on top. Let it stand for 5 minutes, until it's dissolved.

3. In a saucepan over medium-low heat, combine the white nerigoma, soft tofu, brown sugar, ½ cup (125 ml) heavy cream, Kombu Water and the gelatin and stir until the sugar is completely dissolved, about 2 to 4 minutes. Transfer the sesame filling to a food processor and process on medium until smooth and creamy, about 2 minutes.

4. Strain the sesame filling through a fine mesh strainer then pour into the crust. Use a spatula to smooth the top.

5. Cover tightly with plastic wrap and refrigerate for at least 2 hours.

6. Using a stand mixer fitted with a paddle attachment, beat the remaining 1 cup (250 ml) of heavy cream on high speed for 3 minutes. Add the sugar to the bowl and keep beating until stiff peaks are formed. Spoon the whipped cream onto the sesame pie, swirling it with a spatula. Sprinkle the sesame seeds over the whipped cream.

7. Use a knife to cut the pie and serve on dessert plates.

Amazake Panna Cotta with Strawberry Sauce

Amazake is a naturally sweet rice drink with a thick and creamy texture made from fermented rice koji. It's served both hot and cold. As an energy drink during the summer, it helps in recovering from fatigue as it has high levels of natural glucose. It's also known to improve digestion and is a good source of probiotics. There are two types of amazake. In this recipe, I'm using the version made from rice koji, which is sweeter and alcohol-free, so everybody can enjoy this healthy dessert at home.

PREPARATION TIME: 10 minutes
COOKING TIME: 25 minutes
SERVES 4

1 cup (250 ml) amazake
1 cup (250 ml) soy or almond milk
1 tablespoon maple or agave syrup
2½ teaspoons unflavored powdered gelatin
2 tablespoons water
8 strawberries, fresh or frozen, divided
4 mint leaves, to garnish

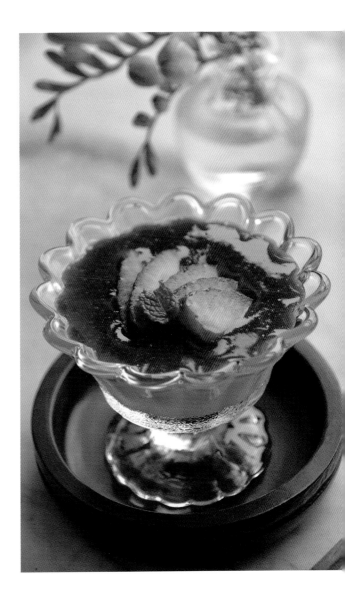

1.   Combine the amazake and the soy milk in a blender and blend well until the mixture is smooth and creamy. Transfer the mixture to a medium saucepan and add the maple or agave syrup. Cook over medium-low heat for 5 minutes.

2.   In a bowl, combine the gelatin with water and add it to the amazake mixture. Stir, dissolving well, for 3 to 5 minutes on low heat. Strain the mixture to remove any lumps, then pour it into four individual cups, each about 4 to 5 oz (100–150 g) in size. Let it cool in the refrigerator for a couple of hours until it's set.

3.   Trim and cut 2 of the strawberries into thin slices.

4.   Put the remaining 6 strawberries in a blender and blend well for 30 seconds or until smooth.

5.   When you're ready to serve, pour the strawberry sauce on top and garnish each cup with the strawberry slices and a mint leaf.

Index

Acknowledgment

To my family, thank you for your support, I couldn't have done this without it.

To Debra Samuels, thanks for helping to bring this book to life.

To Sonya Gropman, thanks for showing me by example how to be a better author.

And to my two amazing children, Jane and Owen, I love you.

Published by Tuttle Publishing, an imprint of Periplus Editions (HK) Ltd.

www.tuttlepublishing.com

Texts and nonarchival photos © 2022 Yumi Komatsudaira

Shutterstock.com photo credits: **Endpapers bottom right** boommaval. **Page 9** kazoka; Dimasranggah; alicja neumiler; JIANG HONGYAN; successo images. **Page 10 bottom left** Brent Hofacker. **Page 11 top** Angela M. Benivegna. **Page 13 bottom** maramorosz. **Page 12 far right below** KOHUKU. **Page 16 top left** norikko; **bottom left** HikoPhotography. **Page 17 top** Dinar Nurnaningsih. **Page 18 top left** Brent Hofacker; **top right** Emily Li. **Page 19 top left** Picture Partners; **top right** Yossi James. **Page 20 from left** somdul; Tamakhin Mykhailo; eye-blink. **Page 21 top, from left** Nishihama; Ear Iew Boo; KOHUKU; Yossi James; **bottom extreme left** Amarita; **bottom extreme right**: istetiana. **Page 26 top left** K321. **Page 27 extreme left** Africa Studio. **Page 29 top left** Pisitphol; **top right** Pum Nin **Page 35 extreme left** yoshi0511. **Page 57 top right** SherSor

Library of Congress Cataloging-in-Publication Data in process

ISBN 978-4-8053-1642-9

TUTTLE PUBLISHING® is a registered trademark of Tuttle Publishing, a division of Periplus Editions (HK) Ltd.

DISTRIBUTED BY

North America, Latin America & Europe
Tuttle Publishing
364 Innovation Drive
North Clarendon, VT 05759-9436 U.S.A.
Tel: 1 (802) 773-8930
Fax: 1 (802) 773-6993
info@tuttlepublishing.com
www.tuttlepublishing.com

Japan
Tuttle Publishing
Yaekari Building 3rd Floor
5-4-12 Osaki, Shinagawa-ku
Tokyo 141 0032
Tel: (81) 3 5437-0171
Fax: (81) 3 5437-0755
sales@tuttle.co.jp
www.tuttle.co.jp

Asia Pacific
Berkeley Books Pte. Ltd.
3 Kallang Sector, #04-01
Singapore 349278
Tel: (65) 67412178; Fax: (65) 67412179
inquiries@periplus.com.sg
www.tuttlepublishing.com

25 24 23 22   10 9 8 7 6 5 4 3 2 1
Printed in China   2209EP

"Books to Span the East and West"

Tuttle Publishing was founded in 1832 in the small New England town of Rutland, Vermont [USA]. Our core values remain as strong today as they were then—to publish best-in-class books which bring people together one page at a time. In 1948, we established a publishing office in Japan—and Tuttle is now a leader in publishing English-language books about the arts, languages and cultures of Asia. The world has become a much smaller place today and Asia's economic and cultural influence has grown. Yet the need for meaningful dialogue and information about this diverse region has never been greater. Over the past seven decades, Tuttle has published thousands of books on subjects ranging from martial arts and paper crafts to language learning and literature—and our talented authors, illustrators, designers and photographers have won many prestigious awards. We welcome you to explore the wealth of information available on Asia at **www.tuttlepublishing.com**.

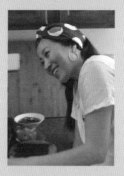

YUMI KOMATSUDAIRA is a recipe developer, food stylist, culinary instructor and the president of K-Seaweed, a leading ocean greens provider. She grew up outside Tokyo, playing—and snacking—in her family's seaweed factory. Now based in New York, she travels to Japan often promoting seaweed and its health benefits.

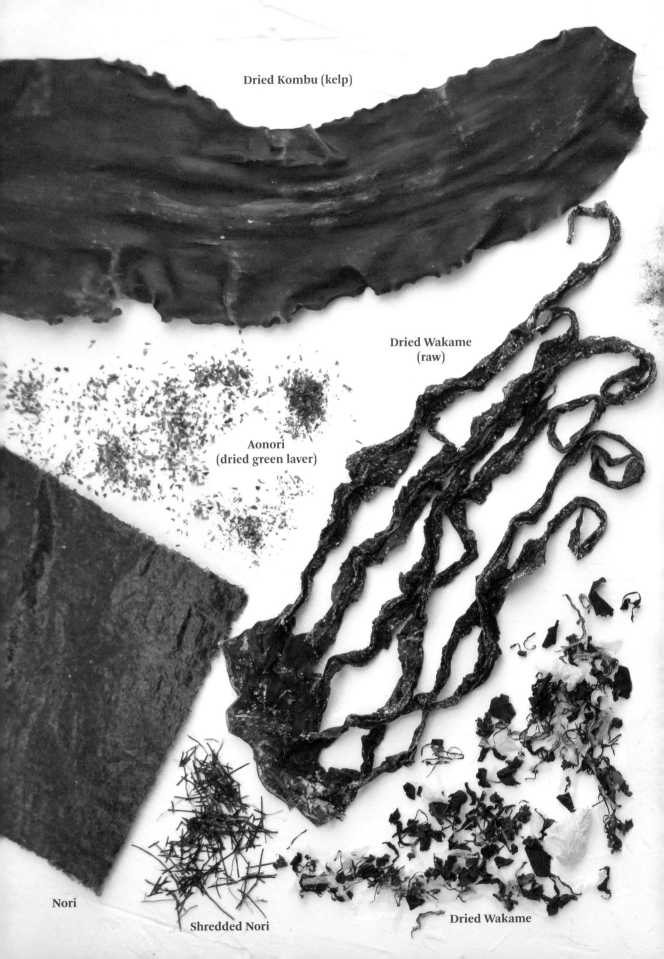

Dried Kombu (kelp)

Dried Wakame
(raw)

Aonori
(dried green laver)

Nori

Shredded Nori

Dried Wakame